Bamboo Shoot

Bamboo Shoot

Superfood for Nutrition, Health and Medicine

Nirmala Chongtham and Madho Singh Bisht

CRC Press
Taylor & Francis Group
Boca Raton London New York

CRC Press is an imprint of the
Taylor & Francis Group, an **informa** business

First edition published 2021
by CRC Press
6000 Broken Sound Parkway NW, Suite 300, Boca Raton, FL 33487-2742

and by CRC Press
2 Park Square, Milton Park, Abingdon, Oxon, OX14 4RN

Library of Congress Cataloging-in-Publication Data

Names: Chongtham, Nirmala, author. | Bisht, Madho Singh, author.
Title: Bamboo shoot : superfood for nutrition, health and medicine / Nirmala Chongtham and Madho Singh Bisht.
Description: First edition. | Boca Raton ; London : CRC Press, 2021. | Includes bibliographical references and index. | Summary: "Bamboo is an ordinary plant with extraordinary properties. Bamboo is an important resource for a healthy planet, and its shoots hold manifold nutritional benefits. Based on 18 years of research, Bamboo Shoot: Superfood for Nutrition, Health and Medicine details health-promoting bioactive compounds found in bamboo and offers practical guidance on how this vegetable, bamboo shoot, is used for food fortification. Bamboo shoots aid in the prevention of cardiovascular disease, cancer, diabetes, hypertension and obesity. Exploring the tradition and culture of bamboo in Asian countries, this book provides information on the science behind the nutritional value of bamboo shoots"-- Provided by publisher.
Identifiers: LCCN 2020020484 (print) | LCCN 2020020485 (ebook) | ISBN 9780367467418 (paperback) | ISBN 9780367470258 (hardback) | ISBN 9781003032939 (ebook)
Subjects: MESH: Bambusa | Plant Shoots | Nutritive Value | Phytochemicals--therapeutic use | Functional Food
Classification: LCC SB317.B2 (print) | LCC SB317.B2 (ebook) | NLM QV 766 | DDC 633.5/8--dc23
LC record available at https://lccn.loc.gov/2020020484
LC ebook record available at https://lccn.loc.gov/2020020485

ISBN: 9780367470258 (hbk)
ISBN: 9780367467418 (pbk)
ISBN: 9781003032939 (ebk)

Typeset in Times
by Deanta Global Publishing Services, Chennai, India

Contents

Foreword ix
Endorsement xi
Preface xiii
Authors xvii
Abbreviations xix

Chapter 1 Introduction 1

1.1 Bamboo for a Healthy Planet 3
1.2 Origin of Bamboo 4
1.3 Bamboo in the Tradition and Culture of Asian Countries 5
1.4 Diversity and Distribution of Bamboo 10
1.5 Bamboo as a Plant 13
1.5.1 Plant Morphology 16
1.5.2 Rhizomes 17
1.5.3 Roots 19
1.5.4 Culms 19
1.5.5 Leaves 21
1.5.6 Shoots 21
1.5.7 Flowering 22
1.6 Multifarious Uses of Bamboo 23
1.6.1 Substitute for Wood in Housing and Building 25
1.6.2 Bamboo-Based Paper and Pulp Industries 26
1.6.3 Bamboo-Based Fibre and Fabric 26
1.6.4 Bamboo as Fuel 27
1.6.4.1 Charcoal 28
1.6.4.2 Gas 29
1.6.4.3 Biofuel 29
1.6.5 Bamboo as Food 29
1.6.5.1 Seeds 30
1.6.5.2 Leaves 30
1.6.5.3 Shoots 31
1.6.6 Bamboo as Medicine 32
1.6.7 Bamboo Salt 33
1.6.8 Miscellaneous 33

Chapter 2 Bamboo as Food and Medicine 37

2.1 Bamboo Shoots as a Nutrient-Rich Food 38
2.2 The Traditional Way of Bamboo Shoot Consumption 47
2.2.1 Fresh Shoots 47
2.2.2 Fermented Shoots 49

2.3 Bamboo as Medicine ... 54
2.3.1 Traditional Knowledge and Practices ... 57
2.3.2 Scientific Documentations about Health Benefits of Bamboo ... 58
2.3.2.1 Anti-Cancer Properties ... 58
2.3.2.2 Anti-Diabetic Properties ... 60
2.3.2.3 Anti-Fatigue Properties ... 61
2.3.2.4 Anti-Obesity Properties ... 61
2.3.2.5 Anti-Microbial Activity ... 63
2.3.2.6 Anti-Inflammatory Effect ... 66
2.3.2.7 Cardioprotective Properties ... 66
2.3.2.8 Hepatoprotective Activity ... 68
2.3.2.9 Immunomodulatory Activity ... 69
2.3.2.10 Bamboo as a Prebiotic ... 69

Chapter 3 Nutrients in Bamboo Shoots ... 71

3.1 Macro-Nutrients ... 72
3.1.1 Protein ... 72
3.1.2 Amino Acids ... 76
3.1.3 Carbohydrates ... 78
3.2 Micronutrients ... 78
3.2.1 Minerals ... 79
3.2.2 Macro-Minerals ... 80
3.2.2.1 Potassium ... 80
3.2.2.2 Calcium ... 80
3.2.2.3 Phosphorus ... 82
3.2.2.4 Sodium ... 82
3.2.2.5 Magnesium ... 83
3.2.2.6 Sulphur ... 83
3.2.2.7 Silicon ... 83
3.2.3 Micro-Mineral Elements ... 84
3.2.3.1 Iron ... 84
3.2.3.2 Zinc ... 85
3.2.3.3 Copper ... 85
3.2.3.4 Manganese ... 85
3.2.3.5 Selenium ... 86
3.3 Vitamin C (Ascorbic Acid) ... 86
3.4 Vitamin E (Tocopherols) ... 87

Chapter 4 Bioactive Compounds in Bamboo Shoots ... 89

4.1 Phenolic Compounds ... 89
4.2 Phytosterols ... 95
4.3 Dietary Fibres ... 98

Chapter 5 Anti-Nutrients in Bamboo Shoots ... 107

5.1 Cyanogenic Glycosides ... 107
5.2 Oxalates ... 110
5.3 Glucosinolates ... 112
5.4 Phytates ... 113
5.5 Saponins ... 114
5.6 Tannins ... 115

Chapter 6 Processing of Bamboo Shoots ... 117

6.1 Harvesting of Bamboo Shoots ... 118
6.2 Pre-Cooking Processing of Shoots ... 120
6.3 Traditional Methods of Bamboo Shoot Processing ... 123
6.3.1 Soaking ... 123
6.3.2 Heat Treatment ... 124
6.3.3 Drying ... 125
6.3.4 Sun-Drying ... 126
6.3.5 Oven-Drying ... 127
6.3.6 Fermentation ... 127
6.3.7 Fermented Shoots ... 128
6.4 Modern Methods of Processing ... 130
6.4.1 Solar-Drying ... 130
6.4.2 Microwave Drying ... 130
6.4.3 Convective Tray-Drying/Hot Air-Drying ... 130
6.4.4 Freeze-Drying ... 131
6.4.5 Osmotic Dehydration ... 132
6.4.6 Canning ... 133
6.5 Processing Methods for Removal of Anti-Nutrients ... 133
6.5.1 Cyanogenic Glycoside ... 133
6.5.2 Effect of Processing on Other Anti-Nutrients ... 135
6.6 Effect of Processing on Nutrient Content ... 136
6.6.1 Protein ... 139
6.6.2 Carbohydrate ... 139
6.6.3 Total Free Amino Acids ... 142
6.6.4 Starch ... 146
6.6.5 Fat ... 146
6.6.6 Ash ... 148
6.6.7 Moisture ... 148
6.6.8 Vitamins ... 148
6.7 Effect of Processing on Minerals ... 150
6.8 Effect of Processing on Bioactive Compounds ... 154
6.8.1 Phenol ... 154
6.8.2 Phytosterol ... 157
6.8.3 Dietary Fibre ... 157
6.9 Organoleptic Properties of Fresh and Processed Shoots ... 159

Chapter 7 Packaging and Shelf-Life Evaluation of Shoots 165

7.1 Bamboo Shoot Packaging 165
7.1.1 Polyethylene Packaging 168
7.1.2 Polyvinyl Chloride Film 171
7.1.3 Vacuum Packaging 173
7.1.4 Modified Atmospheric Packaging 174
7.1.5 Edible Film and Coatings 174

Chapter 8 Bamboo Shoots as Functional Foods and Nutraceuticals 177

8.1 Food Fortification and Functional Foods 178
8.2 Fortifying Food Products with Bamboo Shoots 179
8.2.1 Biscuits/Cookies 180
8.2.2 Nuggets 183
8.2.3 Candies 184
8.2.4 Chips 185
8.2.5 Crackers 186
8.2.6 Pickles 186
8.3 Nutraceuticals 187
8.4 Bamboo Shoots as Nutraceuticals 188
8.4.1 Anti-Oxidant Activity of Bamboo 192
8.4.2 *In-vivo* Studies in Balb/c Mice 196
8.4.3 Effect of Bamboo Shoots on Body and Organ Weight 196
8.4.4 Effect of Bamboo Shoots on the Anti-Oxidant Defense System 197
8.4.5 Effect of Bamboo Shoots on Glucose and Lipid Profile 197
8.4.6 Effect of Bamboo Shoots on Liver Function 199
8.4.7 Effect of Bamboo Shoots on Kidney Function 201

Epilogue 203

Glossary of Scientific Names 207

References 213

Index 239

World Bamboo Organization
9 Bloody Pond Road, Plymouth, MA 02360 USA
www.worldbamboo.net

WORLD BAMBOO

Foreword

I have been aware of the work of Dr. Nirmala Chongtham for over 5 years, as her team at Panjab University, Chandigarh, India, is leading the way in multiple research projects concerning bamboo shoots. This book contains vital information on bamboo as a health food and is very timely. The United Nations Sustainability Goals have provided a roadmap for what the world needs to do to improve life on earth, and this book relates to a few of these paramount goals: SDG 2 (Zero Hunger), SDG 3 (Good Health and Well-being), SDG 4 (Quality Education), SDG 8 (Decent Work & Economic Growth), SDG 9 (Industry, Innovation & Infrastructure) and SDG 15 (Life on Land). The Food and Agriculture Organization has expressed the urgency of need and demand for nutritious food for a growing world population in need of new food resources. Although bamboo shoots are eaten by millions of people every day as a staple, few are aware of the benefits to the human body as a 'superfood'.

Global health crises such as diabetes, heart disease, obesity and cancer threaten human populations, as well as real hunger and malnutrition. Eating bamboo in any form can help reduce the risks and the maladies due to providing anti-oxidants, essential vitamins, and metabolic processes that benefit the human body's defence system. Contemporary chefs will welcome bringing bamboo shoots to new recipes, to new audiences, creating new cuisines.

Agriculturists, farmers, educators, nutritionists, industrial food companies, health food innovators, chefs, foodies and the general public will find information within these pages very revealing and informative.

The array of imagery shows the physical structure of various species of shoots, preparation techniques, other uses of bamboos, as well as enticing prepared dishes that should make anyone want to try bamboo shoots! The Giant Panda has been a symbol of protecting wildlife, and its diet consists primarily of bamboo. We can also see the bamboo shoot as a symbol of protecting human health!

Susanne Lucas, Executive Director (WBO) **email: info@worldbamboo.net**

Endorsement

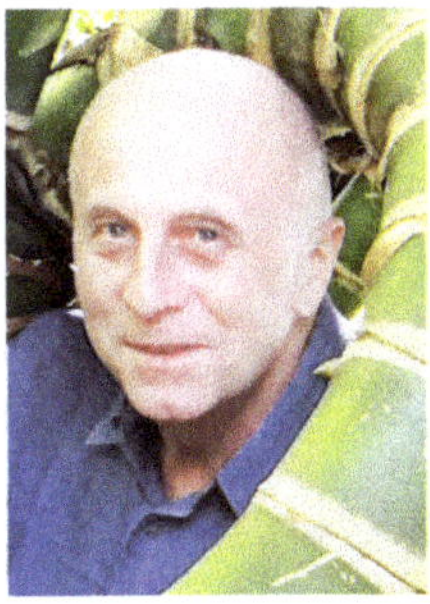

Be careful, the document in your hand is not a book, it's a bomb!

An amazing manifesto about bamboo shoots recognized as a health food of the 21st century. It offers a new perspective of using bamboo for food and medicine as a plant able to help humanity with simplicity and humility. It's an opportunity to imagine and create brand-new products able to answer the big question of a lot of humans living on urban areas (55% of population in 2018, 68% in 2030): 'how to eat safely a food profitable to my spirit, my body and my health?'.

To my humble knowledge, after 32 years on bamboo field, as former president of European Bamboo Society and as president of World Bamboo Organization, in spite of a personal two-metre-long bookshelf dedicated to bamboo books, it's the first time that I'm getting so much information not only about bamboo shoots but also about leaves, rhizomes, roots; processing and cooking of bamboo shoots and its multi-use and benefits to humankind, for eating, for caring, for curing … all that in a single book.

Nirmala Chongtham, one of the best worldwide specialists in bamboo shoots, helps us to discover the nutritional potential of this food rich in protein, carbohydrates, minerals and fibre but low in fat and sugar.

In Chapter 2, the food section, we have the keys to 21 dishes from India and 20 recipes from Philippines to Mexico, via Japan, Vietnam, Australia, China, Indonesia … and even from France.

In the section devoted to health and medicine, we dive into the multitude of uses of this plant and its effects on the main wounds of our time: stress, aging, oxidants, cancer, diabetes and obesity as well as on Alzheimer's, Parkinson's, asthma and many more conditions.

For the discerning and industrious reader, this book opens the door to a number of new products that could fulfil the unmet needs of our contemporaries for the reduction of cholesterol, for the prevention of cardiovascular diseases, for the stabilization of hypercholesterolemia and also, for its potential effects as an aphrodisiac.

For sure it is time for bamboo to be truly recognized for its extraordinary value. Indeed, bamboo is a superfood!

Read it and taste it. Your vision of this plant will enrich your days forever.

Paris, March 21, 2020

Michel Abadie
President
World Bamboo Organization

Preface

Bamboo, an ordinary plant with extra-ordinary qualities, has been associated with mankind since time immemorial. The fossil records indicate the presence of bamboo in Neogene, Paleogene to late Miocene-Pliocene from South America, North America, Europe, Australia and New Zealand to Asia. Bamboo fossil culms and leaves have recently been reported from the late Oligocene and late Miocene-Pliocene sediments of North East India which represent the earliest records of bamboos from India indicating that bamboo probably dispersed to Asia from India after the establishment of land connections between the Indian and Eurasian plates. In Asia, bamboo has been mainly used in East and South East Asia in countries like China, Japan, India, Indonesia and Philippines and it has been an integral part of culture, economy, house construction and household items, livelihood, religions and rituals and is often considered as a symbol of constancy, fidelity, integrity and purity inspiring the emotional and spiritual life and bestowing good luck upon the people. In the 21st century, bamboo is gaining increased attention as an evergreen plant with multiple functions and benefits. It has extremely bright prospects as it can help countries to reach their sustainable developmental goals without any negative impacts on the environment. A plant with tremendous versatility, bamboo plays an important role in soil erosion control, soil remediation and climate change mitigation. Climate change is considered one of the greatest threats facing humanity. Various studies suggest that bamboo forest ecosystems can be leveraged to help mitigate climate change whilst simultaneously providing other important services for human adaptation and development.

In the modern world, much emphasis is given to bamboo as a material for construction and its use as food is given least importance even though for centuries, bamboo has been valued as an important source of food and medicine both for animals and humans. In fact, for some animals like giant panda and golden bamboo lemur, bamboo is the only food. Bamboo shoots are popular vegetables in many Asian countries and their food value and medicinal properties have been documented in ancient medicinal books. In China during the Tang Dynasty, a banquet was incomplete without bamboo shoots and in Japan, bamboo shoot is considered king of forest vegetables. In India, the use of bamboo for medicine goes back to around 10,000 years during the time of *Chawanrishi* when bamboo in the form of *banslochan,* an amorphous substance collected in the culms of some bamboos, was used for making the tonic still popularly known as *Chawanprash.* In the Meetei community of Manipur, planting of bamboo in the courtyard is considered lucky and a symbol of prosperity. Bamboo shoots, both fresh and fermented, are most consumed in the North Eastern region of India. When we started our research on bamboo shoots in 2002, there were very few papers dealing with detailed studies of the nutritive value and health promoting properties of the shoots and we felt that there is a need to highlight these qualities of which many people are not aware. It was this realization that inspired us to write this book on bamboo shoot highlighting its health benefits as a superfood. The book is a compilation of our 18 years of research on bamboo shoots;

10 students have been awarded their PhDs based on this work. Starting with a brief introduction about bamboo and its uses as food and medicine, the other chapters include almost all our research data on the nutrients, bioactive compounds, antinutrients, processing and packaging, fortification of food items with bamboo shoots and bamboo as a nutraceutical. To collect information of edible bamboos and to know about the traditional uses of the shoots as food and medicine, surveys were conducted in the bamboo shoot consuming regions of India to get authentic data. The book has general information about bamboo shoots and their traditional uses followed by scientific studies which validates the ancient hypothesis about the nutritional and health benefits of shoots.

Prof. C. Nirmala would like to thank Dr. M.L. Sharma, Emeritus Professor, Department of Botany, Panjab University, Chandigarh, India, with whom the work on bamboos was initiated. We are also indebted to all our research scholars who painstakingly conducted the research work with full dedication and also helped us in the compilation of the book. Without their work, this book would be incomplete. Thanks to Dr. Vivek Sharma and Dr. Harjit Kaur Bajwa for their assistance from time to time. A special thanks to Dr. Oinam Santosh for the photography, figures and going through the manuscript so meticulously. Financial assistance from Ministry of Food Processing Industries, Department of Biotechnology and University Grants Commission, Government of India to conduct the research work is duly acknowledged. Our heartfelt thanks to Ned Jaquith Foundation and American Bamboo Society, USA and Panjab University, Chandigarh, India for providing financial assistance for writing this book. We also acknowledge the contribution of our bamboo friends Michel Abadie, Ximena Londono, Merdelyn Cassi Lit, Mauricio Mora Tello, Avery Chua and Bryan Benitez McClelland who provided us with photos and bamboo shoot recipes. Special thanks to Mr. Yoshinobu Komatsu, owner, Bamboo Shoot Restaurant UOKA, Japan for providing his recipes and photographs. Thanks to Mr. Arun, Bangalore, India for editing one of the chapters. We also express our gratitude to Prof. Cherla Sastry Professor (Adjunct) Forestry University of Toronto, Canada for his support and guidance. Thanks to everyone in the CRC publishing team, especially Ms. Randy Brehm and Dr. Julia Tanner, who have been so efficient, cooperative and patient.

Prof. Nirmala Chongtham expresses her heartfelt thanks to Susanne Lucas, Executive Director, World Bamboo Organization, USA, for her help and support. Thank you, my dear friend for being there and introducing me to WBO, an amazing platform which brings all bamboo enthusiasts together. Finally, thank you to all those who have been a part of my journey: Dr. Chongtham Priyoranjan, Professor, Department of Economics, Manipur University, Ch. Manoranjan, Chongtham Bijoy, Dr. Satyaranjan Chongtham, Dr. Sandhyarani Nongmaithem, Ms. Monica Chongtham and Mr. Rajesh Irungbam. My reverence to my late parents Mr. Ch. Ibochoubi Singh and Mrs. Ch. Kumudini and grandparents Mr. Wahengbam Radhamohan Singh and Mrs. Guni Devi for introducing me to bamboo, a pure natural resource and, above all, for instilling in me the importance of compassion and empathy.

Nirmala Chongtham
Department of Botany
Panjab University, Chandigarh, India

Madho Singh Bisht
Department of Environmental Studies
NEHU, Shillong, India

FINANCIAL ASSISTANCE

American Bamboo Society

NJF
Ned Jaquith
FOUNDATION

PANJAB UNIVERSITY ★ पंजाब यूनिवर्सिटी ★ ਪੰਜਾਬ ਯੂਨੀਵਰਸਿਟੀ
★ 1947 ★

Authors

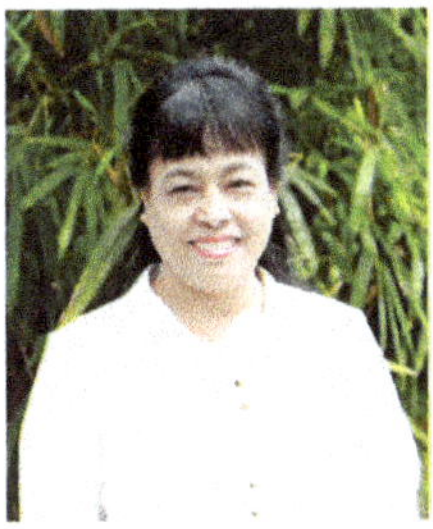

Nirmala Chongtham is presently working as Professor in the Department of Botany, Panjab University, Chandigarh, India. She has been working in bamboo shoot nutrition for the last 18 years and has guided more than 15 PhD students. Born and brought up in Manipur in the north-east region of India, she was introduced to bamboo and bamboo shoots at a very early age. She has surveyed most of the bamboo-growing areas in India focusing mainly on the north-eastern states which is the bamboo paradise of India and where bamboo shoots are part of the traditional cuisine and used regularly in most households as part of daily diet. Her team is working on various aspects of bamboo shoots starting from nutrient and phytochemical analyses, processing and packaging, food fortification with bamboo shoots and phytomodulatory effects of shoots in some non-communicable diseases using animal models. Food products fortified with bamboo shoots have also been developed by her group. She is closely associated with the World Bamboo Organization, USA. In recognition of her work in bamboo, she was appointed World Bamboo Ambassador from India in 2015. As an ambassador, she continues her work in promoting bamboo for environmental and socioeconomic development. She worked as Chair of the Technical Committee, World Bamboo Congress (WBC) 2015 in Korea, Co-Chair in WBC Mexico, 2018, Co-coordinator of the Third World Bamboo Workshop held in Manipur, India in 2019 and is the Chair for the 12th WBC to be held in Taiwan. She has travelled widely and has been invited to deliver lectures and has visited Germany, Belgium, Thailand, Korea, the United States, Mexico, Columbia and Costa Rica among others. Prof. Chongtham has received many project grants from India such as the University Grant Commission, Department of Science and Technology, Department of Biotechnology and Ministry of Food Processing Industries, New Delhi, India for conducting work on bamboo shoots. She has more than 100 research papers in international and national journals to her credit. In recognition of her work, she was awarded a grant by the Ned Jaquith Foundation and American Bamboo Society, USA to continue her work.

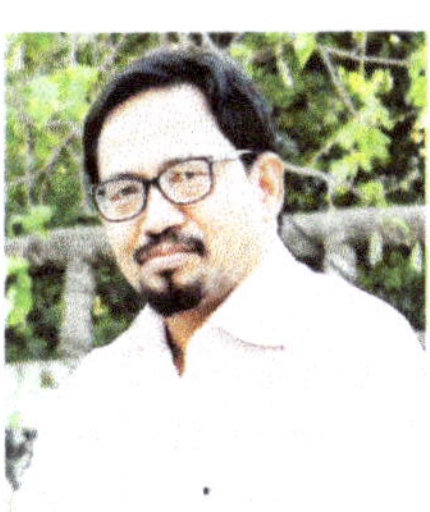

Madho Singh Bisht, Professor in Environmental Studies, North-Eastern Hill University, Shillong, Meghalaya, India, received his PhD in Botany from Delhi University in 1992, and has worked on various aspects of plants including cytogenetics, physiology, biodiversity and food and nutrition. He has worked at various research institutes and universities in India including Indian Agricultural Research Institute (IARI), Delhi, Delhi University (DU), Delhi, G.B. Pant Institute of Himalayan Environment and Development (GBPIHED), Almora and outside India at Osaka Koiku University, Osaka, Japan. For the last ten years, he has been working on the use and application of bamboo in the daily life of the people in north-east India, particularly on bamboo as a health food. He has published a number of research papers and articles on the promotion of bamboo shoots as a health food. The main emphasis is on the fortification of daily food items with various forms of young juvenile bamboo shoots.

Abbreviations

AD	Anno Domini
ADF	Acid detergent fibre
AGS	Adenocarcinoma gastric cell line
ANN	Artificial neural network
AuNPs	Gold nanoparticles
Balb/c	Bagg albino mice
Bax	Bcl2-Associated X protein
BCE	Before common era
Bcl-2	B-cell lymphoma 2
BEX	Bamboo extract
BL	Bamboo leaf
BS	Boiled shoots
BS-9x	Nine-time-baked bamboo salt
BSCP	Bamboo shoot crude polysaccharides
BSDF	Bamboo shoot dietary fibre
BSE	Bamboo shoot extract
BSO	Bamboo shoot oil
BSP	Bamboo shoot powder
BUN	Blood urea nitrogen
C57BL/6J	C57black 6J
cAMP	Cyclic adenosine monophosphate
CD	Cabinet solar dryer
CVD	Cardiovascular disease
d.w.	Dry weight
DF	Dietary fibre
DNA	Deoxyribonucleic acid
DPSD	Double pass solar dryer
e.g.	Exempli gratia (For example)
EBS	Extract from bamboo shavings
ERG	Engineering resources group
etc.	Etcetera
f.w.	Fresh weight
FAO	Food and Agriculture Organization
FBS	Fermented bamboo shoot
FBSM	Fermented bamboo shoot mince
FDA	Food and Drug Administration
FOS	Fructo-oligosaccharides
FSANZ	Food Standards Australia New Zealand
FTIR	Fourier transform infra-red
GB	Glass bottle
GC-MS	Gas chromatography mass spectrometry
GFR	Glomerular filtration rate

HDL	High-density lipoprotein
HDL-C	High-density lipoprotein cholesterol
HDPE	High-density polyethylene
HEK293	Human embryonic kidney cells
Hep3b	Hepatoma cell line
HepG2	Human liver cancer cell line
HFBS	High fat bamboo shoot fibre
HFC	High fat cellulose
HOMA-IR	Homeostatic model assessment of insulin resistance
HPLC	High performance liquid chromatography
i.e.	id est (that is)
IAUC	Incremental area under the curve
ICP-AES	Inductively coupled plasma—atomic emission spectrometry
ICR	Institute of cancer research
IDF	Insoluble dietary fibre
IFN-γ	Interferon gamma
IL-2	Interleukin-2
INBAR	International Bamboo and Rattan Organization
LAB	Lactic acid bacteria
LDL	Low-density lipoprotein
LDL-C	Low-density lipoprotein cholesterol
LDPE	Low-density polyethylene
lig-8	Lignophenol derivative from bamboo lignin
MAP	Modified atmospheric packaging
NBS	Non-bacterial prostatitis
NDF	Neutral detergent fibre
NF-κB	Nuclear factor kappa light chain-enhancer of activated B cells.
NK	Natural killer cells
NMBA	National Mission on Bamboo Applications
NMR	Nuclear magnetic resonance
NSAIA	Non-steroidal anti-inflammatory agent
NSC	Non-structural carbohydrates
OD	Osmotic dehydration
OSD	Open sun drying
P≤0.05	Probability less than or equal to 0.05
PCM	Paracetamol
PCT N-glycan	Plant complex type N-glycans
pH	Potential of hydrogen
POP	Phytosterol oxidation products
Pp-AMP	Anti-microbial peptides from *Phyllostachys pubescens*
RBC	Red blood cells
ROS	Reactive oxygen species
RT-PCR	Reverse transcription polymerase chain reaction
SanSTAGE(TM)	Pure compounds obtained from the bamboo grass leaves; 25% of bamboo grass extract and 75% of dextrin
SB	*Scutellaria baicalensis* root
SBE	*Sasa borealis* extract

SD	Standard deviation
SDF	Soluble dietary fibre
SHRS	Spontaneously hypersensitive rats
Spp.	Several species
SQE	*Sasa quelpaertensis* extract
SS	Soaked shoots
TBARS	Thiobarbituric acid reactive substances
TBS	Tender bamboo shoot
TC	Total cholesterol
TCA8113	Human tongue squamous carcinoma cell
TG	Triglyceride
TNF-α	Tumour necrosis factor alpha
US	Unprocessed shoots
USA	United States of America
USD	United States dollar
USFDA	United States Food and Drug Administration
Var.	Variety
Vit C	Vitamin C
Vit E	Vitamin E
Viz	Videlicet (meaning: namely)
WBP1	Water-soluble polysaccharides 1
WBP2	Water-soluble polysaccharides 2
WDXRF	Wavelength dispersive X-ray fluorescence spectrometry
WEBS	Water phase extract of bamboo shavings
WHO	World Health Organization

CHEMICALS

ABTS	2,2-zino- bis (3-ethylbenzothiazolin-6-sulfonic acid)
ACE	Angiotensin converting enzyme
AgNPs	Silver nanoparticles
ALP	Alkaline phosphatase
ALT	Alanine aminotransferase
AMPK	AMP-activated protein kinase
Asp-Tyr	Asparagine-Tyrosine
AST	Aspartate aminotransferase
AuNPs	Gold nanoparticles
BHT	Butylated 4-hydroxytoluene
C_2O_2	Ethylene dione
$C_6H_{18}O_{24}P_6$	Phytic acid
$CaCl_2$	Calcium chloride
CAD	Cinnamyl alcohol dehydrogenase
CAT	Catalase
CCl_4	Carbon tetrachloride
ClO_2	Chlorine dioxide
CMC	Carboxymethyl cellulose
CO_2	Carbon dioxide

COX-2	Cyclooxygenase-2
DAPI	4,6-diamidino-2-phenylindole
DMBA	7,12-Dimethylben(a)anthracene
DPPH	2,2-Diphenyl-1-picrylhydrazyl
GOT	Glutamic oxaloacetic transaminase
GPT	Glutamic pyruvic transaminase
GPx	Glutathione peroxidase
GR	Glutathione reductase
GSH	Glutathione
GSH-Px	Glutathione peroxidase
HCN	Hydrogen cyanide
HDL	High-density lipoprotein
HDL-C	High-density lipoprotein cholesterol
HFC	High fat cellulose
iNOS	Inducible nitric oxide synthase
KMS	Potassium metabisulphite
LDH	Lactate dehydrogenase
MDA	Malondialdehyde
MTT	3-(4,5-dimethylrhiazol-2-yl)-2,5-diphenyl tetrazolium bromide
NaCl	Sodium chloride
NADPH	Nicotinamide adenine dinucleotide phosphate hydrogen
NaOH	Sodium hydroxide
NO	Nitric oxide
PAL	Phenylalanine ammonia-lyase
PE	Polyethylene
POD	Peroxidase
PPO	Polyphenol oxidase
PVC	Polyvinyl chloride
SGOT	Serum glutamic-oxaloacetic transaminase
SGPT	Serum glutamic-pyruvic transaminase
SNP	Sodium nitroprusside
SOD	Superoxide dismutase
STZ	Streptozotocin
TBA or TBARS	Thiobarbituric acid
WST-1	Water soluble tetrazolium salts-1
XOS	Xylo-oligosaccharides

SYMBOLS

α	Alpha
β	Beta
$	US dollar
%	Percentage
<	Less than
=	Equal to

>	Greater than
±	Plus, or minus
≤	Less than or equal to
≥	Greater than or equal
®	Registered
°N	Degree North
°S	Degree South
°brix	Degree brix
°C	Degree Celsius
°F	Degree Fahrenheit

UNITS

µmol H_2O_2	Reduced/min/mg proteins micromole of hydrogen peroxide reduced in one minute by one milligram of protein
µmol/L	Micromole per litre
cc/m^2	Cubic centimetre per square metre
cfu	Colony forming unit
cm	Centimetre
D	Dalton
g	Gram
g/100 g	Gram per hundred grams
g/kg	Gram per kilogram
GAE/g	Gallic acid equivalent per gram
ha	Hectare
hr	Hour
hrs	Hours
IC_{50}	Half maximal inhibitory concentration of anti-oxidant activity
IU/mg protein	International unit per milligram protein
kg	Kilogram
log cfu/cm^2	In term of logarithm colony forming unit per square centimetre
log cfu/g	In term of logarithm colony forming unit per gram. Log value is used for generating graph so that all big and small values can be expressed in one graph
m	Metre
mg	Milligram
mg CNE/g	Milligram catechin equivalent per gram
mg GAE/100 g	Milligram gallic acid equivalent per hundred grams
mg GAE/g	Milligram gallic acid equivalent per gram
mg QUE/g d.w.	Milligram quercetin equivalent per gram dry weight
mg/100 g	Milligram per hundred grams
mg/100 g f.w.	Milligram per hundred-gram fresh weight
mg/day	Milligram per day
mg/dl	Milligram per decilitre
mg/g	Milligram per gram
mg/kg	Milligram per kilogram
mg/kg b.w.	Milligram per kilogram body weight

min	Minute
ml/l	Millilitre per litre
mM	Millimolar
mm	Millimetre
mmol	Millimole
mmol/L	Millimoles per litre
nmol of NADPH consumed/min/mg protein	Nanomole of nicotinamide adenine dinucleotide phosphate hydrogen consumed in one minute by one milligram of protein
nmol of NADPH oxidized/min/mg protein	Nanomole nicotinamide adenine dinucleotide phosphate hydrogen oxidized in one minute by one milligram of protein
nmol/mg	Nanomole per milligram
Ppm	Parts per million
QUE/g	Quercetin equivalent per gram
Rpm	Revolutions per minute
U/L	Units per litre
W	Watt
w/w	Weight by weight
µg GA/ml	Microgram gallic acid per millilitre
µg/g	Microgram per gram
µg/ml	Microgram per millilitre
µm	Micrometre

ELEMENTS

Ca	Calcium
Ca^{2+}	Calcium ion
Cu	Copper
Fe	Iron
Fe^{2+}	Ferrous ion
K	Potassium
Mg	Magnesium
Mg^{2+}	Magnesium ion
Mn	Manganese
Na	Sodium
Ni	Nickel
P	Phosphorus
S	Sulphur
Se	Selenium
Si	Silicon
Zn	Zinc

AMINO ACIDS

Ala	Alanine
Asn	Asparagine
Asp	Aspartic acid
Cys	Cysteine
Glu	Glutamine
Gly	Glycine
His	Histidine
Ile	Isoleucine
Leu	Leucine
Lys	Lysine
Met	Methionine
Phe	Phenylalanine
Ser	Serine
Thr	Threonine
Trp	Tryptophan
Tyr	Tyrosine
Val	Valine

1 Introduction

Bestow upon us a hundred bamboo clumps.

Rig Veda

This chapter opens with a beautiful quote which is the first direct reference to bamboo in Indian literature in *Rig Veda*, a sacred religious book written in Sanskrit around 1500 BCE and considered to be the oldest compilation of human wisdom (Sastry 2008). Bamboo, referred to as the 'poor man's timber' is projected to become the 'wood and food' of the 21st century. Bamboo is known as 'the plant with a thousand faces' and has played a significant role in human society since ancient times. Today, it contributes to the subsistence needs of over 1 billion people worldwide. Over the centuries, bamboo has fulfilled all human needs, particularly in the East and Southeast Asian region. The plant is intertwined deeply with the daily life of rural populations, as it is an indispensable part of their cultural, traditional, social and economic requirements. Bamboo is a natural renewable resource which can help countries to reach their sustainable development goals; 6 of the 17 sustainable development goals are relevant to bamboo, as they contribute to poverty reduction; food security and improved nutrition; energy; housing and urban development; sustainable production and consumption; climate change; and land degradation. They all contribute to a seventh goal—stronger implementation and partnerships. Most important of all, bamboo can make a positive contribution to women's empowerment, economic growth and technology (Figures 1.1 and 1.2).

Around the world, it is estimated that over 1 billion people live in homes made from bamboo. Bamboo remains the single most important organic building material in Asia, accounting for over 70% of rural housing (INBAR 2007). There are more than 1,500 recorded uses of bamboo, providing jobs to more than 2 billion people worldwide. Due to its various uses and applications in many parts of the world, bamboo is referred to as the 'cradle to coffin plant', 'mankind's best friend', 'miracle grass' and 'green gold'. Buddhists call it the 'blessing of the heavens' (Crouzet 1998). Bamboo has been used for many different purposes, for example, to make a surgical blade, to create shelter, food and medicine, and for bamboo biers and coffins. Even renowned scientists used bamboo in their inventions: Thomas Edison used carbonized bamboo as a filament for his glass lightbulb, and Alexander Graham Bell used a bamboo needle for his first phonograph. Bamboo is a very hardy and adaptive plant and is known for its resilience: in Hiroshima and Nagasaki, after the devastation caused by the atomic bombs, bamboo was the first plant which sprouted (Kynes 2006). Today, bamboo is recognized as an important asset in eradication of poverty and in economic and environmental development, and it remains extremely important as a basic crop and material for rural people living in Asia, Latin America and Africa. In some countries, the processing of bamboo has shifted from low-end crafts and utensils to high-end, value-added commodities such as laminated panels,

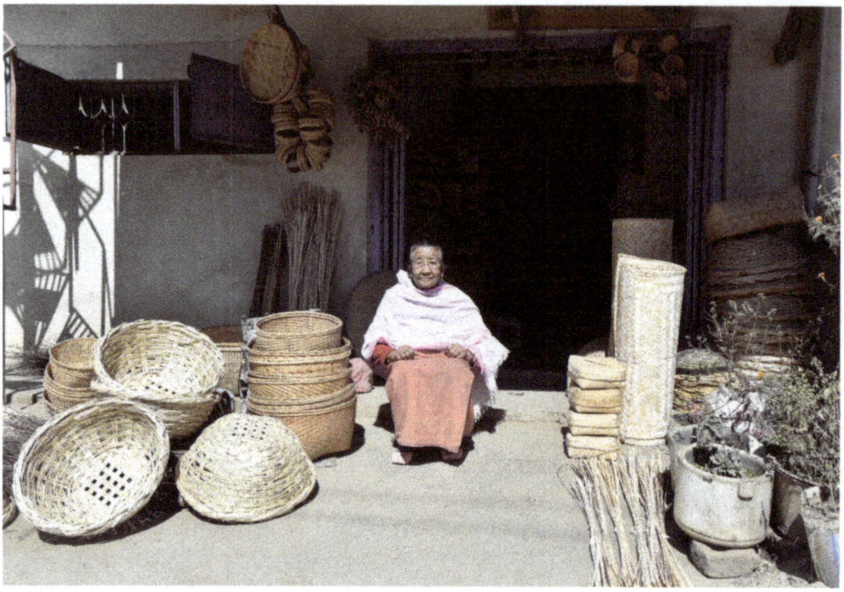

FIGURE 1.1 Women earn a livelihood from bamboo products in Manipur, India.

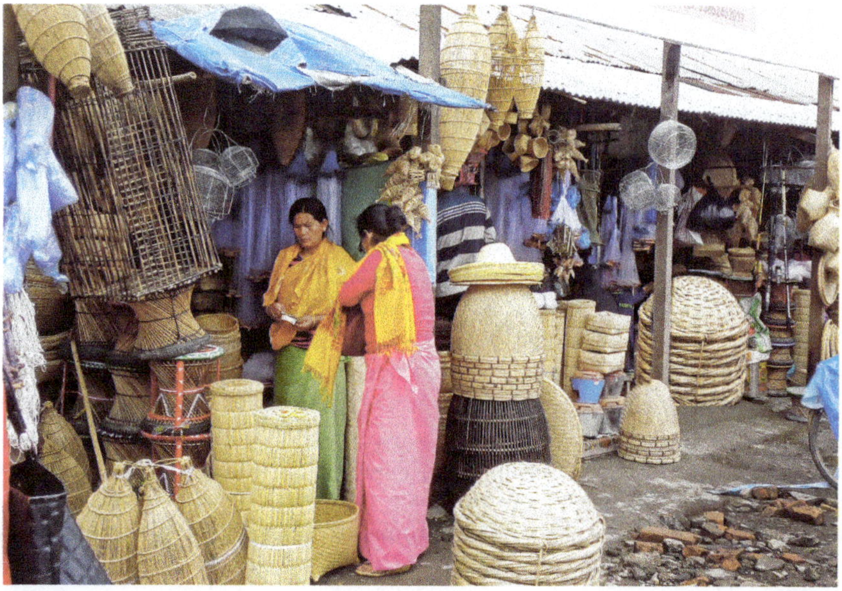

FIGURE 1.2 Bamboo products in the women market or Ima Keithel of Imphal, Manipur, India.

boards, pulp, paper, mats, prefabricated houses, cloth, cosmetics, medicine, fuel and value-added products from bamboo shoots. With its high growth rate, a wide range of applications and the ability to renew easily, bamboo resources are extremely important in the 21st century. In addition to contributing to local economies and the environment, global bamboo industries have rapidly developed in recent years and contributed more than USD 60 billion annually, proving that bamboo forests have the potential to contribute to inclusive and green economic development at both regional and global levels (INBAR 2019).

1.1 BAMBOO FOR A HEALTHY PLANET

Bamboo is a plant with tremendous versatility. Its application not only acts as a wood substitute in a variety of applications but also as an erosion control, soil remediation and climate change mitigation agent. Climate change is considered to be one of the greatest threats facing humanity. The rapid increase in atmospheric CO_2 and global surface temperature since the advent of the Industrial Revolution has motivated many scientists to investigate methods that can securely contain or lessen atmospheric CO_2. Increasing the level of carbon sequestration is one of the important viable options for reducing the total amount of carbon dioxide in the atmosphere and thus mitigating future dangerous climate change related scenarios. The ability of bamboo to provide global environmental services through carbon sequestration is now receiving high levels of interest. Based upon its fast growth rate, high carbon sequestration capability and high annual regrowth after harvesting, bamboo outperforms fast-growing trees in its rate of carbon accumulation and, consequently, climate mitigation has long been an important part of its green credentials (Yiping et al. 2010). According to the Guinness Book of World Records, the fastest-growing plant on earth is bamboo; it grows up to 91 cm (35") per day, which is almost 4 cm (1.5") an hour. The capacity of bamboo for carbon sequestration and oxygen release is 35% higher than those of trees (Zhaohua and Wei 2018). The best part is that the captured carbon by bamboo is not released immediately to the environment and can be used in various ways. Bamboo forests have a high carbon stock potential, especially when the harvested culms are used as durable products. Various studies suggest that bamboo forest ecosystems can be leveraged to help mitigate climate change, whilst simultaneously providing other important services for human adaptation and development. Bamboo forests are potent eco-guardians as they recycle a huge amount of CO_2 (about 14 tons/ha/annum) and minimize pollution by reducing up to 35% carbon dioxide and delivering more oxygen to the environment. Moreover, bamboo consumes high amounts of nitrogen which helps to decrease water pollution. The root and the extensive underground rhizome system, which is mostly concentrated in the upper 30 cm of the soil, enhances its holding capacity, thereby proving very effective in preventing soil erosion. It grows well on steep hillsides, road embankments, on the banks of ponds and streams and can thus prevent land sliding and also is effective in flood control. Bamboo creates a huge biomass and enhances the moisture retention of forests because of its dense leaf litter. The extent of available fertile lands is under increasing pressure from varied causes, including overuse of fertilizers and pesticides, salinization, acidification or alkalization and nutrition depletion. In mountainous areas of Japan, bamboo forests have been reported to play an active role in preventing soil acidification. Bamboo forests have great potential in reclaiming degraded land because of its ability to grow on most soil types. Bamboo can grow even on the marginalized land unsuitable for most crops or in combination with other crops in forestry and agroforestry. Because of its rapid growth and biomass-generating abilities, it can rehabilitate degraded lands at a faster rate and can thus play a key role in achieving recently adopted global restoration targets which include the Bonn Challenge that aims to restore 150 million ha of degraded and deforested land by 2020 and the New York Declaration on Forests to restore 350 million ha by 2030. In recent decades, a rapid increase of metal in agricultural soil due to urbanization and industrialization causes threats to human health when they enter the food chain. Bamboo can also counter the problem of heavy metal contamination as it has a tremendous ability to rapidly accumulate heavy metals from soil and water which can be utilized in purification of contaminated soil and water bodies.

Bamboo is a highly renewable grass that matures in four to five years, whereas a hardwood tree takes almost 60 years to mature. If bamboo is used more often as a building material, it will help save hardwood trees. Moreover, compared to hardwood trees, bamboo can produce 20 times more usable material in a single harvest. Thus, it plays an important role in reducing pressure on forestry resources. The successful use of bamboo in different product lines, ranging from furniture and flooring to paper and packaging demonstrates the high potential for bamboo as a more sustainable alternative material in the production of many products.

1.2 ORIGIN OF BAMBOO

The word *bamboo* has its origins in the ancient Indian name for bamboo, 'Mambu''. The earliest mention of the word from which the present word, 'Bamboo' has been derived is in *The Canon of Medicine*, an encyclopedia of medicine compiled by the Persian physician-philosopher Avicenna (Ibn Sina) and published in five volumes in the 11th century. In this book, the author refers to a medicine called *Tabaxir*, which in Arabic means milk, juice or a liquid in condensed form. Garcia da Orta, a Portuguese physician, herbalist and naturalist working in Goa, India, described many plants from India in his book, *Coloquis dos Simples Drogas da India* in 1563 and mentioned *Tabaxir.* According to Garcia da Orta, local people at that time called this medicine 'Saccar Mambu' (Saccar in Portuguese is sugar and 'Mambu' in the Goan language is the cane or branch of a tree). Gaspard (Caspar) Bauhin, a Swiss botanist, in his book *Phytopinax*, which was published in 1596, used the name *Arundo* for a woody or tree-like reed from India. Later this tree-like reed was found to be a bamboo and was renamed *Arundo arbor.* Bauhin mentioned that the substance derived from Arundo was called *Tabaxir* by Avicenna and the plant-producing *Tabaxir* was called 'Mambu' by Indians. Mambu became *Bambusa*, the basis of the genus *Bambusa* of Linnaeus (1753) and bamboo in English. This *Tabaxir* (*Tabasheer*) of Avicenna is the same as *Banslochan* used by Chyawan Rishi (around 10,000 years ago), an important ingredient in the age-old health tonic *Chyawanprash*. '*Banslochan*' is made up of two words, *'Bans'* and lochan. *'Bans'* means bamboo and is used to make Bansuri or a flute, one of the oldest musical instruments, played by Lord Shri Krishna, the Hindu God. All of these clearly indicate that the words 'Mambu' and 'Bans' are used for naming the same plant that produces a milky substance or juice called *Tabasheer* or *Banslochan*. According to Clark (1997), woody bamboos evolved in the lowland tropics of Gondwanaland during the tertiary period and bamboos dispersed to Asia from India. Srivastava et al. (2019) reported fossil leaves and culms from the late Miocene-Pliocene sediments of Arunachal Pradesh and late Oligocene sediments of Assam in north-east India. The fossil culms are named *Bambusiculmus tirapensis* and *Bambusiculmus makumensis* from the late Oligocene (about 25 million years old) sediments in Arunachal Pradesh and leaves *Bambusium deomarense* and *Bambusium arunachalense* from the late Miocene to Pliocene sediments. Previously, the Yunnan province in China recorded the oldest fossil, but these are less than 20 million years old, clearly indicating that Asian bamboo originated in India and migrated to China. The culm fossils reported from India represent the earliest records of bamboos from Asia, thereby indicating that bamboos probably dispersed to Asia from India after the establishment of land connections between the Indian and Eurasian plates. The fossil records of bamboos also indicate that ancient bamboos diversified in warm and humid monsoonal climates in Asia.

1.3 BAMBOO IN THE TRADITION AND CULTURE OF ASIAN COUNTRIES

Bamboo has been culturally and economically important in many Asian countries. According to an ancient Asian saying, 'A man is born in a bamboo cradle and goes away in a bamboo coffin, everything in between is possible with bamboo'. McClure (1966) wrote that 'Bamboos are everything to some people and something to every person'. In some parts of India, bamboo is also called *Kalpavirksha* (divine tree in Indian mythology fulfilling all the needs and desires) due to its numerous uses in daily life in physical as well as in spiritual form. China is known as the 'bamboo civilized country' from where the bamboo culture spread to neighbouring countries including Korea, Japan and others (Jiayan 2014). In Korea, the remains of bamboo baskets indicate the use of bamboo from 1–2 BCE recorded in the Dahori Tomb at Changwongun, Gyeongsangnam-do. The importance of bamboo in Chinese culture is reflected in the words of Su Dongpo, a revered literary figure of the Song Dynasty (960–1270), who said that without bamboo the people of China would lose their serenity as well as their culture (Yang et al. 2008). The Chinese were the first to appreciate the beauty and utility of bamboo with poets extolling this versatile plant and artists painting it, cherishing its grace and beauty (Tom 1989). Oriental scholars, artists, and epicures have praised the admirable qualities of bamboo in painting, rhymed couplets and lyrical tributes. Shen Kuo (1031–1095), a scientist and polymath from the Song Dynasty (960–1279), based his geological theory of gradual climate change based on the findings of underground petrified bamboo in the dry northern regions of the country. In China, the oldest bamboo item, a plaited bamboo mat discovered in the Gaomiao cultural relic site in central-south China, is 7,400 years old. Bamboo articles were recorded in the oldest Chinese characters inscribed on bone and tortoise shell unearthed from the ruins of the Yin Dynasty (1600–1100 BCE) in Anyang, Henan. During the Zhou Dynasty (1100–300 BCE), small culms were used as fishing-rods, and larger culms were split into slips on which historical events were recorded. Musical instruments were made of bamboo and bamboo shoots were cooked and eaten with fish and meat. In the Jin Dynasty (313–420), more than 200 agricultural implements and everyday items were made from bamboo. In ancient China, bamboo replaced hemp for paper making and became the most common material from 8th century CE. This improved bamboo paper has been graded as the best for Chinese painting and handwriting. In ancient wars, bamboo bows and arrows were effective weapons and the first firearms and missiles were made from bamboo culms after the invention of gunpowder in China.

People from several south-east Asian countries often consider bamboo as a symbol of constancy, fidelity, integrity and purity, inspiring the emotional and spiritual life and bestowing good luck upon the people. Bamboo has always been associated with people of Asian countries from birth to death and there are several folk tales, myths, beliefs and even superstitions associated with bamboo highlighting the intricate relation of this wonderful plant with the culture and tradition of several Asian societies. According to 'The Tale of the Bamboo Cutter', a tenth-century Japanese Monogatari, princess Kaguya was discovered as an infant by a bamboo cutter who split open a bamboo to find her asleep inside. In the Philippines, it is believed that the first man and woman emerged when a bamboo stalk was split into half. In Meghalaya, India, there is a clan called *Nongseij*, which means originating from the bamboo grove. Japan considers bamboo to be a sacred plant and a symbol of long life, while in rural districts of Nepal, bamboo is used for reincarnation ceremonies. An old Vietnamese proverb links the longevity of bamboo to the people of Vietnam: 'When the bamboo is old, the bamboo sprouts appear' signifying the fact that Vietnam will always remain alive because even if the older generation dies, there will always be a younger generation.

For many people, bamboo is a source of inspiration for aesthetic, biological and culinary pursuits. According to Crouzet (1998), bamboo exemplifies the Taoist belief that in facing any present challenge, bending in order not to break will lead to triumph later. The image that characterizes this notion is that the tall bamboo stalks bowed down to the ground from the irresistible force of a storm that nevertheless returns afterward to their fully upright glory. In the Chinese culture, bamboos symbolize gentleness, modesty and serenity and the people consider it as one of the four noble plants along with plum, orchid and chrysanthemum. Because of its durability and its vigorous growth during the cold winter, bamboo is one of the symbols for longevity and is also considered a 'friend of the winter'. The versatile application of bamboo in people's daily lives in Asia was vividly described by Geil (1904) in his book *A Yankee on the Yangtze*, which is a narrative of a journey from Shanghai through the central kingdom to Burma. He wrote:

> A man can sit in a bamboo house under a bamboo roof, on a bamboo chair at a bamboo table, with a bamboo hat on his head and bamboo sandals on his feet. He can at the same time hold in one hand a bamboo bowl, on the other hand, bamboo chopsticks and eat bamboo sprouts. When through with his meal, which has been cooked over

> a bamboo fire, the table may be washed with a bamboo cloth and he can fan himself with a bamboo fan, take a siesta on a bamboo bed, lying on a bamboo mat with his head resting on a bamboo pillow. He might then take a walk over a bamboo suspension bridge, drink water from a bamboo ladle and scrape himself with a bamboo scraper.

In modern days, bamboo is used as industrial raw material for pulp and paper, construction and engineering materials, food and medicine. Many nutritious and active components such as vitamins, amino acids, proteins, phenolic acid, polysaccharide, trace elements and steroid can be extracted from bamboo culm, shoot and leaf, and all these have anti-oxidant, anti-aging, anti-bacterial and anti-viral functions. Due to all these chemical properties of bamboo and its capacity to set right various global problems, there is currently unprecedented interest in bamboo all over the world.

The use of bamboo in rituals of birth and death still persists in some parts of the world. Traditionally, a piece of sharp blade of bamboo is used to cut the umbilical cord of a newly born baby. In the Meetei community of Manipur, India, the sharp blade called *Wakthou* is specifically made from *Bambusa tulda* taking the upper layer of a section of bamboo. Even today, a ritual known as *Epan thaba* is performed six days after the birth of a baby in which the baby is placed on a *Yangkok* or a circular winnowing bamboo fan with a prayer for the good health and long life of the baby (Figure 1.3A and B).

The reason for putting the baby on a circular winnowing fan is because the fan symbolizes the shape of the earth and though given birth by the mother, the baby will be brought up upon the earth. Then the maternal uncle will take a bow and arrows made of bamboo and shoot the arrows in four directions to ward off evil. The coffin for carrying the dead body includes three or five supporting bamboos among the planks on the inner and lower surface of the coffin. A large bamboo hat known as *Yenpak* is placed over the coffin and a *Yangkok* is also carried which also serves as a fan in the cremation process. Four poles of bamboo with bushy top known as *Chanduwa* are erected around the four corners of a funeral pyre. In many tribal communities of India, a dead body is placed on a bamboo mat or beneath a thatched bamboo hut. Then the body is placed inside a large bamboo basket and carried on a bamboo bier to the cremation or burial ground. A bamboo culm is used for keeping water and a prayer is performed after which the water is poured on the ground on completion of the ceremony. This signifies that like the rest of the material world, man is made up of elements that disintegrate after death and dissolve into nature. Bamboo is an indispensable part of the *Karbis*, a hill tribe of Assam, India and there is a popular proverb that says 'A *Karbi* is born with bamboo in his hand and leaves the world holding a bamboo' (Teron and Borthakur 2012). In *Karbi* society, when a mother conceives, the family performs certain rituals in honour of the unborn baby using rice grains wrapped with banana leaves and tied with bamboo. During the lifetime of the person, he/she uses bamboo mat tied to a bamboo culm with bamboo and taken to the cremation ground. Hence, for the *Karbis*, life begins with bamboo and ends with bamboo.

Bamboo is also used in the rituals of some Indian weddings. Four or eight bamboo poles that represent fertility and purity are used for the corners of the wedding canopy with one at the centre. The top of the canopy is covered with green bamboo

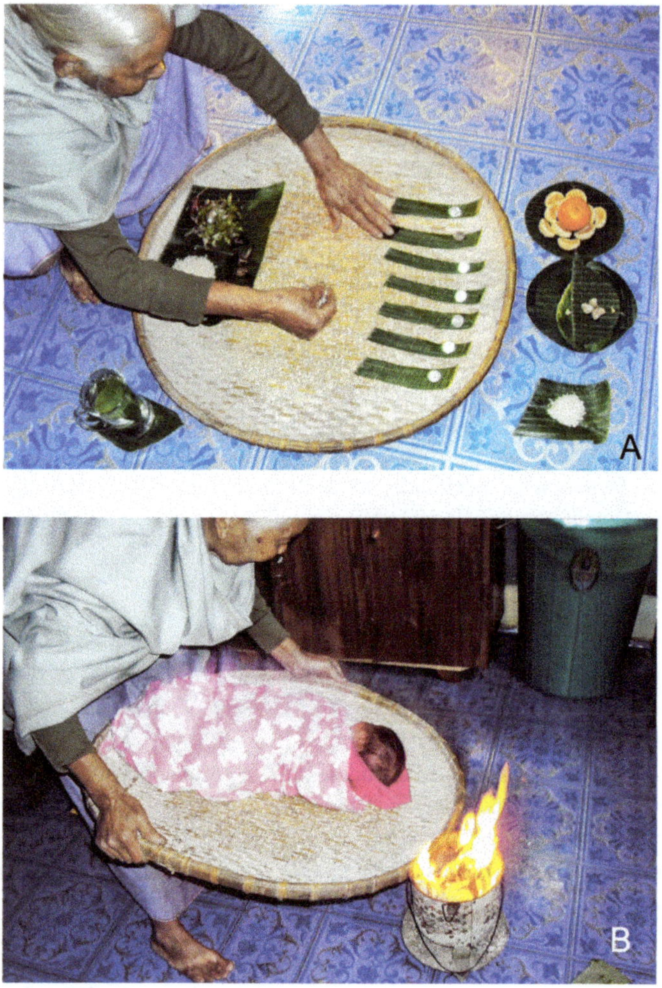

FIGURES 1.3 A and B. A Manipuri *Maibi* (physician) performing rituals for a newly born baby on a bamboo winnowing fan.

leaves and kush grass (*Eragrostis cynosuroides*). This is symbolic of the umbrella which is a symbol of 'respect, prestige and honour'. In the *Khasi* tribe of Meghalaya, it is customary to exchange betel nut and betel leaf between the groom and bride's parties which is only placed in a bamboo basket symbolizing mutual respect. In Manipuri society, on the day of the marriage, the groom's party carries different items such as rice, fruits, fish, vegetables and clothes for the bride in a ceremonial basket (s) made of bamboo called *Phiruk/Phingaruk* (Figures 1.4 and 1.5).

Bamboo has even been revered as a deity and worshiped in many cultures of India and Japan. Japanese people believe that bamboo is a symbol of the Budha (Jiayan 2014). Music played on a bamboo flute is considered spiritual. In Indian culture, the bamboo flute called *Bansuri* (Ban—bamboo and Sur—music) was used

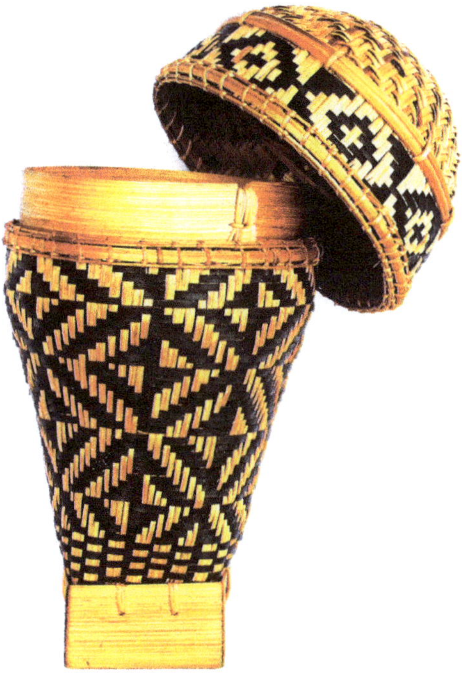

FIGURE 1.4 *Phiruk* or *Phingaruk*, a bamboo basket used during the Manipuri marriage ceremony.

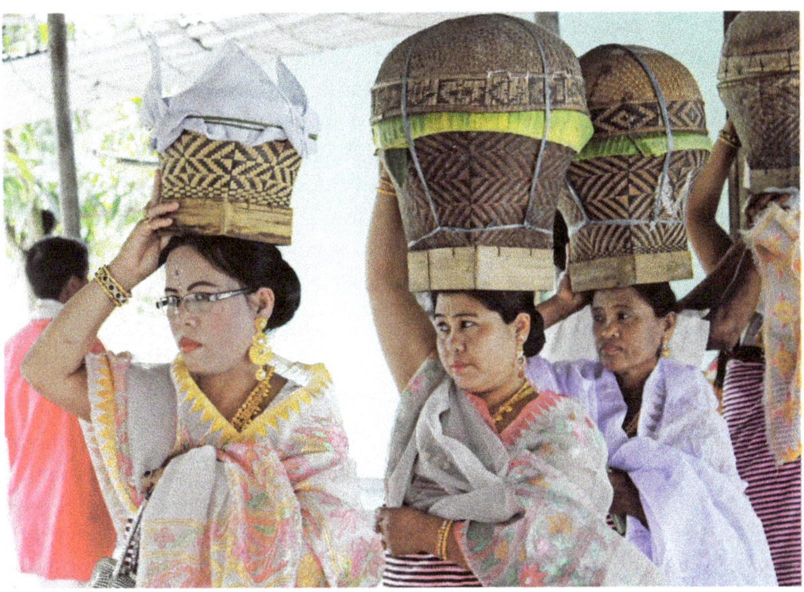

FIGURE 1.5 The groom's party carrying different items for the bride in bamboo containers during the marriage ceremony of Manipuri society.

to play music by Lord Krishna dating from the time of Mahabharata (before the tenth century BCE). In India, the *Mising* tribe of Assam makes a worshiping place or sacrificial altar called *Dobur Uie* from sticks and leaves of *Bambusa tulda* (Sharma and Pegu 2011). Similarly, bamboo is a deity in many societies like in Tripura during Ker Puja and Ganga Puja. In the Meitei community of Manipur, planting a bamboo plant in the courtyard is considered lucky, a symbol of prosperity (Singh et al. 2003). At Karang, an isolated island in Loktak lake of Manipur, people used to put up tall straight bamboo poles with a lovely cluster of small branches and leaves at the tip in their courtyard (Bahadur 2013). These totems signify that the marriageable daughter in the family is engaged to her future husband. The Meitei Hindus in Manipur on the occasion of *Hariuthan* erect tall straight bamboo poles of the longest variety on which circular bamboo rings are fixed. Bamboo has also remained a fascinating material for artists, writers and poets particularly in countries like China, Korea and Japan. There are books like *The Book of Songs* from China; *Leaves Collection*, *Taketori Monogatari* from Japan; and *Bamboo Window*, *Bamboo Forest* from Korea written on bamboo or about bamboo (Jiayan 2014).

Bamboo is considered as a symbol of good fortune and is also associated with bad omen, evil spirits, miseries, calamities, devastations and death in some communities. In Nepal, there used to be a ban on planting bamboo because of the belief that the shadow of a bamboo falling on a person invited *Yamaraj*, the spirit of death. In Bangladesh, when a villager is buried, a small piece of bamboo is hung above the grave to scare away evil spirits (Arens and Beurden 1978). Bamboo is known for causing famine and devastation as in Mizoram state in India and other adjoining areas of India like Myanmar and Bangladesh. Around 90% of the bamboo area in Mizoram is covered with *Melocanna baccifera* which flowers and bears fruits every 30 to 40 years as recorded since 1863 causing famine and devastation of crops by rodents. Another belief is that bamboo impoverishes the soil on which it grows and does not allow anything to grow under it. Similarly, there are a number of beliefs associated with bamboo such as 'those who plant bamboo will die', 'bamboos are the cause of quarrel with the neighbour', 'bamboo should not be planted in front of the house' (Das and Mitchell 2005). Some of these beliefs have valid reasons, for instance bamboo is the fastest-growing plant and if planted in the courtyard, it will spread everywhere and later will be difficult to remove. Bamboo grove also provides very good shelter and breeding ground for rodents and snakes which are also not good for the human settlements.

1.4 DIVERSITY AND DISTRIBUTION OF BAMBOO

Bamboo is a group of perennial giant or small woody evergreen plants belonging to the grass family Poaceae and subfamily Bambusoideae. The most important characteristics which distinguish the majority of bamboos from grasses are their woody perennial habit and peculiar flowering and seedling behavior. Bamboos originated in the paleozoic/mesozoic period in south-east Asia and broadly disseminated through Asia and the Pacific, the Americas and the Caribbean and Africa except for Europe and Antarctica (FAO 2010). It can adjust effectively to a range of climatic and soil conditions including grasslands, coniferous forest, temperate deciduous forests and lowland tropical forests from 46°N and 47°S. Bamboos can develop in an altitudinal range that reaches out from simply over the ocean level up to 4,000 m in the Himalayas and flourishes at a temperature of 8.8 to 36°C, though a few species can even grow in a frosty atmosphere with a temperature of about –20°C. Bamboo favours regions of high precipitation extending from around 1,270 mm to around 6,350 mm.

Estimates of bamboo diversity vary, as the taxonomy of bamboo is one of the most complex because of the infrequent flowering in most of the species and also partly due to various genomic characters. Bamboo has very small chromosomes and a high level of polyploidization (Chongtham et al. 2013). A number of species are known only vegetatively (Triplett et al. 2006, Clark et al. 2015). The earliest bamboo classification was attempted by Munro (1868), who described 170 species under 20 genera (Clark et al. 2015). A global total of 840 species and 49 genera of bamboos were reported by Clayton and Renvoize (1986). According to a later estimate (Ohrnberger 1999), 88 genera and 1,447 species of woody bamboos were described and accepted worldwide. In terms of bamboo diversity, Asia is the leading continent with maximum diversity in China (39 genera and 500 species, Zhu et al. 1994, Keng and Wang 1996), followed by India (18 genera and 128 species, Seethalakshmi and Kumar 1998) and south-east Asia (20 genera and 200 species, Dransfield and Widjaja 1995). In a recent update on the bamboo diversity of India, Sharma and Chongtham (2015) have estimated a total of 29 genera, 148 species and 4 varieties of bamboo in India (both wild and cultivated). The most up-to-date comprehensive and the phylogenetically based bamboo taxonomical system is derived from DNA sequence data in combination with various morphological and anatomical features (Clark et al. 2015). Currently, bamboo encompasses 1,482 species within 119 genera and are classified into three tribes: (1) Arundinarieae: the temperate woody bamboos, albeit some occur in the tropics at higher elevations; 546 species; (2) Bambuseae: the tropical woody bamboos, even some occur outside of the tropics; 812 species; and (3) Olyreae: the herbaceous bamboos; 124 species (Clark et al. 2015). Culms in woody bamboos are highly lignified and are protected by culm sheaths. Herbaceous bamboos, on the other hand, have very weakly lignified culms and lack distinct culm sheaths. Woody and herbaceous bamboos also differ in terms of floral characters and flowering patterns possessing bisexual floral spikelets with gregarious monocarpic flowering whereas herbaceous bamboos have unisexual spikelets with seasonal flowering (Akinlabi et al. 2017). All members of a monocarpic bamboo species flower simultaneously and then die. The underlying mechanism of this mass flowering followed by the mass suicide event in monocarpic bamboos is not clearly understood but it is believed to be species-specific and it normally happens after a fixed interval of time, which may range from 30 to 120 years.

Bamboo is highly adapted to varied climatic and ecological conditions and is distributed throughout the world naturally except in Antarctica and Europe (Figure 1.6). Earlier bamboo was not found in two continents, Europe and Antarctica, but now bamboo is cultivated in many parts of Europe and used for various purposes. The spreading of bamboo plants can be broadly assigned into three major regions, namely Asia–Pacific, America and Africa (Zhou 1998). The greatest diversity of bamboo is found in south-east Asia and South America, where they occur in tropical,

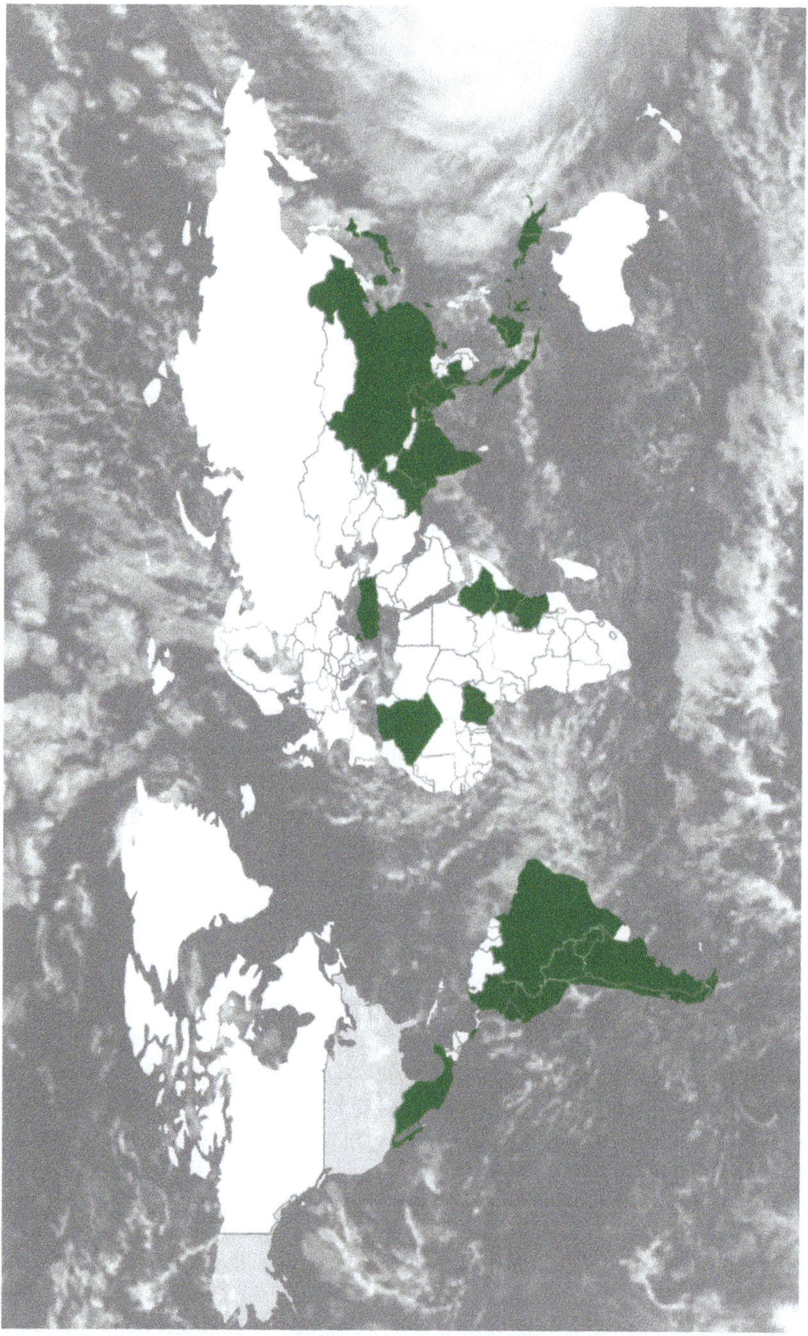

FIGURE 1.6 Global regions with natural abundance of bamboo.

subtropical and temperate regions, while fewer bamboo species are found in Africa in comparison to the other two regions, with the exception of Madagascar, which is rich in endemic genera and species (Zhou 1998, Bystriakova and Kapos 2006). Qiu (1992) reported that almost one thousand bamboo species are found in Asia, predominantly indigenous rather than plantation or introductions. In the whole of Europe, there is not even one native species and from mainland Africa, only three native species are reported. However, a large number of bamboos are now in cultivation in Europe and Africa. Bamboos from China and Japan were introduced in Europe in the early 1800s. *Phyllostachys nigra*, the black bamboo was the first to be introduced in Europe around 1827. At present, over 400 different taxa are cultivated in Europe, 300 of which are temperate bamboos. Many species of bamboo have been introduced into Africa also and now bamboo grows in almost every part of Africa except the Sahara desert. In Africa, countries including Ethiopia, Kenya, Nigeria and Uganda are now the major bamboo growing regions (Lobovikov et al. 2007).

Bamboo covers an estimated area of 37 million hectares, equivalent to nearly 4% of the world's total forest coverage (FAO 2010). Asia is home to the largest acreage of bamboo, about 23.62 million hectares of the total world bamboo area of 37 million hectares, followed by America and Africa (Figure 1.7). In Asia, India has the major acreage of bamboo forests (11.36 million hectares) which is around half of the total bamboo area reported for Asia and China contributes around 70% of total Asian bamboo (Figure 1.8) (FAO 2007). With regard to diversity, Asia leads, with countries such as China having around 500 species of bamboo (Table 1.1). India and Japan have more than 100 species of bamboo.

1.5 BAMBOO AS A PLANT

Bamboos are arborescent or shrubby grasses with varied morphology. They can reach in culm height from a few centimeters like in *Raddiella vanessiae* (Judziewicz and Sepsenwol 2007) to over 40 m and diameter of 3 mm to over 25 cm within 3–4 months (Giant bamboo, *Dendrocalamus giganteus*) Most bamboos grow erect, but

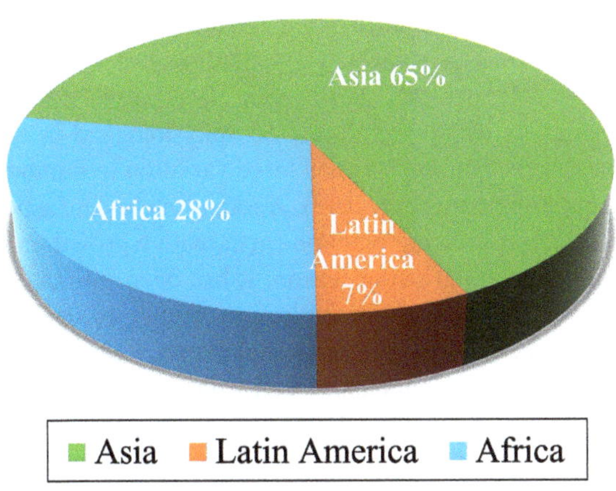

FIGURE 1.7 Distribution of bamboo areas in major regions of the world.

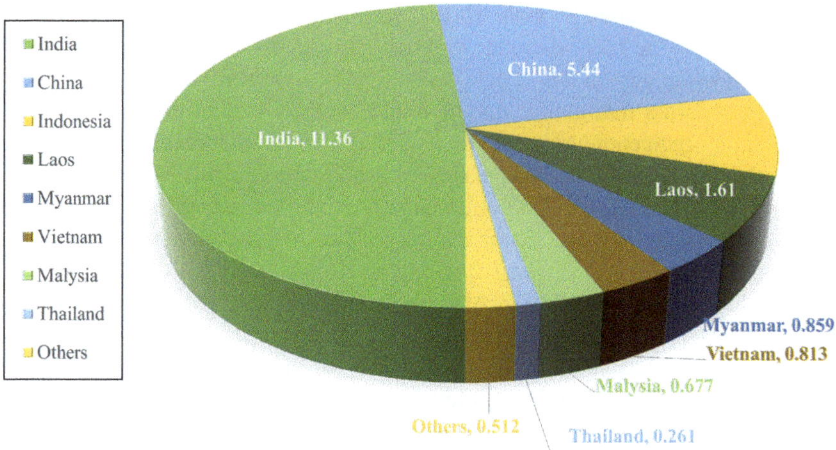

FIGURE 1.8 Bamboo acreage in Asian countries (in million hectares).

some are scrambling stragglers (e.g. *Neomicrocalamus prainii*, *Cephalostachyum capitatum*, *Chusquea* spp.) or vine-like climbers (*Dinochloa* spp.).

Bamboos are divided as running or clumping bamboos based on the growth pattern of underground rhizome producing new shoots or culms above the ground. *Phyllostachys mannii* is running (monopodial) bamboo where the terminal meristem continues to grow and shoots (sprouts) are produced from the sides (Figures 1.9 and 1.10).

Gigantochloa atroviolacea is the clumping (sympodial) bamboo where the terminal meristem produces the shoots and a new meristem or growing point comes from the side of the rhizome (Figures 1.11 and 1.12).

As a plant, bamboo has a number of peculiar characters like long flowering periods, which goes up 123 years in some species or more, vegetative method of propagation and adaptation at diverse climatic and geographical conditions and large-scale variation at the morphological, chromosomal and molecular level (Chongtham et al. 2013). With the result, bamboo identification and classification has always remained a problematic and controversial subject. There are many species or varieties of bamboo which are differently identified in different parts of the world based on a few morphological characters which are mainly eco-physiological in nature. With very small chromosome sizes, bamboo shows a large variation in numbers ranging from $2n = 36$ to $2n = 72$ (Chongtham et al. 2013). Another interesting aspect of bamboo is its growth. It is the fastest-growing plant on earth, with a growth rate of around 100 cm per day during its prime growing season. It has been estimated that a bamboo culm can accumulate 75% of its biomass in just around 40 days during its initial 'explosive' growth stage, facilitated by rapid mobilization of non-structural carbohydrates (NSC) such as soluble sugars and starch from the mother plant to developing culm. After initial growth in height and diameter, it enters the second growth stage, lasting for an average span for three to five years. During this period, culm increases its strength by accumulating dry mass and continued lignification of parenchymatous cell walls until it is mature enough to be harvested for its multiple uses.

TABLE 1.1
Worldwide Distribution of Bamboos along with Area and Stock*

Countries	Bamboo area (1000 ha) 2005	% of bamboo area to forest area 2005	Bamboo stock in million tones	Species
Bangladesh	83	9.5	1	33
Cambodia	29	0.3	-	4
China	5,444	2.8	164	500
India	11,361	16.8	122	119
Indonesia	2,081	2.4	10	118
Japan	154	0.6	-	139
Lao People's Democratic Republic	1,612	10.0	-	13
Malaysia	677	3.2	11	92
Myanmar	859	2.7	18	97
Pakistan	20	1.1	0.21	3
Papua New Guinea	45	0.2	-	25
Philippines	172	2.4	6	21
Republic of Korea	6	0.1	-	5
Sri Lanka	3	0.2	-	10
Thailand	261	1.8	-	36
Vietnam	813	6.3	-	69
Total Asia	**23,620**	**4.4**	**332**	**1284**
Ethiopia	167	6.5	21	2
Kenya	124	3.5	1	1
Nigeria	1,590	14.3	27	-
United Republic of Tanzania	128	0.4	5	4
Uganda	67	1.8	3	2
Madagascar	-	-	-	33
Other African countries	-	-	-	4
Total Africa	**2,758**	**4.1**	**57**	**46**
Brazil	9,300	2.1	-	232
Chile	900	5.6	-	11
Columbia	-	-	-	56
Venezuela	-	-	-	68
Peru	190	0.3	-	35
Ecuador	9	0.1	-	42
Other American countries	-	-	-	190
Total South America	**10,399**	**1.9**	-	**634**
World	**36,777**	**3.2**	**389**	**1964**

*Sources: Bystriakova et al. 2003, Lobovikov et al. 2007.

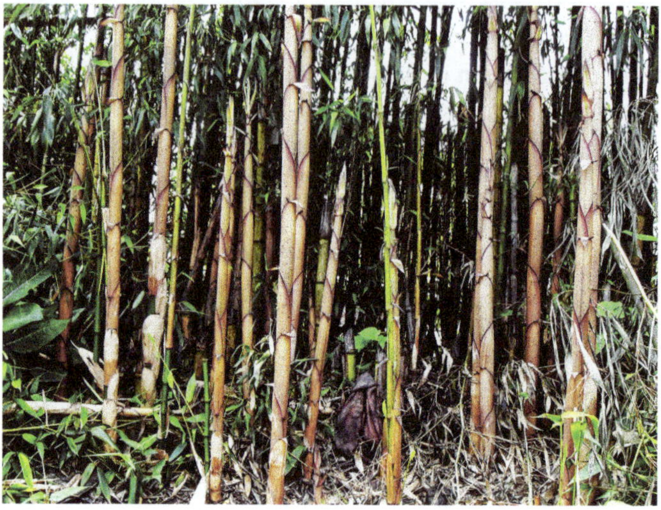

FIGURE 1.9 The growth form of *Phyllostachys mannii*, a monopodial bamboo.

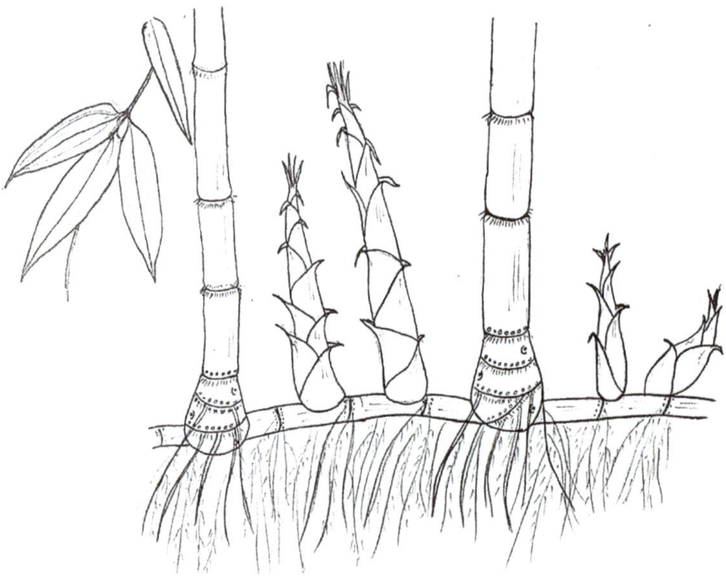

FIGURE 1.10 Diagrammatic representation for the growth form of a monopodial bamboo.

1.5.1 Plant Morphology

Bamboo is a grass, made up of morphological parts like rhizomes, roots, shoots, culms, branches, leaves, flowers and fruits. A bamboo plant consists of two distinct parts: (i) underground jointed rhizomes from which arise the aerial culms and (ii) the above-ground jointed, hollow or solid stem commonly known as culm with its aerial roots, branches and leaves. The rhizome also bears true roots at its nodes. The

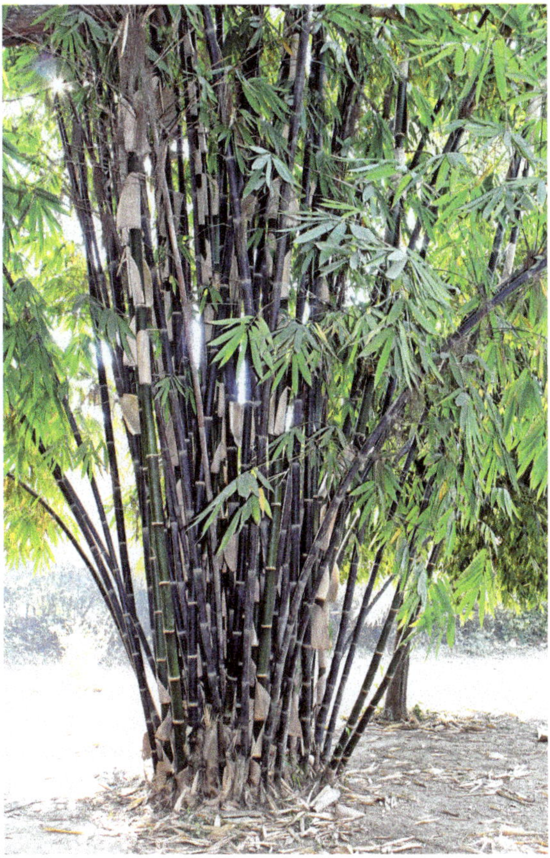

FIGURE 1.11 The growth form of *Gigantochloa atroviolacea*, a sympodial bamboo.

lateral branches arise at the position of nodes on the main culms and these bear foliage leaves (Figure 1.13). The newly formed culms bear another type of leaves called culm leaves or more commonly as 'culm sheaths'. The inflorescence in bamboos may consist of 'true spikelets' or 'pseudospikelets' (McClure 1934, 1966), each made up of various bracts and prophylls enclosing the flowers.

1.5.2 Rhizomes

The rhizome is well developed in bamboo and is the underground, branched portion of the plant from which the aerial culms grow. It spreads to produce an interconnected network from which shoots or new rhizomes arise from its nodes. Together with the roots arising at its nodes, the rhizome anchors the plant firmly to the soil. The rhizome is a segmented axis consisting of two parts: the rhizome proper and the rhizome neck. The rhizome neck is generally relatively short and obconical in shape but in some bamboos, it may be greatly elongated and 'running' type. The rhizome neck has a diameter smaller than that of the parent rhizome from which it arises.

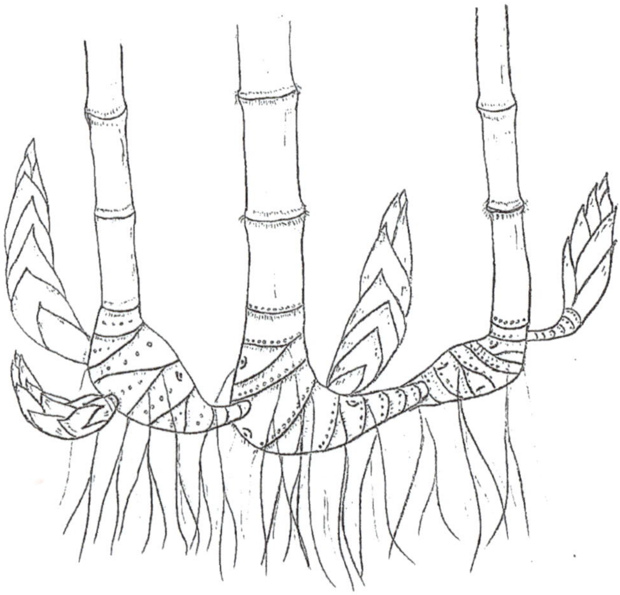

FIGURE 1.12 Diagrammatic representation for the growth form of a sympodial bamboo.

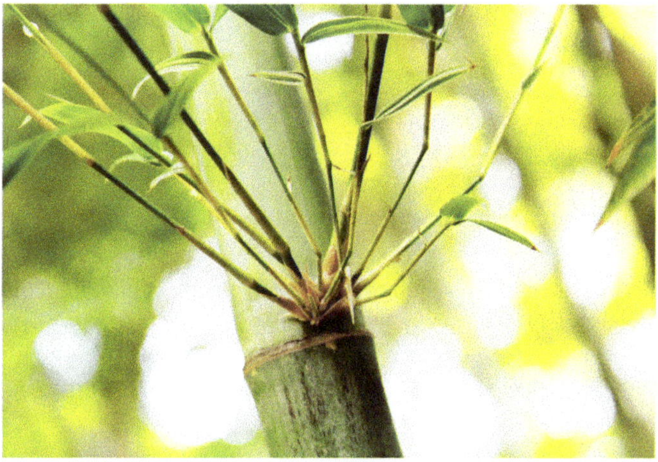

FIGURE 1.13 A bamboo culm showing lateral branching.

The rhizome proper is typically subterranean and possesses roots or root primordia, prophyllate buds (solitary at each node) at all or most of its nodes, and sheaths clothing the rhizomes.

Woody bamboos show the most extreme development of rhizomes, which may be leptomorph (running or monopodial) or pachymorph (clumping or sympodial) or metamorph (having both running as well as clumping type on the same plant). Leptomorph rhizomes are long and slender, typically hollow, cylindrical or subcylindrical, usually with a diameter less than that of culms originating from them. The internodes in such rhizomes are longer than broad, relatively uniform in length, symmetrical or nearly so and typically hollow (rarely solid). Leptomorph rhizomes are common in bamboos of temperate and cold regions and are found in bamboos that do not form clumps (e.g. *Arundinaria* spp., *Phyllostachys* spp., *Chimonobambusa* spp.). Most bamboos with leptomorph rhizomes have the power to spread in open places in incredibly short periods. The length of rhizome between the aerial culms may be as much as 90 cm (3 feet, Gamble 1896). Pachymorph rhizomes, on the other hand, are short and thick, sub-fusiform (rarely spherical), more or less curved (rarely straight) and with a maximum thickness somewhat greater than that of the culm into which they have transformed apically. Lateral buds of pachymorph rhizomes produce only rhizomes and no culms. Pachymorph rhizomes are common in bamboos of warm, tropical regions (e.g. *Bambusa* spp., *Dendrocalamus* spp., *Gigantochloa* spp., *Dinochloa* spp., *Schizostachyum* spp., *Thyrsostachys* spp.).

The culms from pachymorph rhizomes are caespitose and very close to each other so that they are often touching each other, with the result that, as the clump grows older, its centre is raised irregularly above the ground and a mound is formed (e.g. *Dendrocalamus strictus*, *Bambusa bambos*, *B. polymorpha*). In some species of bamboos with pachymorph rhizomes, the culms in a clump are fairly scattered due to long necks of rhizomes (e.g. *Melocanna baccifera*, *Yushania jaunsarensis*). The long necks in pachymorph rhizomes may sometimes be confused with leptomorph rhizomes. In *Melocanna baccifera*, rhizome necks may be as long as 1–1.5 m which helps in the wide spacing of its culms. In *Yushania jaunsarensis*, rhizome necks may be as long as 1 m.

1.5.3 Roots

Bamboos, like grasses, possess an adventitious root system which serves the function of anchorage and absorption. Roots are unsegmented, slender, cylindrical and uniform in diameter throughout and are the vegetative axis of the bamboo plant. The roots arise from the seedling as well as from nodes of rhizomes and culms at the base. Roots in bamboo are fibrous originating from the nodes of rhizomes and lower parts of the culms which mainly function for holding the plants in the soil plus other physiological function of absorption. In some species with pachymorph rhizomes, roots may also develop on the swollen base of primary branches at the lower mid-culm nodes (e.g. *Bambusa vulgaris*, *Dendrocalamus hamiltonii*). In *Chimonobambusa armata*, *C. callosa* and few other species, aerial roots from culm nodes become spiny and afford an easy means of species identification.

1.5.4 Culms

It is the vegetative aerial stem in bamboo and is the most distinguishable part arising from the rhizome and finally grows in size from just 2 cm in some bamboos to 50 m in *Dendrocalamus giganteus* (Figure 1.14). Each culm arises directly from the apex of a rhizome either from the lateral meristem or branches (in leptomorph rhizome) or apical meristem (in pachymorph rhizome). A culm gets its maximum height in

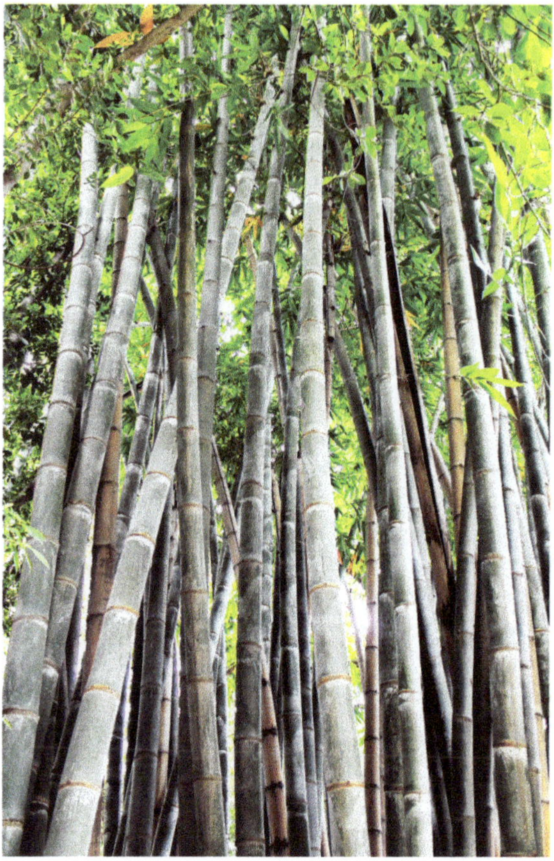

FIGURE 1.14 Culms of *Dendrocalamus giganteus.*

one growing season and fully matures in three to five growing seasons. In habit, the culms vary from erect, erect with pendulous tip, broadly arched, straggling to clambering, nearly straight to strongly zigzag or irregular as found in tortoise bamboo shell. The culms are usually woody, more or less cylindrical, usually hollow (e.g. 'female bamboos' such as *Cephalostachyum pergracile*, *Bambusa polymorpha*) or solid (e.g. 'male bamboos' such as *Dendrocalamus strictus*, *D. membranaceus*, *Bambusa burmanica*, *Gigantochloa albociliata*). The culms are usually cylindrical, rarely partially quadrangular (e.g. *Chimonobambusa quadrangularis*, a native of China). The colour of the culm varies from mostly green to brown, yellow with green strips (*Bambusa vulgaris* var. *vittata*), green with yellow or white strips (*Bambusa affinis*) and jet black as in *Phyllostachys nigra*. Culms in some bamboo-like *Phyllostachys atrovaginata* have a waxy coat on the culm that emits a pleasant fragrance similar to incense and is commonly known as 'incense bamboo'. The repeating units of culm consist of a node, an internode, a bud, branches, leaves and one or more adventitious roots or root primordial. The wall thickness varies from very thin in *Pseudostachyum polymorphum* to very thick with a small lumen as found in *Dendrocalamus strictus*, *Neomicrocalamus mannii*, *N. prainii*. The culm is of main economic value in bamboo used for various purposes.

1.5.5 Leaves

Leaves in bamboos are of two types: culm leaves and foliage leaves. Culm leaves, also commonly known as 'culm sheaths', are borne on the new growing culms where they completely cover and protect the growing shoots. In these leaves, the sheath proper (which corresponds to the petiole of ordinary leaves) represents the greater part of the leaf while the blade is little developed. The culm leaves are usually non-photosynthetic, and their shapes are characteristic of species. The young leaves are food to many animals like the giant panda, golden bamboo lemur, elephants and so on and also considered of high medicinal value in many Asian countries. The leaves have a number of anti-oxidant compounds and are now being promoted as bamboo leaf tea as well.

1.5.6 Shoots

The young emerging vegetative aerial culms are generally called shoots. These miniaturized bamboo culms are tightly covered with overlapping sheaths that have to be removed to extract the edible part. The sheaths are very hard and protect the soft delicate culm or shoot inside. These soft culms are famous food in east and south-east Asian countries. The shooting period and frequency vary from species to species, their size and weight depending on soil nutrients, watering and drainage conditions, temperature, pH and soil fertility and are generally harvested after a growth period of two weeks after emerging out of the ground. When being harvested for edible purposes, care is taken so as not to remove all the new shoots from a clump as this might affect the photosynthetic capabilities of the clump, which in turn will exert an adverse effect on the growth of underground rhizome resulting in less shooting frequency for next growing season. However, recently it has been found that regular harvesting of shoots from a growing stand can actually enhance the shooting frequency in the following growing seasons probably because of the 'over-compensatory' growth of bamboo rhizome in response to harvesting (Katayama et al. 2015).

Bamboo shoots are often characterized into three types depending upon the time of their emergence from the underground rhizome and their harvesting period viz. winter shoots, spring shoots and summer shoots. Winter shoots, which begin their growth from the lateral buds of underground rhizome early in the autumn, are harvested during winters whilst still underground. They are very small and somewhat conical in shape. As the shoots are still underground when harvested, these are super-soft and offer superior taste quality, for example *Phyllostachys edulis*, *P. pubescens*, and so on (Liu 2011). On the other hand, spring shoots refer to shoots that have continued their growth and have emerged from the soil. These shoots have a very soft but actively growing tip region; therefore, for the best results, they are harvested young before they reach the height of 20–25 cm as after that, shoots will start becoming lignified, and lose their edibility. Summer shoots emerge during late summer toward the onset of the monsoon season. In the present day, the bamboo shoot has taken the status of health food and is arousing the interest of scientists, nutritionists and businessmen alike.

1.5.7 Flowering

Most bamboos are monocarpic, that is they flower only once in their lifetime. They are also characterized by the prevalence of long vegetative periods prior to flowering. Some bamboos cease vegetative growth for a short period before switching over to flowering, while others change suddenly from leaf growth to growth of spikelets on a single axis in the middle of a growing season (Figure 1.15).

Bamboos flower both gregariously and sporadically. Most bamboos lose all foliage leaves during flowering. The information available in literature reveals that while some bamboos flower every year, others show a cyclic recurrence of flowering cycles varying from a few years to 120 years or more. The bamboos that flower at long intervals usually exhibit gregarious flowering, which extends to all parts of the plant. The period between two gregarious flowerings for a species over the same area is called its 'flowering cycle' or 'physiological cycle'. This is more or less constant for a species in a given locality but can differ between locations, and between populations with well-marked climatic and soil differences.

The seeds/fruit have a wide range in types, size and weight, varying from husky caryopsis, smaller than the size of a rice kernel and weighing up to 125,000 seeds/kg (*D. polymorpha*) to pear sized, fleshy fruit, weighing up to three to four fruits per kg (*Melocanna baccifera* Figure 1.16). These seeds of bamboo have nutrients slightly higher than rice and wheat (Mitra and Nayak 1972). While humans have been a major consumer of bamboo seeds for centuries, rodents, birds and large animals like bison and elephants too consume bamboo seeds when available. Humans have been major predators on bamboo seed throughout the history of bamboo flowering. *D. strictus* seeds kept over 35,000 people alive during the 1899–1900 drought in the central province of India (Lowrie 1900). Similarly, during the famine, seeds of

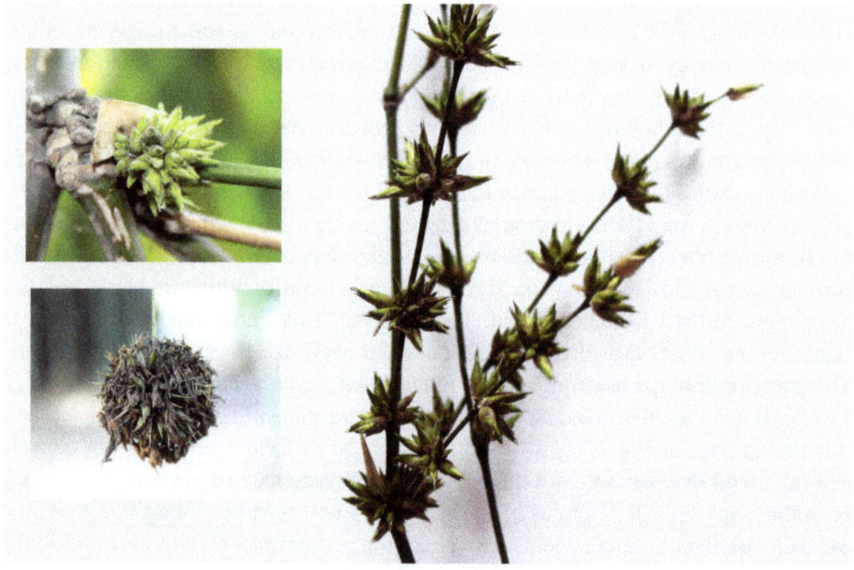

FIGURE 1.15 Flowering in *Dendrocalamus membranaceus*.

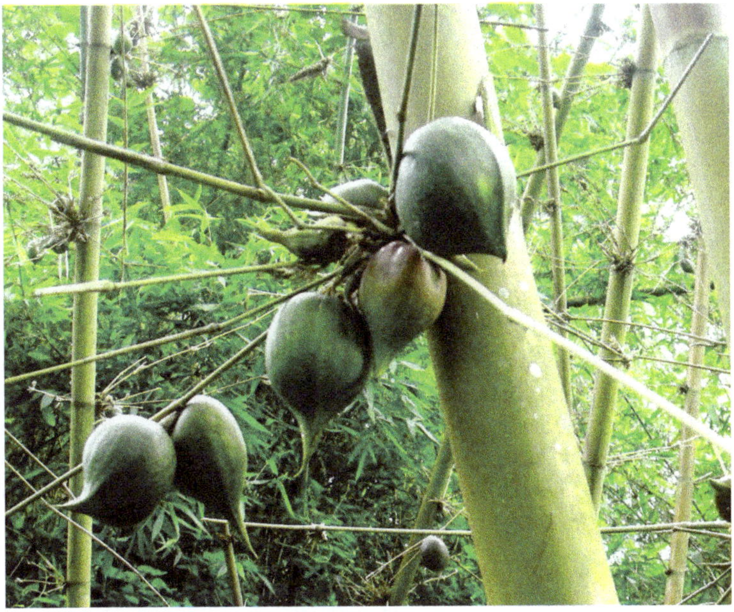

FIGURE 1.16 Seeds of *Melocanna baccifera*.

Chusquea spp. in Chile (Gunckel 1948) and *Sasa* spp. in Japan (Numata 1970) were collected for consumption by the starving people.

In some parts of the world, this gregarious flowering or mast seeding of bamboo is also related to famine and calamity, particularly in the case of flowering of *Melocanna baccifera* in north-east India (Mizoram and Manipur states) and in adjoining hills such as Chin-Hills in Myanmar and Chittagong Hill Tracts in Bangladesh (Adhikari 2013). In fact, the bamboo flowering and then famine became a cause of insurgency and led to the birth of a new state, Mizoram, in India. *M. baccifera*, which flowers after a vegetative growth of 45 to 48 years, produces pear-shaped seeds which are nutritious; this can be a cause of famine and calamity as the seeds are eaten by rodents which multiply in millions and after finishing the seeds of *M. baccifera* move to the agricultural fields and human settlements devouring everything on their way. If the seeds of *M. baccifera* are put to some appropriate use, this type of devastation could be avoided. It is believed that the seed increased the fertility of the rodents leading to the population explosion. Detailed biochemical analysis of the seed would be worth studying to discover the component that can be used to produce fertility drugs.

1.6 MULTIFARIOUS USES OF BAMBOO

Bamboo is one plant in which every part of the plant is used starting from the root, rhizome, leaf, culm leaves, culms and young shoots. Due to the numerous varieties of bamboos and their remarkable ability to adapt to any climatic and soil conditions, there is a bamboo suitable for every application and human need. There are about

3,000 companies around the world involved in the production of numerous bamboo-based products, thus making it an ideal species capable of providing livelihood, food and nutritional security and economic sustainability on account of its manifold uses and industrial applications. Bamboo has over a thousand documented applications from birth to death being used to make cradle and toys for the young children, house for living, utensils in the kitchen, implements for agriculture and fishing, weapons for hunting and defense, musical instrument for entertainment, mats, chopsticks, sports instrument, food and medicine for good health and bier or coffin. However, during the Industrial Revolution of the 19th and 20th century, the invention of materials like steel and plastic pushed bamboo in oblivion and neglect, particularly in the regions where it was once considered to be 'everything for the people'. During this time, negative characteristics of bamboo as an obnoxious weed and massive flowering were considered to be the main causes of famine and disaster in some parts of north-east India and Myanmar. But by the turn of the 21st century, bamboo evolved into a totally new product, seen as the fastest-growing renewable natural resource poised to replace malleable plastic and competitive with the best steel. The numbers of known usages are constantly increasing now, as developments in industrial systems allow processing of bamboo into new shapes and forms. No other product comes close to bamboo in terms of diversity of use. In the modern era, bamboo is gradually replacing wood and is the best material for making hard boards, flooring, corrugated sheets, veneers, panels, wall coverings, architectural moldings and stair systems. Bamboo is posed to play a greater role in the future, due to its being one of the most important sources of top-quality building material, décor product, fibre and fabrics to tough and durable material for the electronics industry in the world. Today, a modern home can be built entirely from bamboo, including all furniture and furnishings (Figure 1.17). It is also utilized as a fuel in the form of charcoal, oil, or gas produced through pyrolysis. Functional foods, nutraceuticals, medicines, cosmetics and various body care products, apparel, furniture and numerous other items made from bamboo are entering the market. The estimated size of the global market in just ten major product lines of

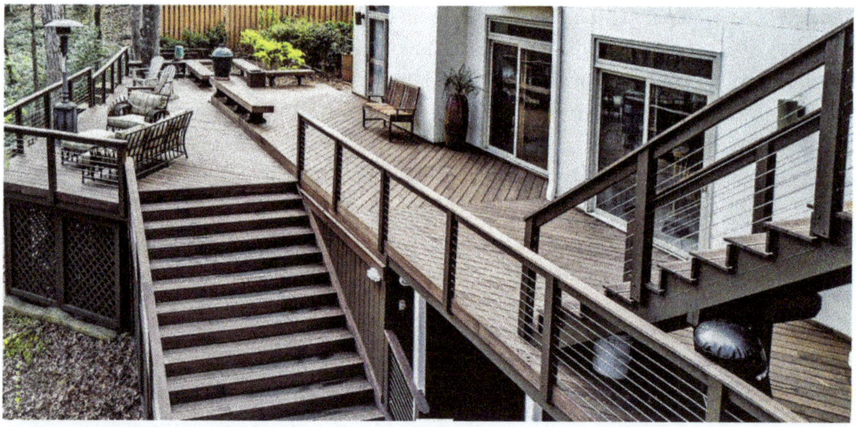

FIGURE 1.17 Bamboo decking and furniture at Atlanta Valley Hall (Courtesy: Avery Chua, President/CEO, dasso XTR).

bamboo was USD 7 billion per annum in 2006, with the potential to grow to USD 17 billion under favourable market conditions. Countries including China, Korea, Thailand and Taiwan have exploited bamboo, their abundant natural resource and have rightly become bamboo economy or 'green economy'.

1.6.1 Substitute for Wood in Housing and Building

Worldwide, there is growing interest in the development of bamboo products as a sustainable, cost-effective and ecologically responsible alternative construction material. Bamboo is a rapidly renewable sustainable resource and has mechanical properties similar to timber. The rapid growth and renewability of bamboo are ideal characteristics for use in construction. Moreover, the tensile and compression strength of a mature bamboo plant is higher than the traditional hard or softwoods. In addition, bamboo wood possesses several times more biomass than other woody species. Thus, bamboo has become the most preferred choice ecologically when it comes to building material and it is gaining popularity as a result of the sustainability trend in modern architecture.

There are three main types of bamboo housing: (1) traditional houses, which use bamboo culms as a primary building material; (2) traditional bahareque bamboo houses, in which a bamboo frame is plastered with cement or clay; and (3) modern prefabricated houses made of bamboo laminated boards, veneers and panels. Experts estimate that over one billion people live in traditional bamboo houses. These buildings are usually cheaper than wooden houses, light, strong and earthquake resistant, unlike brick or cement constructions. New types of prefabricated houses made of engineered bamboo have certain advantages. Large-scale modern buildings made of bamboo can be seen worldwide, ranging from private residences, lodges, offices to airports (Figure 1.18). As bamboo's technical construction qualities become better

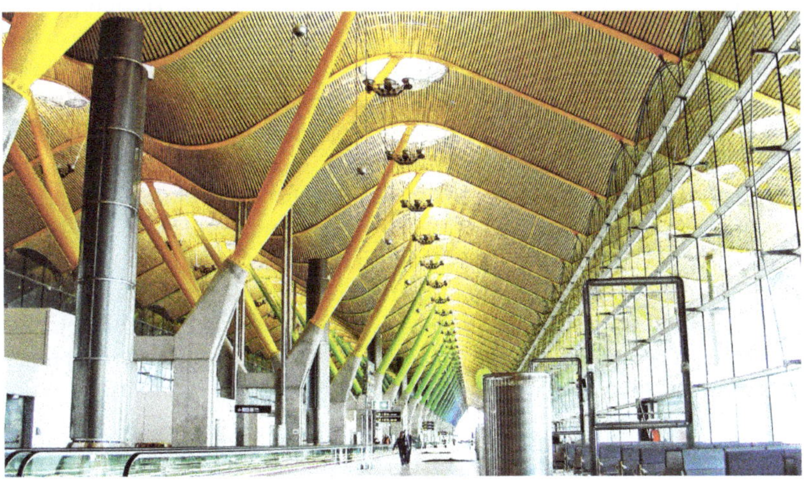

FIGURE 1.18 Madrid International Airport constructed using bamboo. (Courtesy: Avery Chua, President/CEO, dasso XTR).

and bamboo buildings meet the standards of construction and building, bamboo will be accepted more. Building with the whole bamboo is challenging. For one thing, it is round, so its cylindrical shape requires special joinery considerations. Bamboo culms have size and surface variabilities, as well as their characteristic segmentation and nodes. Bamboo must be properly cured and treated for many applications.

Use of bamboo panels, laminated bamboo floorings, ply bamboo, bamboo veneers, bamboo mats and so on is rapidly gaining popularity in house construction, furniture manufacturing and the handicraft industry. Bamboo can also be used as a strip board, medium density board, sticks of varying descriptions and uses, roofing, partitions, doors and window frames and so on. Various types of bamboo boards and panels have advantages over wooden boards due to their rigidity and durability. Bamboo flooring is gaining worldwide popularity over the wooden floor due to its smoothness, brightness, stability, high resistance, insulation quality, flexibility, soft natural luster and natural gloss and elegance of bamboo fibre. The use of bamboo in composite panels and boards overcomes differences in quality related to the culms and allows the production of homogenous products. Bamboo decking has become very popular with its attractive look and a long life span (Figure 1.17). Bamboo decks are made from compressed, thermally treated bamboo strips. The extreme stability of the material ensures a very durable bamboo terrace. In the near future, engineered bamboo will replace wood, steel and concrete in many building and construction work.

1.6.2 Bamboo-Based Paper and Pulp Industries

Bamboo is a rapidly growing plant with good fibre qualities and is widely employed in paper industries throughout the Asian region. Several bamboo-producing countries, such as China and India, use bamboo in pulp and paper. Bamboo pulp which first came to prominence for paper making during the reign of the Han Dynasty (206 BC–AD 220) of China, continues to be the preferred non-wood raw material for paper mills because of its superior quality and easy availability. The morphological characteristics of bamboo fibre yield paper with a high tear index, similar to that of hardwood paper. The quality of the paper may be improved by refining the pulp. Bamboo paper has practically the same quality as paper made from wood. Its brightness and optical properties remain stable, while those of paper made from wood may deteriorate over time. The tensile stiffness is somewhat lower when compared to softwood paper. The strain strength is between that of hardwood and soft wood papers. The pulp and paper industry processes huge quantities of lingo-cellulosic biomass every year. The technology for pulp manufacture is highly diverse and numerous opportunities exist for the application of microbial enzymes. The carbonized bamboo fibre which once powered Edison's incandescent lamps now fuels highly efficient super-capacitors with practical applications in various electric appliances such as elevators, high capacity cranes, trains and other futuristic transport systems.

1.6.3 Bamboo-Based Fibre and Fabric

The development of processed bamboo fibre, textile and apparel products provide a noteworthy opportunity for providing sustainable textiles. For clothing and apparel, bamboo is considered to be one of the best materials particularly for newborns and infants as bamboo fibre are anti-fungal, anti-microbial and good absorber of moisture and body odour. Bamboo fibre is very smooth, strong and lustrous. A large number of products made from bamboo fibre are available such as shirts, scarfs, towels, undergarments, hankies and so on. The use of bamboo fibre for apparel is a 20th-century development initiated by several Chinese companies. Successful extraction of bamboo fibres and the use of modern bleaching chemicals to produce white fibres led to the creation of commercially available bamboo fabrics that were successfully marketed to the United States and other developed countries.

There are two ways to process bamboo to make into a fabric: mechanically or chemically. The fibre extracted by the mechanical way is often referred to as 'natural' or 'original' bamboo fibre and more or less the same manufacturing method used to produce ramie. It is made by crushing the woody parts of the bamboo plant and then use natural enzymes to break the bamboo walls into a mushy mass so that the natural fibres can be mechanically combed out and spun into yarn. This is essentially the same eco-friendly manufacturing process used to produce linen fabric from flax or hemp. Bamboo fabric made from this process is sometimes called bamboo linen. Very little bamboo linen is manufactured for clothing because it is more labour-intensive and costly. Chemically manufactured bamboo fibre is a regenerated cellulose fibre similar to rayon or modal and is sometimes called bamboo rayon because of the many similarities with rayon during manufacturing and feels while wearing. Most bamboo fabric that is the current eco-fashion rage is manufactured by the chemical process (Rayon process) by 'cooking' the bamboo leaves and woody shoots in strong chemical solvents such as sodium hydroxide (NaOH—also known as caustic soda or lye) and carbon disulfide by the process of hydrolysis alkalization combined with multi-phase bleaching. This is basically the same process used to make rayon from wood or cotton waste by-products.

Recently, nanotechnology has been introduced to manufacture bamboo charcoal fibre that improves the performance of textiles. In this process, bamboo charcoal is turned into nanoparticles which are then embedded into natural or synthetic polymers to form fibre that is woven or knitted into fabric form (Nayak and Mishra 2016). It has been reported that the resulting fabric is enhanced with performance qualities such as odour absorption, low surface resistivity, anti-bacterial and anti-fungal property, thermal regulation, prevention of static electricity buildup and so on. Not all attributes are proved with sufficient scientific evidence. More scientific research is needed to prove these facts specially, the benefits of health-related effects.

1.6.4 Bamboo as Fuel

Generally, bamboo biomass comprises 40–45% cellulose, 25–35% hemicellulose and 15–30% lignin, which can be converted into low molecular weight compounds including alcohol and biofuel. Through pyrolysis, bamboo can be converted into three valuable products: bamboo charcoal, oil and gas. Changing the pyrolysis parameters like temperature and oxygen can lead to the development of different products.

1.6.4.1 Charcoal

Also known as 'black diamond', bamboo charcoal is produced from pieces of bamboo harvested at least after five years and is burned in ovens at temperatures ranging from 800 to 1200°C (pyrolysis process). Bamboo charcoal is an excellent fuel for cooking and barbequing and is traditionally used as a substitute for wood charcoal or mineral coal (Figure 1.19). As early as 1486 CE, bamboo charcoal was used in various ways due to its tremendous extraordinary properties. The charcoal has a porous structure, is a rich source of minerals, emits health beneficial infrared rays, helps to maintain humidity equilibrium and dissipates electromagnetic waves. What makes this charcoal so amazing is the carbonization process which creates a product with an enormous surface area to mass ratio which has a high ability to attract and hold (adsorption) a wide range of materials, chemicals, minerals, humidity, odours and harmful substances. Due to these properties, bamboo charcoal is used for protection from electromagnetic waves, odour and humidity protection and for the production of cosmetics and health care products and other by-products. Moreover, bamboo charcoal products can be processed and turned into activated charcoal products that have applications in both traditional and high-tech industries. The adsorption properties of bamboo charcoal can be improved to become a perfect absorbent when the charcoal is further activated either thermally or chemically and hence, they are utilized in a solar cell as the electrode, adsorbent for water purification and electromagnetic wave absorber. The calorific value of bamboo charcoal is almost half that of oil of the same weight, better and cheaper than those of wood charcoal. China is a leader in bamboo charcoal production. At present, Japan, the Republic of Korea and Taiwan are the main consumers, but its importation is rapidly expanding in Europe and North America. There are three main reasons contributing to the success of bamboo charcoal in international trade: (i) bamboo grows faster and has a shorter rotation compared with tree species; (ii) the calorific value; and (iii) absorption properties

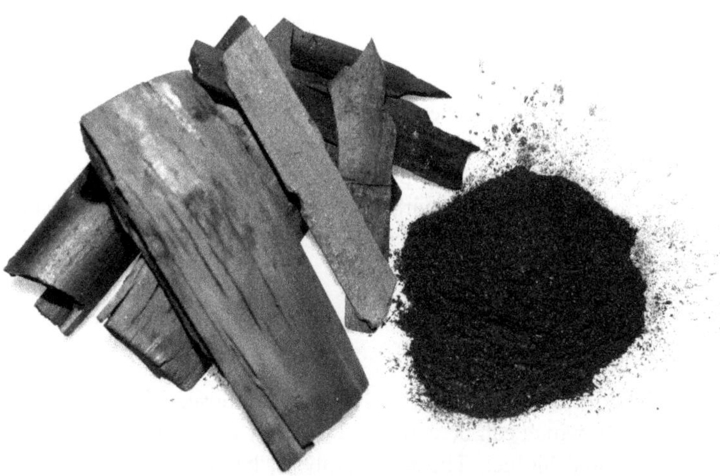

FIGURE 1.19 Bamboo charcoal from *Phyllostachys mannii.*

of bamboo charcoal. Bamboo charcoal products are also gaining popularity with consumers and, hence, the future of bamboo charcoal is bright.

1.6.4.2 Gas

Bamboo can also be converted to gas for the generation of power and heat. Gasification is a thermochemical conversion of bamboo biomass into a gas at a temperature of 750–1200°C. The gasification units require a small proportion of raw material and produce 15% of the biomass as a by-product in the form of high-grade charcoal. A 100 Kw gasifier requires 1,000 tonnes of raw material and produces 130 tonnes charcoal per annum. The produced gas includes combustible (methane, hydrogen and carbon dioxide) and non-combustible (carbon dioxide, nitrogen, etc.) gases. The combustible gases from bamboo (around 40%) are used as fuel for various purposes.

1.6.4.3 Biofuel

The global increase in energy consumption, depletion of fossil fuel reserves and concerns about climate change have urged the development of sustainable liquid biofuels is an urgent necessity due to concerns regarding energy security, oil price volatility and environmental pollution. Moreover, it can reduce carbon footprint better compared to an equivalent area of woody plants. They are the highest biomass producers among other bioenergy plants in terms of tons of dry weight per acre per year. In recent years, the huge consumption of petroleum-based fuels has led to increased demand for alternative energy sources. Biofuel production from lignocellulosic biomass is a green and effective technology targeting the alleviation of the dependence on fossil fuels for meeting energy demands. Currently, renewable fuels such as biodiesel, biohydrogen, biobutanol and bioethanol are obtained by utilizing waste agricultural biomass and lignocellulosic biomass. Lignocellulosic biomass could be used as a low-cost raw material and an alternative for second-generation biofuel production. Current know-how on biofuels production from lignocellulosic biomass includes sequential processing of the biomass for delignification and saccharification in order to obtain reducing sugar-rich broth which is ultimately utilized for fermentation. Bioethanol from lignocellulosic biomass can be utilized for clean and renewable energy production. Moreover, it is an economical process and large quantities can be obtained from a low-cost substrate. Ethanolic biofuel obtained from renewable resources has attracted lots of research in the past few decades to replace petroleum-based fuels. Bamboo is a promising renewable feedstock for ethanol production because of its high growth rate and high content of holocellulose. Countries including China and India that have large bamboo resources have started producing ethanol from bamboo. Bamboo is also used as a feedstock for the production of bioethanol after dilute acid pretreatment and enzymatic saccharification.

1.6.5 Bamboo as Food

Bamboo is an important source of food both for humans and animals. Amongst animals, two species rely upon it entirely. Both the endangered giant panda (native to China) and the golden lemur (native to Madagascar) feed almost exclusively on various parts of the bamboo plant. The parts which are used as food are seeds, leaves and young shoots.

1.6.5.1 Seeds

Seeds of *Bambusa arundinacea* is utilized as a food grain by the *Kani* tribe of Kanyakumari district, Tamil Nadu, India (Kiruba et al. 2007). The seeds are locally known as *Mungil-arisee* in the Tamil language that means bamboo rice. For consumption, the seeds are boiled in water just like rice and consumed with fish curry and vegetables by indigenous people as a substitute for rice. The seeds are also used to prepare *Mungil-arsee-dosa* and *Mungil-arsee-pongal* which is a sweet dish made with the seeds and some additives like milk, jaggery and so on. The seed grain can also be used to make cakes. *Mulayari-payasam*, a dessert made of bamboo rice is very popular in Kerela, one of the southern states of India. With a wheat-like texture, this creamy and rich sweet delicacy is good for health too. The seeds not only provide food but also help to empower and improve the economy of the tribal women as the excess seeds are sold to the adjoining areas. It is believed that the seeds of *B. arundinacea* enhance fertility and so there is a demand for the seeds in the pharmaceutical industry to manufacture drugs to improve fertility. In China, aromatic short-grain white rice has been infused with chlorophyll from young bamboo leaves. As the rice is milled, the chlorophyll is added, giving the rice grains a green colour.

1.6.5.2 Leaves

Young bamboo leaves, shoots and culms are a favourite meal for animals such as panda, lemurs and elephants. Bamboo leaves are also used as a source of fodder for goats, sheep, yaks, cattle and chicken. In fact, bamboo lemur and giant pandas live almost exclusively on bamboo (Figure 1.20). Bamboo lemur, considered to be one of the most endangered species on earth, is a cat-sized primate living on the island of

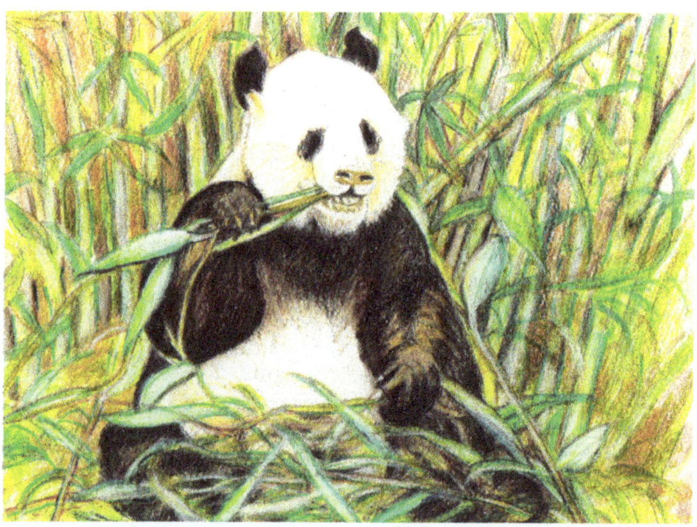

FIGURE 1.20 Bamboo as food for pandas.

Madagascar. They almost exclusively eat a single species of bamboo, including the woody trunk, known as culm. But they prefer the more nutritious and tender bamboo shoots and use their specialized teeth to gnaw on culm only when necessary during the dry season. Bersalona (2015) conducted an experiment by feeding chickens on an organic diet containing fresh bamboo leaves and observed that there was an increase in body weight by as much as 70% more than those fed on standard organic diets. The results suggest that the fibre in the bamboo leaves enlarges the digestive tract and enables the chickens to consume more and to grow faster. Chicken in the experimental group was 70% heavier than the chickens in the control group by the 56th day. Thus, leaves can be conveniently used as fodder for livestock.

For humans, bamboo leaves are commonly used as wrapping material rather than consuming it completely. In China, in the dragon boat festival (*Duan-Wu-Day*), it is mandatory to eat rice dumplings called *Zong-zi*. Sticky rice dumplings with a basic savory filling of pork, chestnut, egg and dried mushroom are wrapped in dried bamboo leaves into a pyramid shape. Bamboo leaves are also used to line the pan for cooking rice cakes, meat patties and other dishes. In southern Taiwan, rice is boiled with bamboo leaves as it imparts a strong aroma. In Japan, dumplings known as *Chimaki* similar to *Zong-zi* are eaten on 5 May to celebrate Children's Day. Bamboo leaves are also used to prepare different types of sushi. Bamboo belly rolls are also prepared by rolling pork belly in bamboo leaves that add flavor to the rolls. The leaves have now become very popular for preparing bamboo tea. For some time, bamboo leaf tea has been considered a delicious and healthy drink in Asian countries, and it is now available to Europe and the United States. It is devoid of theine and caffeine and is rich in protein, calcium, iron, magnesium and is recommended for various pharmaceutical applications particularly stomach pain. In Korea, the leaves are ground and used in making ice cream.

1.6.5.3 Shoots

The delicious and crispy bamboo shoots have been quite a favourite of people of Asian countries (Figure 1.21). Liang Shiqui, a famous modern Chinese writer, describes Beijing cuisines of 'stewed shrimps and winter bamboo shoots' and 'ham with stewed

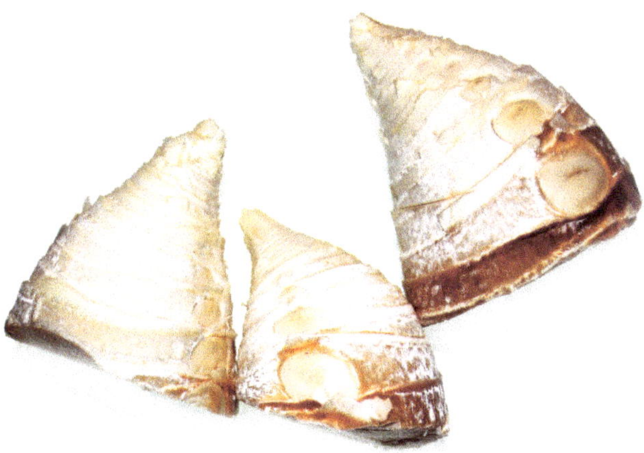

FIGURE 1.21 Edible soft and crunchy peeled shoots of *Bambusa balcooa*.

winter bamboo shoots' (Tom 1989). Bamboo shoot is the young, immature, tender, extending culm with a long tapered apical part, which grows from the nodes of the underground rhizome of bamboo plants throughout the rainy season. The edible portion of shoot comprises of rapidly dividing meristematic cells and is generally enclosed in protective non-edible culm sheaths of various colours, for example black, brown, yellow, orange, green and purple, depending on the bamboo species. The edible shoots are usually harvested when they are about 20–30 cm in height and, if not harvested, would mature into the tall bamboo plant within three to four months. In India, young shoots mostly appear from May to September. However, there are some species like *Chimonobambusa callosa*, the shoots of which sprout up to November. The shoot size and weight depend upon the species and are also affected significantly with several factors like location, depth, pH, climate, rainfall, temperature and soil conditions. The shoots are free from residual toxicity as they grow without the application of hazardous fertilizers or pesticides. Since ancient times, the shoots have its utilization as food and medicine in China and south-east Asian countries and because of its dietary qualities, it is recognized as a treasured dish in the Tang dynasty of China. A detailed account of the bamboo shoot as a food is given in Chapter 2.

1.6.6 Bamboo as Medicine

The use of bamboo for medicine and health in some societies is very old. In ancient Indian literature, it is said that 'bamboo by nature is laxative, frigid, seminal, curative, palatable, bladder purifier and full of astringent juice. It splits cough, subsides bile and cures leprosy, blood flux, wounds and swellings. In China, the medicinal properties of bamboo shoots were recorded in the book *Compendium of Materia Medica*, a pharmaceutical compilation written in the Ming dynasty (1368 to 1644): 'It's slightly cold, sweet, nontoxic and it quenches thirst, benefits the circulatory system and can be served as a daily dish' (Yuming and Jiru 1998). All parts of the bamboo plant, such as rhizomes, culms and bark shavings, resin, shoots, leaves, and seeds, have clinical applications. Culm shaving of *Bambusa breviflora* is used to clear phlegm in the lungs. Now it has been observed that leaves, which are generally discarded, are the best source of a number of anti-oxidants and bioactive compounds. Several in-vitro experiments on animals have confirmed important biological and medicinal properties of bamboo *in-vivo* leaves extracts such as anti-oxidant, anti-microbial, anti-inflammatory, anti-ulcer, anti-helminthic and anti-diabetic (Muniappan and Sundararaj 2003, Lu et al. 2005, Wang et al. 2012, Bajwa et al. 2017). In India, the first recorded use of bamboo as a medicine and health tonic dates back more than 5,000 years. The first reported use of *Banslochan* (also called *Tabasheer*), a siliceous substance that accumulates in the culms of some bamboo species, was in the preparation of a tonic called *Chyawanprash* named after the sage *Chyawan*, who is believed to have prepared the recipe for the tonic. *Banslochan* is used in Ayurvedic medicine system since ancient times as a cooling tonic and aphrodisiac and in asthma, cough and other debilitating diseases (Chongtham and Bisht 2017). According to ancient Chinese medicinal books, the consumption of young shoots helps in improving digestion, relieving hypertension, sweating, preventing cardiovascular diseases and cancer. The medicinal properties of bamboo are described in detail in Chapter 2.

1.6.7 Bamboo Salt

Bamboo salt also known as *Jukyeom* originates from Korea (Figure 1.22). It was originally developed by Korean doctors and monks almost 1,000 years ago as a folk medicine remedy for various types of illnesses. This bamboo salt is made by putting sea salt into a three-year-old bamboo culm internode, the ends are sealed with natural yellow clay rich in minerals. The culms are then roasted for about 10 hrs in a furnace with pinewood being used as fuel at a temperature of between 1000°C and 1500°C. This procedure is repeated one to ten times so that the salt gains higher medical effectiveness. The salt that is baked nine times is called purple bamboo salt because of the purple hue that results from the numerous repeated roasting, and it has the highest medical efficacy. This bamboo salt contains more than 70 minerals due to leaching of minerals from bamboo, pine tree resin and the yellow clay. The main minerals are calcium, phosphorus, magnesium, iron, copper, potassium, zinc and sulfur. This makes the salt highly alkaline (pH 10.5) and is claimed to be anti-allergic, anti-diabetic, anti-cancer, anti-obesity and anti-inflammatory and is also used in dental treatment, as preventive care for *Salmonella enteritidis*, as a reducer for chemotherapy side-effects and treatment for arthritis. It has been introduced to the North American market as a salt that has anti-cancerous and anti-viral properties. At the same time, it has been labeled as a wonder beauty product that can effectively treat acne and boost the youthful glow in the skin when used as a facial and body scrub.

1.6.8 Miscellaneous

Bamboo is a beautiful plant that can be used aesthetically for outside décor, ornamental landscapes and to make perfect screens for privacy. The sturdy culms are utilized for making a range of products such as decorative items, cutlery, toys, chopsticks, tableware, packaging materials, beverages and health care products (Figures 1.23, 1.24 and 1.25). Bamboo vinegar, a by-product of the bamboo carbonization process contains

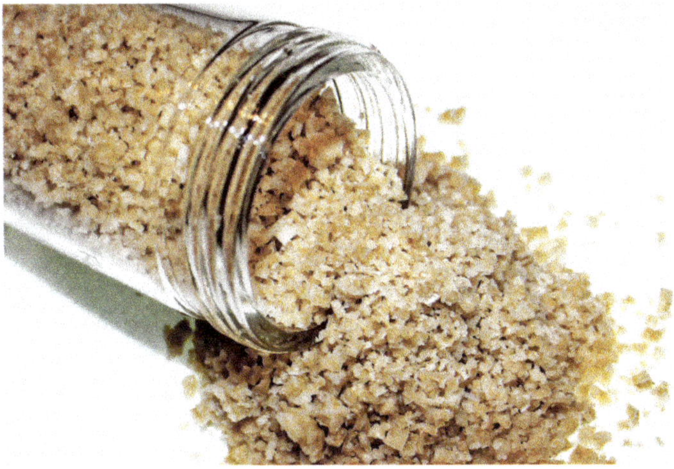

FIGURE 1.22 Bamboo salt.

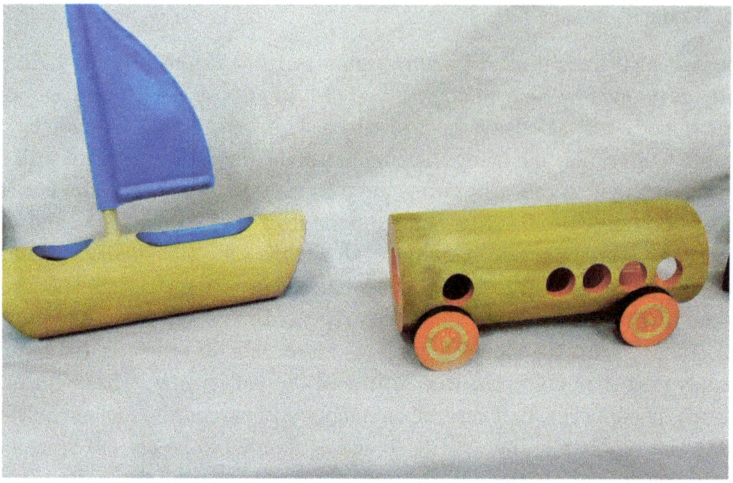

FIGURE 1.23 Bamboo toys.

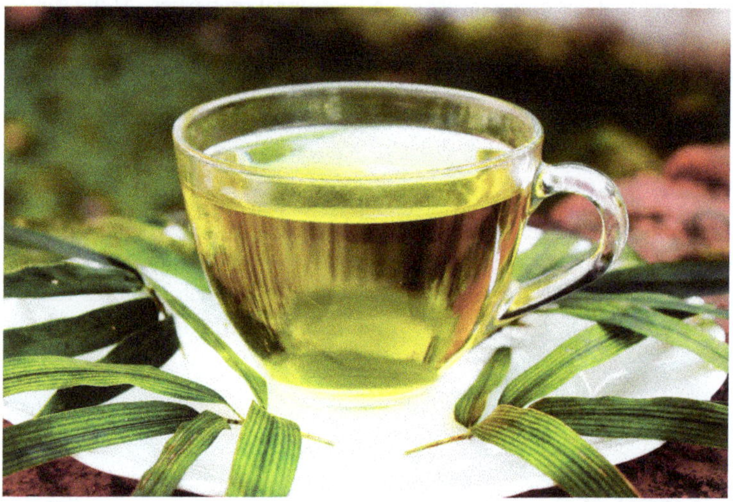

FIGURE 1.24 Bamboo leaf tea.

around 20% organic matter which can be further used in the manufacturing of several organic solutions such as acetic acid, formic acid, butyric acid and methyl alcohol, etc. having immense industrial applications. Bamboo bikes are now becoming popular as it addresses climate change, poverty, rural-urban migration and youth unemployment by creating jobs for young people, especially women (Figure 1.26). Some car companies are experimenting with bamboo, which could be used to build and reinforce some features of their new cars. Soon, some surfaces inside their vehicles could be made from a combination of plastic and bamboo to create a super-hard material. Composite bamboo charcoal-knitted fabric bullet-proof vests have been developed.

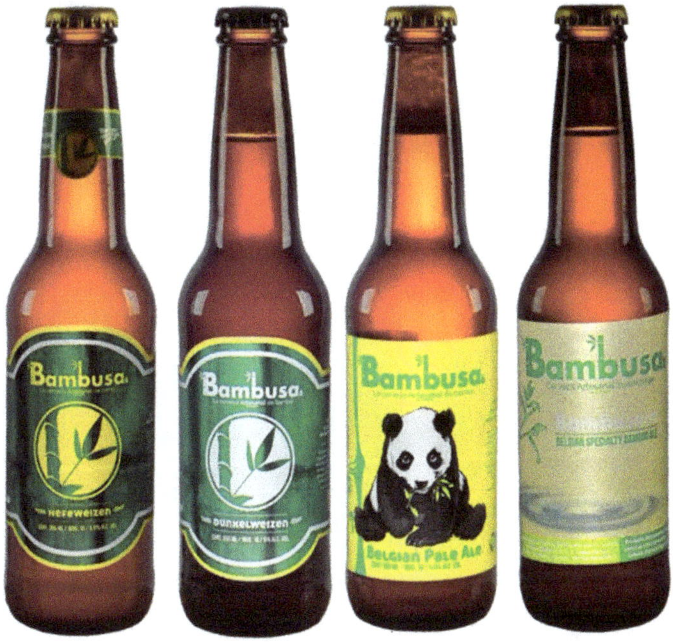

FIGURE 1.25 Bamboo beer. (Courtesy Mauricio Mora, Founder and CEO, Bamboo Liquid Innovations, Mexico.)

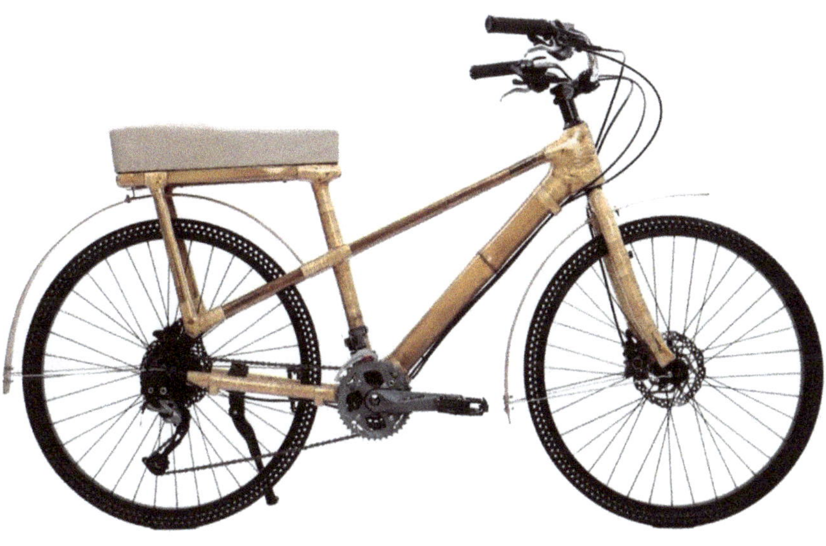

FIGURE 1.26 Bamboo cycle (Courtesy: Bryan Benitez McClelland, Founder, Bambike, Philippines).

Thus, bamboo is a marvellous resource that provides a myriad of benefits for billions of people. Development of bamboo resources is economically assisting impoverished people while at the same time stabilizing erodible slopes and flood-prone watersheds. The ability to substantially accentuate rapid growth through intensive management for commercialization purposes magnifies its many benefits.

2 Bamboo as Food and Medicine

Food assurance to every single individual of the world is a Magna Carta for human development as food provides all essential nutrients for healthy growth and development of human beings. According to Ayurveda, food is for body, soul and mind. Acharya Charaka (200 to 400 BCE) evidently mentioned that food helps in maintaining good health and prevents the occurrence of diseases, besides providing the basic nutrition to the body. Similarly, Hippocrates (500 BCE), Greek Physician and Father of Modern Medicine said, "Let food be thy medicine and medicine be thy food". From a total of 250,000 recognized plant species, only 7,000 have been utilized for human sustenance and out of these only three crops—wheat, rice and maize provide 50% of plant-derived calories. At present, more than 800 million people are chronically hungry and undernourished and 2 billion people are deficient in one or more micronutrients (FAO 2017). To increase food security and meet the global demand for food which is going to increase by 60% by 2050 due to high population growth; there is a need to promote food diversity and utilization of neglected and underutilized plants that are nutritional. Plant biodiversity offers a rich source of naturally existing nutrients that provide dietary diversity and also provide food, nutrition, health and economic security. Bamboo is one such common agro-forestry multipurpose plant, which is highly popular in several Asian countries but is lesser known for its edibility and nutritional potential in India except for north-eastern regions and some parts of central and south India.

Bamboo is a complete food to some animals and health food and medicine to man. Folk tales, stories, dramas and cultural activities of many regions depict the use of bamboo as food by animals and humans. Bamboo is not only the true gourmets for some animals like the giant panda, red panda, bamboo lemur, elephants and many other herbivores, but a delicacy and healthy food for humans. According to an ancient story from the state of Mizoram, India, village people used to watch a tortoise every year appearing and eating bamboo shoots only during the sprouting season of bamboo and sleep for rest of the year. This lead the people to believe that bamboo shoots must be healthy food as tortoise survives the whole year just eating bamboo shoots (Bisht et al. 2012). The use of bamboo as food dated since early civilization and mainly in places where edible bamboos were commonly found and people tried their own methods to consume the shoots. The Chinese in the tropical belt are thought to be the first to utilize bamboo as a vegetable. According to Marden (1980), Chinese value bamboo shoots for food because of their crisp texture and subtle flavour. As Chinese civilization spread to Japan, Burma, Thailand and Vietnam, the food value of bamboo shoots also spread. In the Philippines, the Malaya Peninsula races from Indonesia must have brought with them some edible bamboo species. The exotic tasty bamboo shoots also provide a means for boosting food and nutritional security in remote areas. Bamboo shoots are also consumed in many parts of India using different forms like fresh, dried and fermented shoots to prepare curries, chutneys and pickles. In the 21st century, bamboo shoots are being recognized as a health food being used to prepare many food products and in pharmaceutical preparations. Asian countries like China, Thailand and Taiwan are the main exporters of bamboo shoots in the world market.

2.1 BAMBOO SHOOTS AS A NUTRIENT-RICH FOOD

Bamboo shoots have a long history of being used as a source of both food and medicine in China and Southeast Asia. A traditional forest vegetable in China for more than 2,500 years, bamboo shoots are not only delicious but are also rich in nutrients and rank among the five most popular healthcare foods in the world. The juvenile shoots are not only delicious but are now proved to be rich in nutrient components, mainly proteins, carbohydrates, minerals and fibre and are low in fat and sugars. In Japan, the bamboo shoot is called the 'King of Forest Vegetables'. In China, knowing the nutritional value and delicious taste, people considered bamboo shoots a treasured dish in the Tang Dynasty (618 to 907) and there was a saying that "there is no banquet without bamboo". The properties of bamboo shoots were recorded in the *Compendium of Materia Medica*, a pharmaceutical text written during the Ming dynasty (1368 to 1644), with the following words: "It's slightly cold, sweet, non-toxic and it quenches thirst, benefits the liquid circulatory system and can be served as a daily dish" (Yuming and Jiru 1998). In India, bamboo shoot has been used as food since long in the north-east region of India as well as in many parts of the country. Consumption of tender shoots is confined mainly to the north-eastern states of India where they are part of the traditional cuisine. Earlier, it was also a solution for food security in the dense forest and remote areas during the lean period. Presently, though the shoots are consumed more like a vegetable by local people, they are made available to others as a delicacy in up-scale markets and specialty restaurants. Hence, bamboos are no longer considered as "poor man's timber" but they form a "rich man's delicacy". The shoots are not only used as fresh vegetables but are also processed and preserved in many forms such as dried, fermented, salted, pickled, water-soaked and canned. Bamboo shoots are gastronomic treats whether used fresh or in fermented or roasted form. The shoots are organic vegetables free from residual toxicity as they grow without the application of hazardous fertilizers or pesticides. Correlations between the consumption of bamboo components and generally improved health status have been observed but lacked scientific validation. Now, many scientific studies have also proved the health benefits of bamboo shoots leading to an increase in its popularity. The global export value of bamboo shoots and shoot-based products has also increased substantially in recent years owing to huge demand from areas such as Europe, the United States, Japan and so on, reaching USD 276 million (Figure 2.1A). China tops the list of countries exporting shoots worth USD 240.9 million whereas Japan is the largest importer, importing shoots worth USD 160.4 million annually (INBAR 2012) (Figure 2.1B). These figures are expected to increase in the coming years with further promotion of capacity building in shoot-based industries in major bamboo shoot producing countries such as China, India, Taiwan, Indonesia and so on.

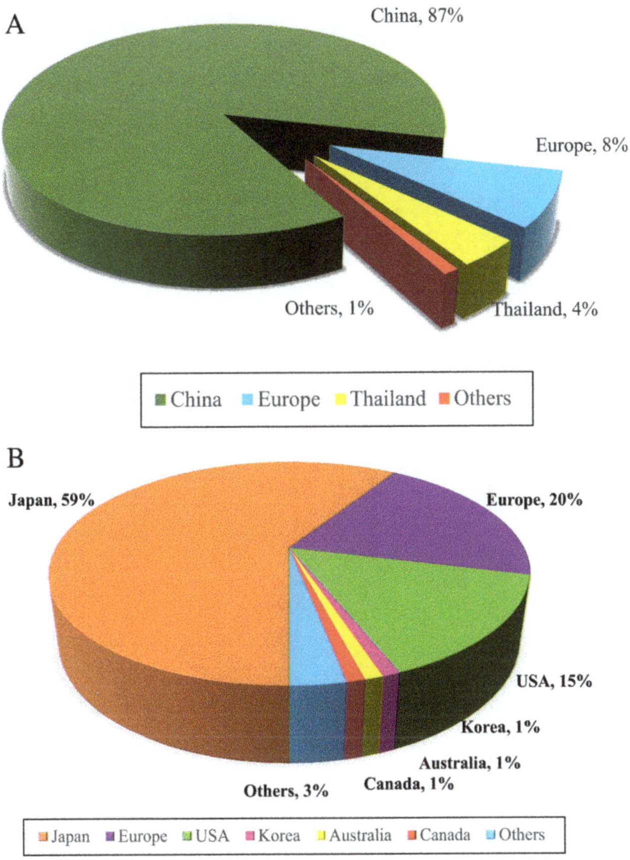

FIGURES 2.1 A. Major exporters and B. importers of bamboo shoots (INBAR 2012).

Most bamboo species produce edible shoots but around 200 species are commonly grown or utilized for their shoots as listed in Table 2.1. While conducting studies on a superior variety of shoots in China, Maoyi (1998) recommended *Bambusa blumeana*, *Dendrocalamus asper*, *D. latiflorus* and *Phyllostachys pubescens* as highest priority species for shoot production in China on the basis of the weight of harvested shoot and weight of edible portion. In India, popular species whose shoots are consumed include *Bambusa balcooa*, *B. tulda*, *Dendrocalamus giganteus*, *D. hamiltonii*, *D. hookerii*, *D. longispathus*, *D. sikkimensis*, *Melocanna baccifera*, *Phyllostachys mannii*, *Schizostachyum dullooa* and *Teinostachyum wightii*. Similarly, species of *Arundinaria aristata*, *A. hirsuta*, *Bambusa arundinacea*, *B. glaucescens*, *B. khasiana*, *B. longispiculata*, *B. nutans*, *B. polymorpha*, *B. tulda*, *B. vulgaris*, *Cephalostachyum capitatum*, *C. fuchsianum*, *C. pergracile*, *Dendrocalamus brandisii*, *D. giganteus*, *D. hamiltonii*, *D. hookerii*, *D. longispathus*, *D. strictus*, *Melocanna baccifera*, *Oxytenanthera albociliata*, *Pseudostachyum polymorphum*, *Sinobambusa elegans* were considered most suitable for the production of bamboo shoots in

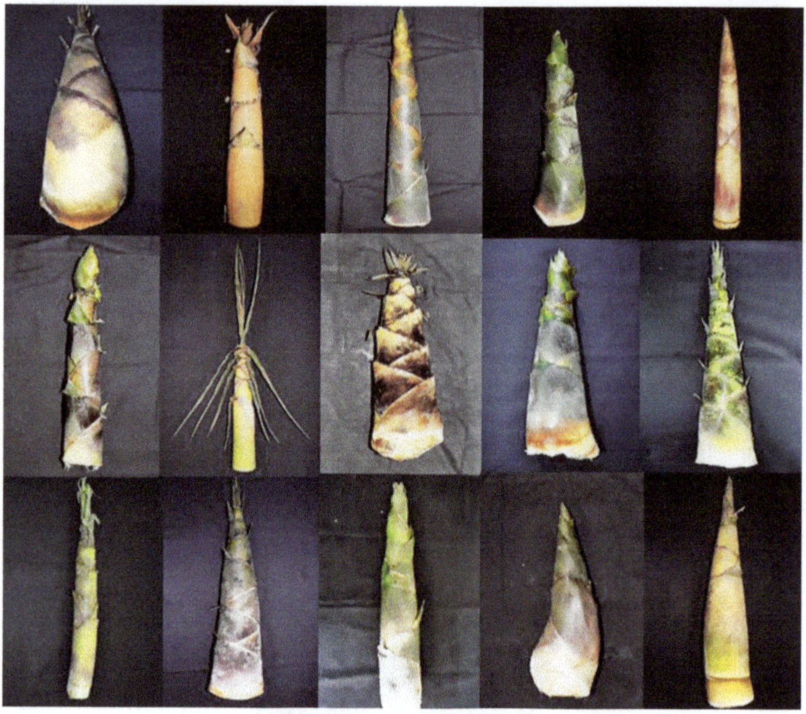

FIGURE 2.2 Physical appearance and shape of bamboo shoots of different species.

south India (Shanmughavel 2004). Devi (2018) carried out a study of edible bamboos of Manipur, India. A survey was carried out in 16 districts of Manipur and it was reported that 15 bamboo species belonging to the genera *Bambusa, Dendrocalamus, Cephalostachyum, Chimonobambusa* and *Melocanna* are mainly used for edible purposes.

New culms or juvenile shoots in bamboos usually develop with the beginning of the monsoon season during which the young edible shoots are harvested. The typical 'shooting season' of a species rarely exceeds two months. This period can be extended by modifying the cultivation and management practices. Shoots of different species vary in shape, size, weight and diameter (Table 2.2). The shoots can be conical, cylindrical, spear or bullet-shaped and small, medium or large in size (Figure 2.2). Three species viz. *Dendrocalamus giganteus, D. latiflorus* and *D. sikkimensis* have a large-sized shoot with a basal diameter ranging from 37 cm to 48 cm. Edible portions are highest in *Chimonobambusa callosa* (67.66%) and least in *Melocanna baccifera* (33.33%). Shoots of some bamboos such as *Phyllostachys edulis, C. callosa, M. baccifera* are small and sweet in taste and considered a delicacy in countries such as China, Japan, India and so on, whereas in some other bamboos such as *D. hamiltonii, Bambusa tulda* and so on the shoots are bitter in taste and need processing before consumption.

TABLE 2.1
List of Edible Bamboo Species Worldwide

Species	Country	References	Monopodial/Sympodial
Acidosasa edulis, A. hirtiflora, A. lingchuanensis	China	Li and Kobayashi 2004	Monopodial
Arundinaria aristata, A. hirsuta	India	Shanmughavel 2004	Monopodial/sympodial
Bambusa arundinacea, B. balcooa, B. bambos, B. blumeana, B. cacharensis, B. edulis, B. glaucescens, B. khasiana, B. kingiana, B. longispiculata, B. manipureana, B. merrilliana, B. mizorameana, B. multiplex, B. nana, B. nutans, B. oldhamii, B. oliveriana, B. pallida, B. philippinensis, B. polymorpha, B. tulda, B. tuldoides, B. vulgaris	Australia, Bhutan, Brazil, China, India, Indonesia, Japan, Nepal, Puerto Rico, Pakistan, Philippines, Sri Lanka, United Republic of Tanzania, Taiwan, Thailand	Shanmughavel 2004, Seethalakshmi and Kumar 1998, Bhatt et al. 2003, 2005, NMBA, 2009, Badwaik et al. 2015, Premlata et al. 2015, Yudodibroto 1985, Tripathi 1998, Poudyal 2006, Tandug and Torres 1985, Li and Kobayashi 2004, Hinsui et al. 2008, Caasi-Lit and Punzalan 2015, Waikhom et al. 2013, Dattagupta et al. 2014, Scurlock et al. 2000, ERG 2005, Singh et al. 2003, Chongtham et al. 2011, Anantachote 1985, Kumbhare and Bhargava 2007, Saini et al. 2015, Kleinenz et al. 2000, Jeyaram et al. 2009, Kennard and Freyre 1957, Bhargava et al. 1996, Chongtham et al. 2007, Lantican et al. 1985, Vivekanandan 1985	Sympodial
Bashania fangiana	China	Li and Kobayashi 2004	Sympodial
Cephalostachyum capitatum, C. fuchsianum, C. pergracile	India	Shanmughavel 2004, Premlata et al. 2015	Sympodial
Chimonobambusa angustifolia, C. armata, C. grandifolia, C. callosa, C. hejiangensis, C. hookeriana, C. lactistriata, C. marmorea, C. microfloscula, C. neopurpurea, C. pachystachys, C. szechuanensis, C. szechuanensis var. *flexuosa,, C. utilis, C. yunnanensis*	India China, Japan, Nepal	Li and Kobayashi 2004, Seethalakshmi and Kumar 1998, Waikhom et al. 2013, Premlata et al. 2015, Chongtham et al. 2011, Yuming et al. 2004, Poudyal 2006	Monopodial

(*Continued*)

TABLE 2.1 (CONTINUED)
List of Edible Bamboo Species Worldwide

Species	Country	References	Monopodial/Sympodial
Chimonocalamus delicates, C. dumosus, C. dumosus var. *pygmaeus, C. fimbriatus, C. longiligulatus, C. makuanensis, C. montanus, C. pallens, C. tortuosus*	China	Li and Kobayashi 2004, Yuming et al. 2004	Sympodial
Chusquea culeou	Argentina, Chile, Patagonia	Ladio and Lozada 2000, Londoño 2001	Sympodial
Dendrocalamopsis beecheyana, D. beecheyana var. *pubescens, D. bicicatricata, D. daii, D. edulis, D. oldhamii, D. stenoaurita, D. validus, D. vario-striata*	China	Li and Kobayashi 2004	Sympodial
Dendrocalamus asper, D. farinosus, D. brandisii, D. fugongensis, D. giganteus D. hamiltonii, D. hamiltonii var. *edulis, D. hookeri, D. latiflorus D. longispathus D. manipureanus D. membranaceus, D. pachystachys, D. semiscandens D. sikkimensis, D. stocksii D. strictus D. tibeticus, D. yunnanicus*	China, India, Indonesia, Japan, Nepal, Philippines, Puerto Rico, Taiwan, Thailand, Bhutan, Myanmar, Pakistan, Sri Lanka, Bangladesh	Kennard and Freyre 1957, Yudodibroto 1985, Scurlock et al. 2000, ERG 2005, Li and Kobayashi 2004, Poudyal 2006, FAO 2007, Kumbhare and Bhargava 2007, Chongtham et al. 2007, Caasi-Lit and Punzalan 2015, Seethalakshmi and Kumar 1998, Shanmughavel 2004, Vivekanandan 1985, Bhatt et al. 2003, 2005, Chongtham et al. 2008, NMBA 2009, Premlata et al. 2015, Anantachote 1985, Bajwa et al. 2016, Stapleton 1994, Premlata et al. 2015, Lantican et al. 1985, Yuming et al. 2004, Waikhom et al. 2013, Tripathi 1998, Jeyaram et al. 2009, Chandramouli and Viswanath 2015, Saini et al. 2015	Sympodial
Drepanostachyum spp.	Nepal	Jackson 1987	Sympodial

(Continued)

TABLE 2.1 (CONTINUED)
List of Edible Bamboo Species Worldwide

Species	Country	References	Monopodial/Sympodial
Fargesia angustissima, F. brevissima, F. canaliculata, F. denudata, F. dracocephala, F. edulis, F. emaculata, F. ferax, F. fractiflexa, F. fungosa, F. jiulongensis, F. lincangensis, F. mairei, F. murielae, F. nitida, F. oblique, F. orbiculata, F. pagyrifera, F. pauciflora, F. pleniculmis, F. porphyea, F. qinlingensis, F. robusta, F. rufa, F. scabrida, F. tenuilignea, F. utilis, F. yulongshanensis, F. yunnanensis	China	Li and Kobayashi 2004	Sympodial
Gigantochloa albociliata G. atter G. felix, G. levis, G. ligulata G. pseudoarundinaria G. rostrata	China, India, Thailand, Indonesia, Philippines, Puerto Rico	Anantachote 1987, Seethalakshmi and Kumar 1998, Li and Kobayashi 2004 Yudodibroto 1985, Caasi-Lit and Punzalan 2015 Kennard and Freyre 1957, Lantican et al. 1985, Bhatt et al. 2004	Sympodial
Guadua angustifolia G. sarcocarpa	Colombia, Ecuador, India, Panama, Puerto Rico, Venezuela Amazonian Peru, Brazil, Bolivia	Kennard and Freyre 1957, Londoño 2001, Viswanath et al. 2012, Chandramouli and Viswanath 2015, Londoño and Peterson 1991	Sympodial
Indosasa angustata, I. glabrata, I. ingens, I. patens	China	Li and Kobayashi 2004	Monopodial
Melocalamus compactiflorus, M. indicus	India	Medhi et al. 2014	Monopodial

(Continued)

TABLE 2.1 (CONTINUED)
List of Edible Bamboo Species Worldwide

Species	Country	References	Monopodial/Sympodial
Melocanna baccifera, M. bambusoides	India, Puerto Rico	Kennard and Freyre 1957, Bhargava et al. 1996, Bhatt et al. 2003, 2005, Shanmughavel 2004, Premlata et al. 2015, Singh et al. 2003, Jeyaram et al. 2009	Sympodial
Oxytenanthera albociliata *O. parvifolia*	India	Shanmughavel 2004, Medhi et al. 2014	Monopodial
Phyllostachys acuta, P. amarus, P. angusta, P. arcana, P. atrovaginata *P. assamica, P. aurea* *P. aurita, P. bambusoides* var. *castillonis, P. bissetii, P. concave, P. dulcis, P. elegans, P. fimbriligula, P. glauca* var. *variabilis, P. heteroclada, P. incarnata, P. iridescens, P. kwanglsiensis, P. makinoi, P. mannii, P. meyeri, P. edulis P. flexuosa, P. glauca, P. heterocycla, P. mitis, P. nidularia, P. nigra,* *P. nigra* var. *henonis,* *P. nuda, P. parvifolia,* *P. platyglossa, P. praecox, P. prominens, P. propinqua, P. pubescens, P. rigida, P. rivali,* *P. robustiramea, P. rubromarginata, P. rutila, P. sulphurea, P. tianmuensis, P. virella, P. viridiglaucescens, P. viridis, P. vivax, P. yunhoensis*	China, India Indonesia, Japan, Java, Nepal, Pakistan, Philippines Republic of Korea, USA, Taiwan	Li and Kobayashi 2004, Lu et al. 2009, Tamang and Tamang 2009, Guoging 1985, Lantican et al. 1985, Yudodibroto 1985, Poudyal 2006, FAO 2007, Seethalakshmi and Kumar 1998, Diver 2001, Bhatt et al. 2005, Scurlock et al. 2000, Kim et al. 2007a, Lu et al. 2009, Yang et al. 2015, ERG 2005	Monopodial

(*Continued*)

TABLE 2.1 (CONTINUED)
List of Edible Bamboo Species Worldwide

Species	Country	References	Monopodial/Sympodial
Pseudostachyum polymorphum	India	Shanmughavel 2004	Sympodial
Pseudosasa longiligula	China	Li and Kobayashi 2004	Monopodial
Pseudoxytenanthera bourdillonii	India	Seethalakshmi and Kumar 1998	Sympodial
Qiongzhuea communis, Q. macrophylla, Q. rigidula, Q. tumidinoda	China	Li and Kobayashi 2004, Yuming et al. 2004	Amphipodial
Schizostachyum annulatum, S. capitatum, S. dullooa	India	Li and Kobayashi 2004	Sympodial
	China	Jeyaram et al. 2010	
S. funghomii, S. pingbianensis		Bhatt et al. 2004	
		Yuming et al. 2004	
Sinarundinaria elegans, S. hirsute, S. hookeriana, S. intermedia	India	Seethalakshmi and Kumar 1998, Shanmughavel 2004	Sympodial
Teinostachyum wightii	India	Bhatt et al. 2005, Jeyaram et al. 2009	Sympodial
Thamnocalamus aristatus, T. falconeri	India, Bhutan	Seethalakshmi and Kumar 1998, Noltie 2000	Sympodial
Thyrsostachys oliveri, T. regia T. siamensis	India, Taiwan, Thailand	Seethalakshmi and Kumar 1998, Chongtham et al. 2011, Scurlock et al. 2000, ERG 2005	Sympodial
Yushania brevipaniculata. Y. cava, Y. crassicollis, Y. glauca, Y. lineolata, Y. mitis, Y. oblonga, Y. qiaojiaensis	China	Li and Kobayashi 2004	Sympodial

TABLE 2.2
Shoot Morphology and Edible Percent of Young Shoots of Some Edible Bamboos

Species	Shape	Size	Length (cm)	Basal Circumference (cm)	Weight (kg)	Edible Portion (%)	Inedible Portion (%)
Bambusa balcooa	Conical	Medium	33.00 ± 1.58	29.20 ± 3.42	1.30 ± 0.12	58.46	41.54
B. cacharensis	Cylindrical	Medium	32.20 ± 3.27	26.00 ± 1.87	0.84 ± 0.11	48.81	51.19
B. manipureana	Cylindrical	Medium	34.60 ± 1.52	25.80 ± 1.30	0.96 ± 0.15	53.13	46.87
B. nutans	Conical	Medium	31.00 ± 1.41	33.00 ± 3.24	1.34 ± 0.15	59.70	40.30
B. tulda	Cylindrical	Small	32.80 ± 3.35	23.80 ± 2.95	0.72 ± 0.12	51.39	48.61
B. vulgaris	Cylindrical	Medium	32.60 ± 1.14	27.00 ± 1.00	1.12 ± 0.13	52.68	47.32
Cephalostachyum capitatum	Cylindrical	Small	32.20 ± 0.84	12.00 ± 1.00	0.27 ± 0.10	55.56	44.44
Chimonobambusa callosa	Spear shaped	Small	34.00 ± 2.35	13.40 ± 0.55	0.28 ± 0.02	67.86	32.14
Dendrocalamus giganteus	Conical	Large	28.75 ± 1.24	48.10 ± 1.48	1.85 ± 0.10	62.70	37.30
D. hamiltonii	Conical	Medium	36.40 ± 3.51	28.10 ± 1.67	1.22 ± 0.19	59.02	40.98
D. hookeri	Conical	Medium	31.40 ± 2.19	26.00 ± 1.00	0.82 ± 0.08	52.44	47.56
D. latiflorus	Bullet-shaped	Large	32.54 ± 4.84	40.25 ± 3.23	1.92 ± 0.79	64.06	35.94
D. longispathus	Conical	Medium	40.80 ± 3.03	23.40 ± 1.52	0.83 ± 0.08	48.19	51.81
D. manipureanus	Conical	Medium	42.40 ± 3.05	26.50 ± 3.08	1.04 ± 0.32	55.77	44.23
D. membranaceus	Conical	Medium	36.66 ± 2.08	30.33 ± 2.30	1.28 ± 0.10	62.50	37.50
D. sikkimensis	Bullet-Shaped	Large	30.20 ± 2.68	37.00 ± 1.58	1.82 ± 0.28	61.54	38.46
Melocanna baccifera	Cylindrical	Small	28.40 ± 2.61	14.60 ± 1.14	0.33 ± 0.02	33.33	66.67
Phyllostachys mannii	Spear shaped	Small	41.74 ± 11.39	11.66 ± 2.88	0.20 ± 0.05	47.00	53.00

2.2 THE TRADITIONAL WAY OF BAMBOO SHOOT CONSUMPTION

2.2.1 Fresh Shoots

Fresh shoots have a crisp, crunchy taste and sweet flavour with a unique taste. They are mostly used in making appetizing soups, delicious snacks, hot curries, spicy stir-fries, attractive salads, pickles, chutneys, aromatic fried rice, spring rolls and other stewed and fried dishes. Shoots are also used as an extender, as they take on the flavour of the ingredients in which it is cooked. The most common preparation involves boiling the shoots in stocks, soups, or salted water for use in assorted dishes. The sap of young stalks tapped during the rainy season is simply made into a soft drink in China (Yang et al. 2008).

Consumption of bamboo shoots is mainly concentrated in south-east Asia, where they are popular ingredients in the local cuisine. China has the largest bamboo shoot industry producing approximately 1.3 million metric tons of fresh bamboo. Worldwide, more than 2 million tons of bamboo shoots are consumed annually of which about 1.3 million tons are produced in China alone. In China, where the use of bamboo shoots as a vegetable dates back to the Han Dynasty (202 BCE–220 CE), shoots were used in dumplings, soups, salads, noodles and gravies. The popularity of Chinese restaurants worldwide gives an opportunity for people in many countries to taste this bamboo vegetable. In India, however, despite the fact that it is the second largest producer of bamboos after China, not much importance has been given to the use of bamboo shoots as food due to lack of awareness of the edible characteristics of the shoots. Bamboo shoot consumption is very popular in north-eastern regions of India. In Manipur, fresh shoots are used to make dishes such as *Usoi-ooti* and *Usoi-kangsu* (Table 2.3 and Figure 2.3). Canned and preserved bamboo shoots currently dominate international trade, but due to increased consumer demand for non-processed food, it is projected that the share of fresh shoots will significantly increase in the near future.

People consume fresh bamboo shoots in various forms. In order to use the shoots as vegetables, the hard sheaths have to be removed to extract the soft edible portion. In the Philippines, bamboo shoots have been part of the traditional and favourite dishes, being among the basic ingredients of many special dishes in different parts of the country (Caasi-Lit 1999). Bamboo shoots are called by several names such as *Labong*, *Rebung*, *Dabung* and *Tambo* and popular dishes are *Ginataang-labong* and *Dinengdeng-na-labong*. In Indonesia, bamboo shoots known as *Rebung* and are made into several traditional cuisines including *Gulai-rebung*, *Lumpia-semarang* and *Sayur-lodeh* (Ningtyas et al. 2014, Sukenti 2014). Bamboo shoots are called *No-mai* in Thailand and are used in stir-fries, soup such as *Tom-kha-kai* curries such as *Kaeng-tai-pla* as well as Thai salads. In Singapore, people consume bamboo shoots in the form of canned or frozen (Pan 1995). *Jiang-sun* is a widely consumed traditional food in Taiwan made with bamboo shoots (Chen et al. 2010). In Bangladesh, tribal collect bamboo shoots from natural forest and use them as a major food item during the rainy season. They also collect bamboo seeds to make cakes (Banik 1997).

TABLE 2.3
Traditional Bamboo Shoot Recipes from North-East India

Bamboo Shoot Recipe	State	Method of Preparation
Rawtuai-bawl (non-veg)	Mizoram	Boiled bamboo shoots (*Phyllostachys mannii*) mixed with fermented pork and spices
Rawtuai -bawl (veg)	Mizoram	Bamboo shoots (*Phyllostachys mannii*) boiled and mixed with green chillies and leaves of small beans
Rawtuai -rep	Mizoram	Sun or fire dried bamboo shoots (*Phyllostachys mannii*) soaked in water and then mixed with either fermented pork or green chillies and leaves of small beans
Rawtuai-kan	Mizoram	Boiled bamboo shoots (*Melocanna baccifera*) fried with oil and other spices
Rawtuai-bai	Mizoram	Fresh shoots of *Melocanna baccifera* chopped soaked in water and boiled with some rice with a pinch of sodium-bicarbonate
Usoi-ooti	Manipur	Sliced bamboo shoots *(Bambusa nutans)* and dried pea soaked in water overnight then boiled with a pinch of sodium-bicarbonate
Usoi-kangsu	Manipur	Overnight water-soaked bamboo slices boiled with potato and mixed with fried fermented fish and dried chillies
Soijin-eronba	Manipur	Fermented bamboo shoots boiled with potato and mixed with fermented fish and dried chillies
Ngakra-soijin-thongba	Manipur	Fermented bamboo shoot (*Soijin*) and catfish (local breed) cooked with oil and spices
Mia-gudhog	Tripura	Fresh bamboo shoots washed and cooked with various vegetables and fermented fish and smashed; chilli, onion and garlic used for taste
Mia-mosho	Tripura	Boiled bamboo shoots used for making chutney with fermented fish and chillies
Mia-chachiew	Tripura	Boiled bamboo shoots cooked either with rice powder, dried pea or dal (pulses) with a pinch of sodium-bicarbonate
Mia-mweiborog	Tripura	Boiled bamboo shoots with vegetables, fish, chillies and onion
Moiya-koshak-shidal	Tripura	Fermented bamboo shoots with fermented fish (*shidal*)
Chakkhoi	Tripura	Fermented bamboo shoots with vegetables
Moya-chakhoi	Tripura	Shoots of non-bitter bamboo soaked in hot water (five mins) dried in sun and consumed with other vegetables
Perok-ikung	Arunachal Pradesh	*Ikung* (fermented) bamboo shoots prepared with fried chicken and spices or boiled with chicken and spices
Yekdin-ikung	Arunachal Pradesh	*Ikung* (fermented) bamboo shoots fried or boiled with pork and other spices
Engo-ikung	Arunachal Pradesh	*Ikung* (fermented) bamboo shoots boiled with fish and spices
Itting-oying	Arunachal Pradesh	Fresh bamboo shoots cut into small pieces and boiled and prepared with vegetable or added with chicken or pork
Ib-oying	Arunachal Pradesh	Dried bamboo shoots prepared with fish, chicken or pork

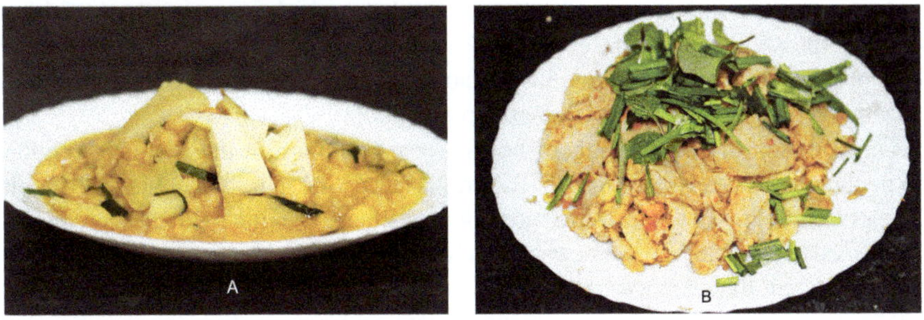

FIGURE 2.3 Fresh bamboo shoot dish from Manipur, India: A. *Usoi-ooti*, B. *Usoi-kangsu*.

In India, although bamboo shoot consumption is most popular in the north-east regions, it is also part of the traditional cuisine of several states such as Andaman and Nicobar Island, Karnataka, Kerala and Odisha. In the Diyun region of Arunachal Pradesh, the Chakma people utilize fresh bamboo shoots, known as *Bashchuri* in the local dialect, as a seasonal delicacy. In Nagaland, bamboo shoots are commonly known as *Bas-tenga* and they are cooked and eaten as a fresh food item or fermented for a variety of culinary uses. Almost all the tribes of the region relish bamboo shoot and have their own recipes and method of using bamboo shoots as food or flavouring agent. In Jharkhand, India, bamboo shoots are known as *Sandhana* and are used to make curries and pickles. The bamboo shoots are used as a special dish *Kanile* in the Malnad region of Karnataka and are also used as a pickle. Bamboo has been an integral part of the tribes of South Gujarat. Apart from using bamboo for household uses, its shoots are used to make delicious curry.

According to species or variety of bamboo, the shoots are consumed fresh, dried or fermented and people have developed culinary art and processing methods of shoots for food with respect to the species or variety available in their areas (Table 2.3). Species whose shoots have a sweet taste are generally preferred fresh, whereas species with shoots having bitter taste are generally fermented or dried. Shoots of *Phyllostachys mannii*, *Melocanna baccifera* and *Chimonobambusa callosa* are mostly consumed fresh as the shoots of these species have less cyanogenic glycosides and hence are not bitter in taste. In Manipur, fresh bamboo shoots are cooked with fresh or dry fish. *Usoi-ooti* and *Ushoi-kangshu* of Manipur, *Rawtuai-bai* of Mizoram, *Mia-gudhog* of Tripura are some of the important recipes prepared from fresh shoots of bamboo. In Western Ghats in India, edible bamboo species are extensively used as snacks, fried foodstuff and curries. In Sikkim, *Tama,* a non-fermented bamboo shoot curry is very popular among the people.

2.2.2 Fermented Shoots

Traditionally, various fermented bamboo shoot products are consumed in the world. Fermentation is one very important technique that is extensively followed in the north-east region of India to increase the shelf life of bamboo shoots, make it more palatable and easier to store and handle. Fermentation not only decreases the level of anti-nutrient cyanogenic glycosides in bamboo shoots but also increases the nutritional and health benefits. The fermentation of bamboo shoots by different methods is also associated with a unique group of microflorae which increases the nutritional value of the shoots (Jeyaram et al. 2009). The fermentation process increases the level of proteins, vitamins, essential amino acids and various bioactive compounds (Sarangthem and Singh 2003, Chongtham et al. 2011).

Fermentation of young bamboo shoots is very common in the north-east region, particularly in states like Manipur, Tripura, Arunachal Pradesh and Meghalaya and there is a number of methods of fermentation which are specific to the tribe, region or species/variety of bamboo. Some tribes such as *Khasi*, *Garo* and *Jaintia* of Meghalaya mainly ferment the chopped bamboo shoots by immersing them in a container filled with water. By this method, shoots can be preserved for more than one year. The fermented shoots develop a sour taste and at the same time maintain the crunchiness which is relished by the local people. The people of Meghalaya mainly prefer the shoots of *Dendrocalamus hamiltonii* for fermentation by this water method. The Adi tribe of Arunachal Pradesh ferment the bamboo shoots in a bamboo basket covered with *Ekkam* (*Phrynium pubinerve*) leaves. In Manipur, bamboo shoots are fermented by the *Meetei* people either in an earthen pot or in a bamboo basket. *Soibum, Soidon* and *Soijin* are types of fermented bamboo shoot, that are delicacies of the Manipuri people and eaten as pickle and curry mixed with fermented fish (Table 2.3). *Eronba* is a popular dish prepared with these fermented shoots (Figure 2.4).

Some of the *Naga* tribes of Nagaland ferment bamboo shoots in a conical bamboo basket which bears a hole at the bottom to collect the exudates from fermented shoots. The exudate is used for flavouring various food items year-round. Various tribes (*Debbarma, Uchoi, Chakma*) of Tripura state also ferment bamboo shoots, mainly in earthen pots. The fermented products are called *Moiya-koshak* (*Debbarma* and *Uchoi* Tribes), *Medukeye* (*Chakma* Tribe) or *Melye-amiley* (*Chakma* tribe). Ethnic people living in Sub-Himalayan regions, Nepal and Bhutan prepare and consume a variety of domesticated and wild bamboo shoots and their fermented products (Tamang and Tamang 2009). Fermented bamboo shoot products of the Eastern hills of Nepal and Bhutan are known as *Mesu*. Use of *Mesu* as a pickle and as a base

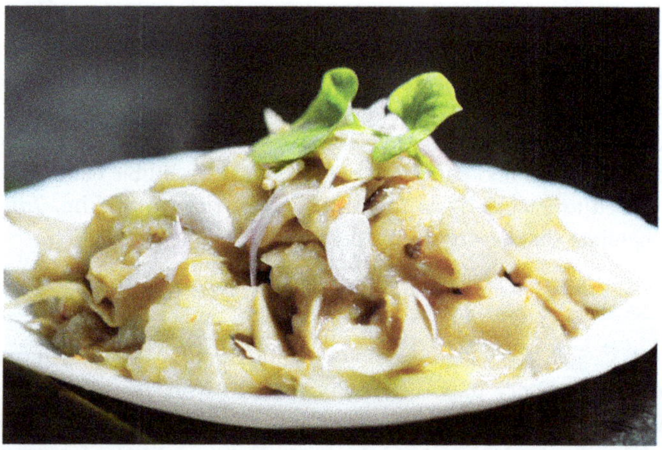

FIGURE 2.4 *Soibum eronba*, a fermented bamboo shoot recipe of Manipur, India.

in curries is a conventional dish among the *Nepalis*, *Bhutias* and the *Lepchas* of the Darjeeling hills and Sikkim. A similar fermented bamboo shoot product called *Naw-mai-dong* or *Nor-mai-dorng* is consumed in Thailand (Phithakpol et al. 1995).

The sap of young shoots collected during the rainy season is fermented to prepare *Ulanzi* (a sweet wine), which is used by Chinese as a delicious liquor (Qing et al. 2008). In Central India, the young shoots are grated and fermented to prepare *Kardi* or *Amil,* a sour vegetable soup. In the region, the bamboo shoots are fermented, dried, ground into a powder and used as a garnish called *Hendua,* which is commonly preferred liquor among the tribal people (Panda and Padhy 2007). In Nepal, bamboo shoots are fermented with turmeric and oil and cooked with potatoes to prepare an item called *Alu-tama*. Different countries have their own unique method of preparing the bamboo shoots as shown in Table 2.4 and Figures 2.5 and 2.6.

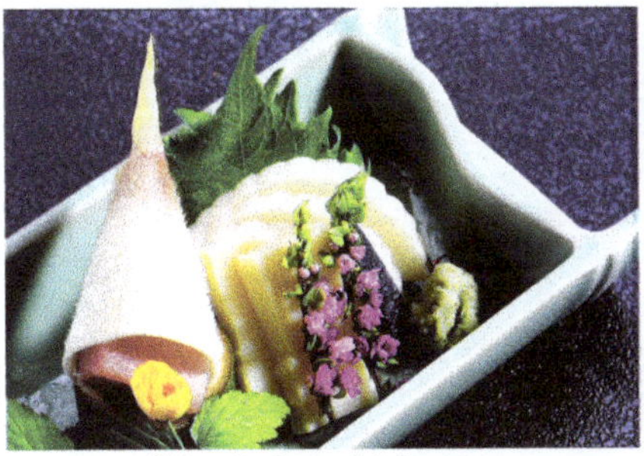

***Takenoko-kagamini*, Japan**
(Courtesy: Yoshinobu Komatsu)

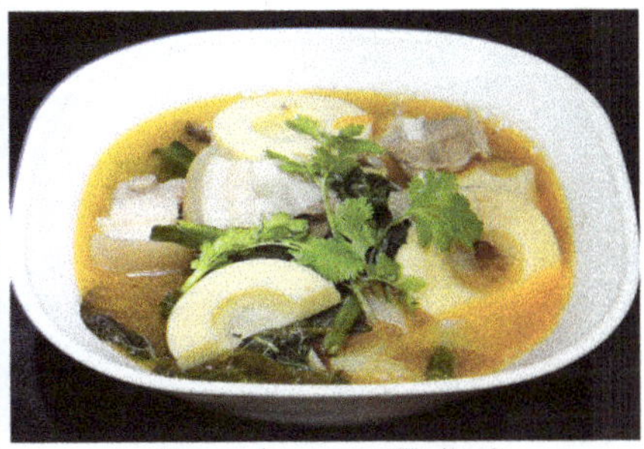

***Naw-mai-moo-nam*, Thailand**

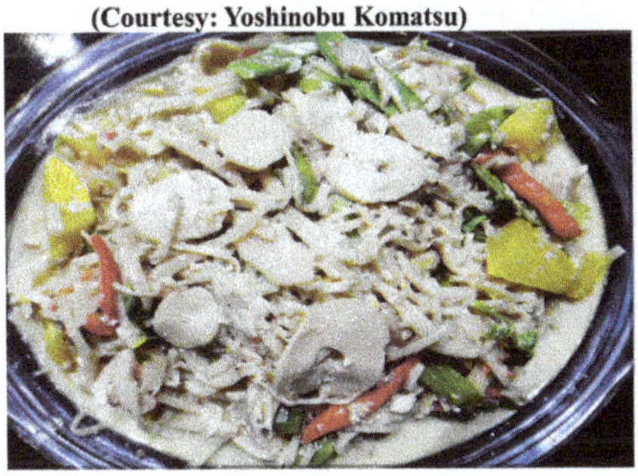

***Ginataang-labong*, Philippines**
(Courtesy: Merdelyn Cassi-Lit)

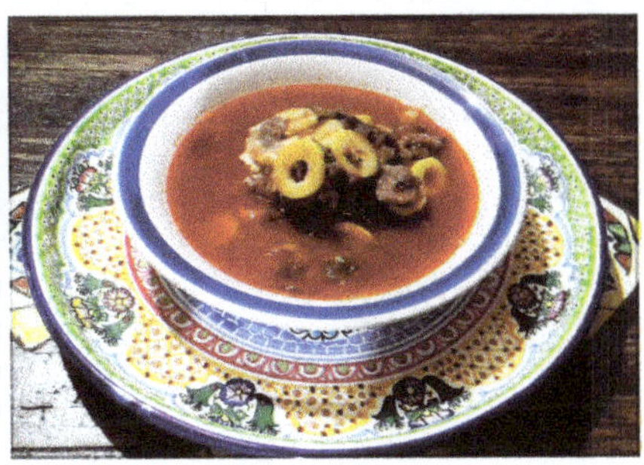

***Chilpozo*, Mexico**
(Courtesy: Mauricio Mora Tello)

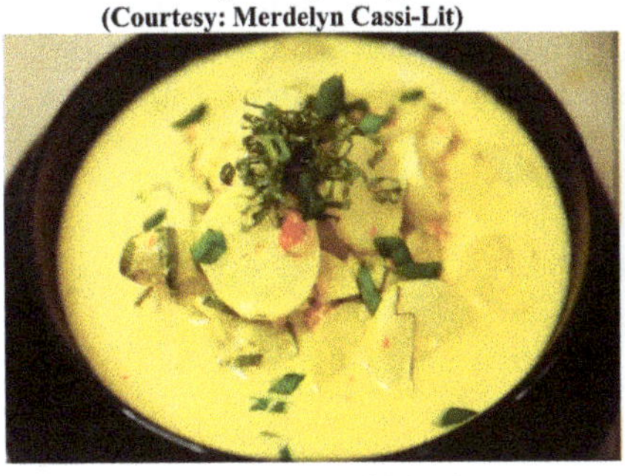

***Masak-lemak-rebung*, Malaysia**
(Courtesy: Avery Chua)

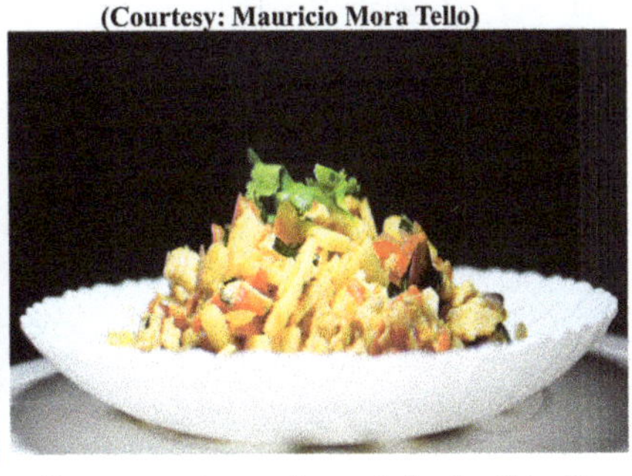

***Huevos-revueltos-con-brotes-de-bambu*, Colombia**
(Courtesy: Ximena Londono)

FIGURE 2.5 Bamboo shoot recipes from different countries.

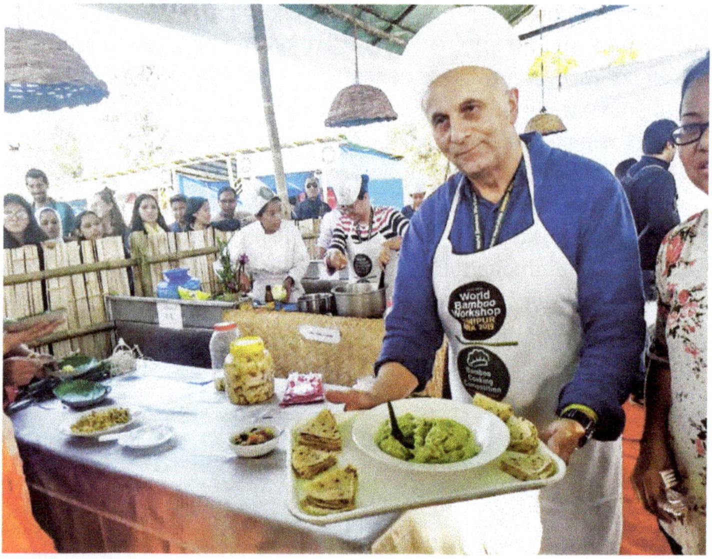

FIGURE 2.6 *President-greenboo*, a bamboo shoot recipe prepared by Michel Abadie (France), President, World Bamboo Organization during the World Bamboo Workshop 2019, Manipur, India.

TABLE 2.4

Bamboo Shoot Recipes of Some Countries

Country	Dish Name	Ingredients/Preparation
China	*Lumpia* (Chicken Bamboo shoot Spring Roll)	A savoury snack made of thin crepe pastry skin called 'lumpia wrapper' enveloping a mixture of savoury fillings consisting of chopped vegetables (carrots, cabbages, green beans, bamboo shoots and leeks) or minced meat (chicken, shrimp, pork or beef)
Japan	*Takenoko-kagamini*	Simmered bamboo shoots cooked in seaweed dashi (stock) and seasonings such as soy sauce, mirin, sake and sugar. When dried bonito flakes, or katsuobushi, is added, this dish is known as *Takenoko-no-tosani*
	Yaki-takenoko	Slices of fresh bamboo lightly marinated and grilled
	Takenoko-gohan	Slices of boiled bamboo shoot cooked with rice and soy sauce
Laos	*Kaeng-naw-mai* or *Soup-naw-mai*	A green stew made with bamboo shoots
	Khao-lam	A sweet sticky rice dish made with red beans, coconut, coconut milk and sugar prepared in bamboo

(Continued)

TABLE 2.4 (CONTINUED)
Bamboo Shoot Recipes of Some Countries

Country	Dish Name	Ingredients/Preparation
Thailand	*Kaeng-tai-pla*	A thick, spicy vegetable curry with turmeric, a sauce made from fish innards (*Tai-pla*) and shrimp paste, containing roasted fish, bamboo shoots and eggplant
	Yam-no-mai	A salad made with strips of boiled bamboo shoots, shallots, herbs, fish sauce, lime juice and chillies
	Soop-naw-mai	Shredded bamboo shoots boiled in wild Thai leaves with hot lime sauce
	Naw-mai-moo-nam	A soup made with bamboo shoot, pork and herbs
Vietnam	*Bún-măng-vịt*	Bamboo shoots and duck noodle soup
Indonesia	*Gulai-rebung*	Sliced thinly and boiled with coconut milk and spices
	Sayur-lodeh	Bamboo shoot and mixed vegetables in coconut milk
Nepal	*Tama*	Fermented bamboo shoots cooked with potato and black-eyed beans
Philippines	*Ginataang-labong*	Bamboo shoot (*Labong*) with coconut milk and chillies
	Dinengdeng-na-labong	Bamboo shoot (*Labong*) in fish bagoong with string beans, saluyot and tinapa
Myanmar	*Myahait-hkyain-hainn*	Bamboo shoots boiled in water after which they can be cooked with curry powder, rice powder and so on
Australia	Bamboo hummus	Traditional hummus recipes are made with chickpeas, but this modern version is based on bamboo. It still has that punch of garlic and lemon
Korea	*Sup-normai*	Spicy bamboo shoot salad
Mexico	*Chilpozo*	Bamboo shoots with pork and mushroom
	Aguachile	Bamboo shoots with shrimp, cucumber, lime juice and spices
	Chilahaute	Bamboo shoots mixed with a blend of sesame seeds beans, pepper, chayote and wrapped in corn husk and steamed
Malaysia	*Masak-lemak-rebung*	Grated ginger, garlic, red peppers, green chillies, shallots are boiled in water; lemon grass, ginger leaves and bamboo shoots are added, stirred until dry; coconut milk is added followed by salt and sugar
France	*President-greenboo*	Boiled bamboo shoots mixed with avocado, garlic, ginger and spices in a mixer grinder; add salt to taste and serve with naan, bread or tacos
	Bamboo shoot and mushroom	Boil sliced bamboo shoot and mushroom and fry in oil or butter; add already cooked white or black beans and salt to taste; garnish with garlic slices and parsley
Colombia	*Huevos-revueltos-con-brotes-de-bambu*	Diced bamboo shoots, tomato and onion mixed with eggs and sautéed in oil or butter

However, consumption of bamboo shoots in the traditional way is gradually declining and traditional cuisines are being replaced or modified due to the non-availability of traditional food items, change in taste or difficulty in processing. The diversification of food away from traditional products and in convergence with western style is responsible for changes in the whole food system. Factors such as income, food prices, individual preferences and beliefs, cultural traditions, as well as geographical, environmental, social and economic factors have all influenced changes in diet, both on an individual and on an international level. Attempts are being made to develop new food items from bamboo shoots that will be easily available throughout the year and cater to the taste buds of the present generation. The development of contemporary food items from bamboo shoots is described in Chapter 8.

2.3 BAMBOO AS MEDICINE

Bamboo plays a significant role in traditional Asian medicine and their therapeutic applications have been well described in all the ancient Pharmacopoeias of the world. The medicinal applications of bamboo were first mentioned around 10,000 BCE, when therapeutic applications of bamboo sap and stem shavings were described. All parts of the bamboo plant such as rhizomes, culms and bark shavings, resin, shoots, leaves and seeds have clinical applications. On the basis of the knowledge of their therapeutic applications, bamboo has been used for medicinal purposes and many beneficial effects of bamboo leaves, shoots, shaving and oils on metabolic disorders and cardiovascular diseases have been reported. In ancient Chinese medicine, leaves were used as a component to reduce the energy of 'fire' (related to inflammation) and treat hypertension, arteriosclerosis and cardiovascular disease (Yaun 1983). Bamboo is considered cooling, calming and phlegm resolving and is used for epilepsy, fainting and loss of consciousness in feverish diseases and a variety of mental disorders that develop with aging. Bamboo shoot decoction is used for treating infections, cleaning wounds, maggot infected sores and ulcers. In Java, sap from shoots is used for curing jaundice. Culm shaving of *Bambusa breviflora* is used to clear phlegm in the lungs. A decoction of fermented leaves was used to treat fevers (Yang 2002). Following traditional practices, there was continuous usage of bamboo in modernized Chinese medicine such as *Zhu Li Kou Fu Ye*, an extract of bamboo leaves inhibiting inflammation in the throat. The important biological and therapeutic properties of bamboo leaf extracts including anti-oxidant, anti-microbial, anti-inflammatory, anti-helmintic, anti-diabetic and anti-ulcer have been confirmed by several *in-vitro* and *in-vivo* experiments. According to Chinese medicinal books such as *Ben Chao Qui Zheng, Ben Jing Feng Yuan, Yao Pin Hua Yi and Jing Yue*, bamboo shoots are beneficial to human health notably by promoting the peristalsis of the stomach and the intestine, helping digestion, preventing and curing cardiovascular disease and cancer and promoting the excretion of urine (Lu et al. 2010). Bamboo medicinal applications were first mentioned in India around 10,000 years ago for preparing *Chyawanprash*, a health tonic prepared from a number of herbs, including bamboo-manna (*Tabasheer or banslochan*) to impart youth, beauty and longevity. *Chyawanprash* is named after Rishi, or a sage by the name of *Chyawan*, who was the first person to prepare this tonic and he regained his youthfulness and vitality with the use of this herbal tonic. It is now famous in the world for its anti-stress and anti-aging properties and there are several versions of the original *Chyawanprash* (Figure 2.7).

Ayurveda, the ancient Indian system of medicine recommends bamboo and its products such as *Banslochan* (*Tabasheer*) and *Sitopaladi-churna* for treatment of various ailments (Table 2.5). *Tabasheer* or *Banslochan* has been used since ancient times as a cooling tonic and aphrodisiac and in asthma, cough and other debilitating diseases. It is a siliceous secretion found in the culms of bamboos and occurs in fragments or masses, about an inch thick. *Tabasheer* may be chalky, translucent or transparent with a specific gravity ranging from 2.16 to 2.19. It has a colour of pumice and sometimes appears bluish white with no taste. It is mainly composed of silicic acid (up to 96.9%) with above 1% of organic matter. The residue obtained on ignition contains 99% silica with traces of iron, calcium, alum and alkalies. A bamboo-derived Ayurvedic remedy, *Sitopaladi-churna* is prescribed for pleurodynia, intercostal neuralgia, cold cough associated with bronchitis, pneumonia, tuberculosis, viral respiratory infection, digestive impairment and pharyngeal or chest congestion. In Tibet, it is used for the treatment of various lung diseases. It is a powder made with tabasheer as the main ingredient, plus small amounts of long pepper, cardamom and cinnamon in a base of sugar. In ancient literature of India (*Bhavprakash Nighantu*), it is written that "Bamboo by nature is laxative, frigid seminal curative, palatable, bladder purifier and full of astringent juice. It splits cough, subsides bile and cures leprosy, flux, wounds and

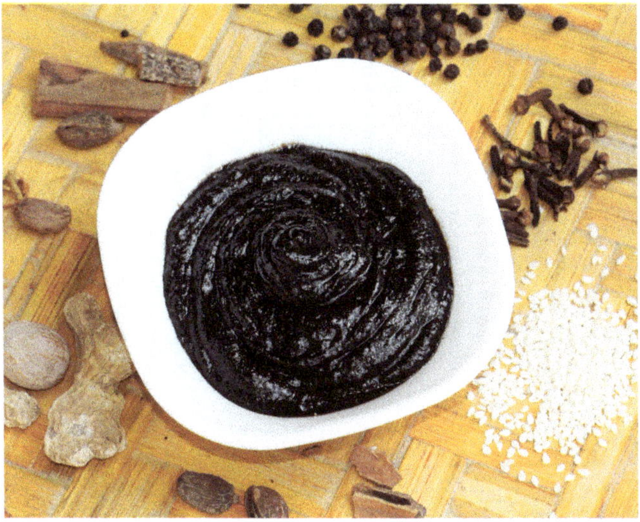

FIGURE 2.7 *Chyawanprash*, a health tonic with banslochan from bamboo as one of the ingredients.

TABLE 2.5
Bamboo in Traditional Medicinal Systems

Name	Constituents/Ingredients	Health Benefits
	Bamboo in Ayurveda, Tibetan and Unani Traditional Medicines	
Tabasheer	Siliceous secretion often called bamboo-manna or bamboo silica found in the hollow internodes of various species of bamboos. *Tabasheer* may be chalky, translucent, or transparent, mainly composed of silicic acid (up to 96.9%) with above 1% of organic matter.	Acts as a stimulant, astringent, febrifuge, relieving asthma, cough, cooling tonic, anti-spasmodic and aphrodisiac.
Sitopaladi-churna	Powder made with *Tabasheer* as the main ingredient, plus small amounts of long pepper, cardamom and cinnamon in a base of sugar.	A popular remedy for the common cold, sore throat, sinus congestion, tuberculosis, coughs and other lung diseases.
	Bamboo in Chinese Traditional Medicine	
Chenjin-wan	Bamboo shaving and *Tabasheer*, arisaema, citrus, hoelen, salvia, silkworm, chrysanthemum, apricot seed, ophiopogon, biota, fritillaria, ginger.	For phlegm mist obstructing the orifices yielding symptoms of insomnia, restlessness and blurred vision.
Gualou-zhishi-tang	Bamboo shaving and sap, fritillaria, platycodon, trichosanthes seed, chih-shih, citrus, saussurea, licorice, scute, gardenia and so on.	For reducing thick phlegm that is difficult to expectorate.
Jupi-zhuru-tang	Bamboo shavings, citrus, pinellia, licorice, hoelen.	Relieving phlegm.
Qinghuo-ditan-tang	Bamboo shaving and tabasheer, arisaema, citrus, hoelen, salvia, silkworm, chrysanthemum, apricot seed, ophiopogon, biota, fritillaria, ginger.	For phlegm mist obstructing the orifices yielding symptoms of insomnia, restlessness and blurred vision.
Qinggong-tang	Bamboo leaf, ophiopogon, scrophularia, rhino horn, forsythia, lotus plumule.	Fever with dryness, penetrating to the pericardium, with delirium.
Qingluo-yin	Bamboo leaf, lotus leaf, luffa, mirabilitum, dolichos flower, lonicera.	Fever with light-headedness, blurry vision, or headache.
Xiaoer-qizhen-dan	Tabasheer, arisaema, cinnabar, realgar, scorpion, croton seed.	For phlegm, wheezing, coughing.
Zhuye-shigao-tang	Bamboo leaf, gypsum, pinellia, ophiopogon, ginseng, licorice, oryza.	Fever with dryness, irritability and insomnia.

swellings" (Tewari 1992). In Chinese traditional medicine, bamboo is generally considered cooling, calming and phlegm resolving and is incorporated in many traditional formulas to treat lung and stomach heat, febrile disease and correct up flowing *Qi* (a fundamental concept in traditional Chinese medicine referring to the energy flow in a living being). Leaves are the part of the plant which is triggering the most intensive interest possible because the leaves comprise a significant portion of the total biomass of the plant, are easy to harvest and process and can be obtained as a waste of bamboo timber industry. Now it has been observed that leaves, which are generally discarded, are the best source of a number of antioxidants and bioactive compounds.

2.3.1 Traditional Knowledge and Practices

Various traditional practices and approaches using bamboo shoot as a base plant for medication still prevail in different communities. Fermented bamboo shoot if mixed with crushed leaves of *Allium porrum* Linn and chilli is also used to cure influenza. The paste made can also be applied to treat fungal infection (Changkija 1999). The decoction of tender shoots of *Bambusa nutans* is applied to wounds and poisonous bites. The shoots are also boiled in water and the soup is taken in cases of stomach ulcers. Tender shoots of *Bambusa tulda* are boiled in water and the soup is taken in cases of poxes and other skin diseases and the paste is applied on poisonous bites and injuries. Young bamboo sprouts and leaves are used as a blood purifier and for the treatment of leprosy. *Kani* tribe of Kanyakumari district from Tamil Nadu consumes seeds of bamboo (mostly from *Bambusa arundinacea*) with a belief that it enhances their fertility and reproductive ability (Kiruba et al. 2007). *Kandha* tribe of Kalahandi district, Odisha uses fermented shoots of *Dendrocalamus strictus* to cure constipation (Panda and Padhy 2007). The juice of *D. strictus* has been reported to be used as an anti-inflammatory agent near joints, as astringent and eardrops and in cooling and healing of cuts (Ramakrishnappa 2002). Valkosen (2001) reported that bamboo shoots mixed with garlic cloves are effective in the treatment of pigs against *Ascaris suum*. The sap of bamboo shoots has been found to contain hydrocyanic acid lending to anti-septic and larvicidal properties. Many female Burmese migrant workers have been reported to use bamboo shoots or sticks with traditional Chinese medicine to penetrate their genital areas to abort the foetus (Ruenkaew 2009). A heavy dose of pepper with bamboo shoots or decoctions of tender shoots with palm jaggery was used to bring about abortions (Chaveerach et al. 2006). Boiled bamboo shoot or pickle is served as an appetizer. Bamboo shoots are used to ease labour and the expulsion of the placenta by inducing uterine contractions. A poultice of the shoots is often used for cleaning wounds and healing infections (Panee 2015). Bamboo shoot decoction taken along with honey is used to treat respiratory disorders. A high level of acetylcholine, an important neurotransmitter in the cholinergic nervous system of vertebrates and insects, has been detected in the upper portion of bamboo shoots (Horiuchi et al. 2003). In Indonesia, bamboo sprouts are used in a pharmaceutical preparation to treat abdominal pain and jaundice, whereas a decoction of bamboo sprouts along with coconut palm tree is used to treat insomnia (Elliott and Brimacombe 1987).

The use of bamboo as medicine by local communities of East Africa has also been well documented (Ogunjinmi et al. 2009). Using the traditional knowledge, pharmaceutical preparations of bamboo-like bamboo salt, bamboo vinegar, bamboo extracts and bamboo silica and so on for the treatment of various health-related problems are now gaining importance.

2.3.2 Scientific Documentations about Health Benefits of Bamboo

Supporting traditional practices, modern research has scientifically validated most of the health claims of bamboos and it is still attracting a great deal of interest from researchers to unearth even more potential health benefits (Gong et al. 2016, Chongtham and Bisht 2017, Ying et al. 2017, Bajwa et al. 2018, 2019a). Biomedical investigations on health beneficial effects of different parts and species of bamboo have been carried out since 1960s and a wide range of protective effects of bamboo-derived products have been documented such as protection against oxidative stress, inflammation, lipotoxicity, cancer and cardiovascular disease. The earliest scientific documentation of potential medicinal use of bamboo was published in the early 1960s (Sakai et al. 1963). Several *in-vitro* and *in-vivo* experiments on animals have confirmed important biological and medicinal properties of bamboo extracts such as anti-oxidant, anti-cancer, anti-microbial, anti-inflammatory, anti-ulcer, anti-helminthic and anti-diabetic (Muniappan and Sundararaj 2003, Lu et al. 2005, Wang et al. 2012) which are discussed next.

2.3.2.1 Anti-Cancer Properties

Cancer is a major cause of disease mainly in developed countries associated with aging of population and lifestyle. A cure for advanced cancer remains a long way off and it is now recognized that cancer prevention is very important and the search for anti-cancer agents from plants has attracted great interest. Different parts of bamboo, mainly leaves and shoots are known to have anti-cancer properties. Hiromichi (2007) isolated an anti-tumour agent from bamboo shoots of *Phyllostachys bambusoides* that was highly effective for the treatment of malignant tumours. An alcoholic extract was administered to cancer-induced Balb/c mice. Tumour growth was suppressed without impairing body growth demonstrating excellent anti-tumour growth.

Akao et al. (2004) isolated a highly bioactive lignophenol derivative lig-8 that exhibits potent activity to suppress apoptosis induced by oxidative stress in human neuroblastoma SH-SY5Y cells. Apoptosis is an active, energy-dependent process through which living cells initiate their own death. Clinical evidence show that disturbed apoptosis cell death is associated with certain diseases such as cancers and immune-insufficiencies. Apoptosis is also considered to be the major death mode of neurons in a neurodegenerative disorder such as Parkinson disease, Alzheimer disease and Huntington disease. Lig-8 protects human neuroblastoma cells (SH-SY5Y) from hydrogen peroxide-induced apoptosis by preventing caspase-3 activation via either caspase-8 or caspase -9. Thus lig-8 is a promising neuroprotector that affects the signalling pathway of neuronal cell death and could delay the progress of neurodegenerative diseases.

Anti-cancer effects of bamboo salt were studied on Human Cancer Cells and on Buccal Mucosa Cancer in mice by Park et al. (2013). In-vitro anti-cancer effects were investigated using MTT assay in HepG2 human hepatoma cells, AGS human gastric adenocarcinoma cells and TCA8113 human tongue carcinoma cells. The growth inhibitory rate of bamboo salt (9X baked) determined by MTT assay was up to 65% compared to sea salt which showed a lower inhibitory effect ranging from 20% to 29%. Bamboo salt significantly ($p < 0.05$) induced apoptosis, up-regulated expression of Bax and down-regulated Bcl-2 expression. The bamboo salt also significantly down-regulated inflammation-related genes of iNOS and COX-2. The ICR mice buccal mucosa cancer model was established by injecting the mice with U14 cells. Following the injection, the wound at the injection site was smeared with salt samples. It was observed that the tumour volumes for the group treated with bamboo salt were smaller than those from the other samples. The buccal mucosa tissues of bamboo salt group mice showed an increase in Bax and a decrease in Bcl-2, iNOS and COX-2 expressions by RT-PCR and Western blot compared with the other treated samples.

Sasa sinensis popularly known as Kumaizasa bamboo is used in traditional medicine in Japan. The leaf extract of this bamboo obtained under vigorous steam conditions at high temperature and high-pressure show immune-potentiating and radical scavenging effects and administration prior to carcinogen exposure or tumour inoculation significantly suppresses tumour incidence and tumour growth and prolongs survival (Seki and Maeda 2010). The extracts obtained by this method (vigorous extract) contained a larger quantity of β-glucan (150-fold) and phenolics (2.5-fold) compared to the conventional hot-water extract. Furthermore, the vigorous extract also exhibited more potent anti-tumour activity against mouse sarcoma S-180 than the conventional hot-water extract when given orally at 0.1%w/w in the diet. In conclusion, dietary supplements of the vigorous extract suppress, in a dose-dependent manner, the carcinogenesis and growth of DMBA-induced breast cancer. These results strongly suggest the potential of this vigorous bamboo leaf extract as a tumour suppressive and cancer preventive food supplement.

Advancements in metal nanoparticle synthesis using plant extracts and their anti-cancer activity have received significant attention in recent years. The metallic silver nanoparticles of *in-vitro* grown leaf samples of *B. arundinacea* and *B. nutans* showed anti-tumour activities against human prostate cancer lines and normal cell lines (Kalaiarasi et al. 2015). Leaves of Kumaizasa bamboo extracted in hot water at 100, 121 and 196°C significantly increases the immune-stimulating activity which induces activation of NK cells, macrophages and induces IL-2, IL-12 and IFN-γ in tumour-bearing mice. Activation of these cells suggests the anti-tumour efficacy that is mediated by immunoprotiation (Seki et al. 2010). The green approach for the synthesis of gold nanoparticles (AuNPs) using leaf extract of *Sasa borealis* was reported by Patil et al. (2017). The synthesized AuNPs were tested for toxic effect on HEK293 cells and anti-cancer activity on human gastric adenocarcinoma cell line (AGS cells) by WST-1® assay and was confirmed by 4,6-diamidino-2-pheynylindole dihydrochoride (DAPI) staining. The *S. borealis*-mediated AuNPs have good activity as an anti-cancer agent and it will be beneficial in cancer therapeutics.

hypertension (high blood pressure) and hyperlipidemia (high levels of fats in the blood that can lead to narrowing or blockages of blood vessels). These are major risk factors for cardiovascular disease and cardiovascular related mortality. Obesity is also associated with cancer, disability and a reduced quality of life, and can lead to premature death. The causes include an increased intake of energy-dense foods and a decrease in physical inactivity due to the sedentary nature of work and changes in modes of transport (Eti et al. 2016).

Yang et al. (2010) studied the effect of *Sasa borealis* leaf extract on inflammatory cytokines and insulin resistance in high-fat diet-induced obese mice. After 12 weeks, mice administered with 5% of leaf extract showed decreased body weight and adipose tissue deposition compared to untreated mice. The decrease in glucose, insulin, IAUC, HOMA-IR, TNF-α, IL-6 and leptin levels was also noted. These results proved that *S. borealis* leaf extracts contained anti-obesity compounds. An anti-obesity effect of leaf extracts of *Sasa veitchii* and *S. quelpaertensis* were investigated on high-fat diet-induced obese mice by Kang et al. (2012) and Yoshioka et al. (2017b). *S. quelpaertensis* leaf extract (SQE) was administered for 70 days that not only decreased the body weight, adipose tissue weight, serum cholesterol and triglycerides but also reduced serum levels of several enzymes along with deposition of lipid droplets in the liver when compared to untreated mice. It was concluded that the anti-obesity effect of SQE is mediated by the activation of AMPK in adipose tissue.

Anti-obesity effects of bamboo salt have been evaluated compared with purified salt and solar salt by oral administration in a diet-induced obesity model using C57BL/b mice (Park et al. 2014). Compared to other salts, bamboo salt significantly reduced body weight, food efficiency ratio and weights of epididymal adipose tissue and liver in high-fat-diet-fed mice. Furthermore, expression of adipogenic factors was suppressed thereby suggesting that bamboo salt may suppress obesity by downregulating adipogenesis. Ju et al. (2015) evaluated anti-obesity effects of bamboo salt by oral administration in a diet-induced obesity model using B57BL/6 mice Compared with other salts, BS-9x significantly reduced body weight, food efficiency ratio and weight of epididymal adipose tissue and liver in high-fat diet fed mice. Hence, the administration of BS prevented obesity by suppressing adipogenesis.

Liu et al. (2016) examined the methanolic extract of *B. textilis* and observed antioxidant and anti-obesity effects in-vivo when tested in a high fat diet rat model. The leaf extract was found to significantly decrease the levels of TC, TG and LDL-C in the serum and effectively increase serum HDL-C concentration. It also revealed that the leaf extract increases the activity of SOD and GSH-Px and decreased the level of Thiobarbituric Acid Reactive Substances (TBARS) in the high-fat-diet-fed rat model thereby preventing cells from free radical disturbances by scavenging ROS. The experiment clearly indicated that the anti-obesity effect is closely related to the influence of the cholesterol level and the reduction of oxidative stress. Kim et al. (2007b) also reported anti-obesity activity of *Sasa borealis*.

Li et al. (2016) have reported that bamboo shoot fibre prevents obesity in mice by modulating gut microbiota. They performed a six-week study on C57BL/6J mice fed on high-fat diet with different fibre types including cellulose (HFC), bamboo shoot fibre (HFBS) and several other commonly consumed fibres. Results showed that the HFBS group exhibited the lowest weight gain among all diet groups and had improved lipid profiles and glycemic control compared with the HFC group. As revealed by 16S rRNA gene sequencing, loss of diversity in the gut microbiota induced by the HFC diet was largely prevented by the HFBS diet. Moreover, compared with the HFC diet, the HFBS diet resulted in markedly increased relative abundance of Bacteroidetes and strong inhibition of Verrucomicrobia, two divisions strongly correlated with body weight. This study provides evidence of a quality difference among different types of dietary fibres and shows that bamboo shoot fibre is the most effective in suppressing high-fat diet-induced obesity, thus indicating that bamboo shoot fibre is a potential prebiotic fibre which modulates the gut microbiota and improves host metabolism.

The anti-obesity effects of several different combinations of extracts prepared from bamboos, *Phyllostachys pubescens* leaf (BL) and *Scutellaria baicalensis* root (SB), were investigated using a high-fat diet-induced obese mouse model. Body weight, weight of adipose tissues, size of adipocytes, levels of glucose, leptin and adiponectin and lipid profile in serum and fat accumulation in liver were investigated (Kim et al. 2016). It was found that a mixture comprising of two parts BL and one-part SB is the most effective in anti-obesity as indicated by reduction in body weight gain, total mass of adipose tissue and the size of adipocyte. Chromatographic separation of the mixture revealed the presence of two compounds, iso-orientin and baicalin. Anti-obesity activity of bamboo shaving polysaccharides (BSP) was investigated against high diet-induced obese mice (Chen et al. 2018). It was evidenced that BSP modulates the gut microbiota and hence could be used as a potential prebiotic or functional food against obesity, insulin resistance and chronic inflammation in obese individuals.

Goh et al. (2019) induced mouse 3T3-L1 cell with a mixture of dexamethasone, 3-isobutyl-1-methylxanthine and insulin to the cell media. The cells were then treated with different extracts of bamboo culm (hot water, ethanol, methanol) for 4 to 13 days. Ethanolic and methanolic extracts treated samples elevate the expression of genes involved in adipogenesis size of adipocytes and adipocyte triglyceride contents indicating that bamboo extract helps in preventing obesity.

2.3.2.5 Anti-Microbial Activity

Anti-microbial substances are widely used in food, pharmaceutical and cosmetic industries. In cosmetics, preservatives protect the formulation during the production and the use by the consumers. Food is easily affected by micro-organisms like bacteria, yeast moulds during processing and preservation and can lead to spoilage and human disease. In the food industry, these additives can improve organoleptic characteristics of food, such as colour, smell and taste, in addition to the protection of food during production, storage and consumption. The growing microbial resistance to existing drugs has generated the need for the pharmaceutical industry to search for new molecules that can be used as preservatives, antibiotics and disinfectants. This factor associated with the toxicity of certain additives and the consumer appeals for the reduction in synthetic substances, encourage the search for alternative solutions. Bamboo can be one of the alternative sources due to the presence of compounds such as polyphenols, carotenoids, flavonoids, terpenoids, alkaloids, tannins, saponins and minerals that have anti-microbial and anti-oxidant activity. The tribal people of Tamil Nadu, India, have long used the young shoot and seeds of *B. arundinacea* as food and to treat several diseases (Thamizharasan et al. 2015). Leaves, roots, shoots and seeds are known to possess, anti-inflammatory, anti-diabetic, anti-ulcer, anti-oxidant and astringent activity. The seed is acrid, laxative and believed to be beneficial in strangury and urinary discharge (Soni et al. 2013, Rathod et al. 2011). Anti-bacterial and antifungal efficiency of *Bambusa arundinacea* seed extracts were examined using hexane, acetone and hydroethanol as solvents and tested against human pathogens such as *Enterococcus faecalis, Staphylococcus epidermidis* and *Pseudomonas aeruginosa* using disc diffusion method. Hexane and acetone extracts showed significant activity against all micro-organisms and could thus be a possible source to obtain new and effective compounds to treat bacterial and fungal infections.

Improvement in the shelf life of the product can have an important economic impact by reducing losses to spoilage and by allowing the products to reach distant markets. It is well known that bamboo extracts have multiple biological activities among which a prominent one is anti-bacterial activity (Lu et al. 2006, Zhang et al. 2010). The anti-bacterial activity of bamboo was known since ancient times from the fact the culm sheaths or bamboo shoot skin has been traditionally used for packaging food. It is used as a preservative container to maintain the taste of tea in China and as packaging material for rice balls and meat in Japan (Tanaka et al. 2013). Bamboo has been utilized as a wrapping material for foods such as meat, sushi and candy (Nishina et al. 1991). An anti-bacterial compound 2, 6-Dimethoxy-p-benzoquinone which can be used as an anti-bacterial agent in food, medicine, cosmetics and so on was isolated from the bark of *Phyllostachys heterocycla* var. *pubescens* and identified by HPLC.

Fujimura et al. (2005) isolated two novel anti-microbial peptides designated Pp-AMP1 and Pp-AMP2 from shoots of *Phyllostachys pubescens* which had anti-microbial activity against pathogenic bacteria and fungi using chitin affinity chromatography. Anti-microbial activity was assayed for the following bacteria and fungi *Erwinia carotovora, Agrobacterium radiobacter, A. rhizogenes, Clavibacter michiganensis, Curtobacterium flaccumfaciens, Fusarium oxysporum* and *Geotrichum candidum.* Yasin et al. (2013) synthesized silver nanoparticles using bamboo leaves which offer an improvement over synthetic or chemical methods as it is cost-effective and environmental friendly. Anti-bacterial silver nanoparticles were synthesized using bamboo leaves of *Phyllostachys aurea* and were tested by disc diffusion method on *E. coli* and *Staphylococcus aureus.* AgNPs synthesized from bamboo leaves exhibited great anti-microbial activities against the bacterial cultures.

Anti-microbial activities of different extracts (aqueous, acetone, ethanol, methanol, petroleum ether and n-hexane) from leaves of *Bambusa bambos, B. vulgaris, B. arundinacea* and *Dendrocalamus asper* against Gram-positive and Gram-negative bacteria including *E. coli, Acinetobacter* spp., *Streptococcus* spp., *Enterococcus* spp., *Citrobacter* spp., *Klebsiella* spp., *Lactobacillus* spp., *Pseudomonas aeruginosa* and *Staphylococcus aureus* was evaluated using well and disc diffusion method (Owokotomo and Owoeye 2011, Mulyono et al. 2012, Sandhiya et al. 2013, Wasnik and Tumane 2014, Kalita et al. 2010). Results revealed that the extracts were very effective compared to the standard antibiotics. Owokotomo and Owoeye (2011) fortified orange and pineapple juices with aqueous leaf extract of *Bambusa vulgaris.* Anti-microbial screening showed that the bamboo's leaf extract was active against *Lactobacillus* spp. Fortification of orange and pineapple juices with the bamboo leaf extract enhanced the inhibitory effect against *E. coli* and *Lactobacillus* spp. Bamboo leaf has also been reported as a potent natural source to manage rice blast disease as the leaves of *Phyllostachys pubescens* inhibit mycelial growth of rice blast fungus *Pyricularia grisea* (Toan et al. 2018). Several active compounds such as flavones, glycosides, phenolic acids, coumarin lactones, anthraquinones and 2, 6-dimethyoxy-p-benzoquinone have been isolated from bamboo leaves and shoots. Tanaka et al. (2013) have reported that the dichloromethane extract from bamboo shoot skin of *Phyllostachys pubescens* inhibits the growth of *Staphylococcus aureus* and *Escherichia coli.* The active constituents were identified as stigmasterol and dihydro-brassica-sterol by NMR and mass spectrometry establishing the large possibility that bamboo shoot skins which are discarded during processing of the shoots can serve as a raw ingredient for producing anti-bacterial compounds. Water phase extract of bamboo shavings (WEBS) by super critical carbon dioxide extraction was evaluated for its anti-microbial action against a wide range of food borne and food spoilage pathogens (Zhang et al. 2010). The WEBS exhibited anti-microbial activity against *Staphylococcus aureus*, *Bacillus subtilis*, *Escherichia coli*, *Aspergillus niger*, *Penicillium citrinum* and *Saccharomyces cerevisiae* indicating that WEBS may be useful in controlling food borne and food spoilage pathogens and serve as natural food preserver. Jankowsky et al. (2018) worked out the anti-bacterial potential of various solvent leaf extracts (aqueous, ethanolic, methanolic, hexane and acetone) of *Bambusa arundinacea*, *B. balcooa*, *B. bambos*, *B. vulgaris*, *D. asper* and *D. hamiltonii* against bacterial strains of *Bacillus subtilis*, *Escherichia coli*, *Enterococcus faecalis*, *Enterobacter aerogenes Staphylococcus aureus*, *Klebsiella pneumoniae*, *Lactobacillus* spp., *Staphylococcus epidermidis* and *Pseudomonas aeruginosa.* They reported that the leaf extract was particularly effective against most bacterial pathogens and thus can be used as a natural source of anti-microbial agents in the development of new drugs.

Tao et al. (2018) analyzed the anti-microbial activity of three major components of essential oils—tricosane, cedrol and hexadecanoic acid from leaf extracts of *Phyllostachys heterocycla* cv *pubescens* against common food related micro-organisms *Bacillus subtilis*, *Escherichia coli*, *Pseudomonas fluorescens*, *Saccharomyces cerevisiae* and *Flavobacterium* spp. Results showed that the extracts had the highest bacteriostatic effect of *Flavobacterium* followed by *P. fluorescens.* Using the data from cellular constituents, fatty acid profiles and atomic force microscope observations, authors concluded that the anti-microbial components of bamboo leaf essential oils act by disrupting the membrane integrity of the microbes thus inhibiting their growth (Tao et al. 2019). Anti-fungal potential of leaf extracts from *Bambusa vulgaris* and *Dendrocalamus strictus* against the strains of *Aspergillus fumigatus*, *A. niger*, *Candida albicans*, *C. glabrata* and *C. tropicalis*, *Trichoderma viride* and *Verticillium albo-atrum* have been studied by Owolabi and Lajide (2015), Patil and Rothe (2016) and Ambika and Rajagopal (2017).

2.3.2.6 Anti-Inflammatory Effect

Inflammation is a pathophysiological response of living tissue to injuries that leads to the local accumulation of plasmatic fluids and blood cells. Although it is a defence mechanism, the complex events and mediators involved in the inflammatory reaction can induce, maintain, or aggravate many diseases. Bamboo has been used in Indian folk medicine to treat various inflammatory conditions. Muniappan and Sundararaj (2003) validated that the anti-inflammatory effect of the methanol extract of the leaves of *Bambusa arundinacea* against carrageenin-induced as well as immunologically induced paw oedema and also its anti-ulcer activity in albino rats when compared to the standard drugs. They also proved that combination of methanol extract and phenylbutazone (Non-Steroidal Anti-inflammatory Agent, NSAIA) was more effective than when they were used individually. They concluded that the combination of methanol extract of *Bambusa arundinacea* with modern medicine (NSAIAs) can result in a very potent anti-inflammatory drug.

Anti-inflammatory and wound healing effects of leaves of *B. vulgaris*, *Sasa quelpaertensis* and *P.edulis* have been evaluated (Shin et al. 2003, Hwang et al. 2007, Wedler et al. 2014, Kim et al 2015). Hwang et al. (2007) provided scientific evidence to the traditional use of *Sasa quelpaertensis* leaves for the treatment of inflammation-related diseases and revealed that hot-water extract of *S. quelpaertensis* could ameliorate inflammation-related diseases by suppressing nitric oxide production in pathological event. Carey et al. (2009) have shown that methanolic extract of *Bambusa vulgaris* possesses anti-inflammatory activity against various anti-inflammatory tests that include formaldehyde-induced paw edema, acetic acid–induced vascular permeability, cotton pellet-induced granuloma and carrageenan-induced peritonitis in albino rats.

Anti-inflammatory and anti-adipogenic effects of methanol extract and ethyl acetate fraction of *Sasa coreana* Nakai leaf was reported by Yang et al. (2017). Several flavonoids were identified including orientin, isoorientin and vitexin which inhibited liposaccharide induced nitric oxide production in macrophages indicating that *Sasa coreana* leaves is a potential therapeutic agent for the prevention of inflammation and obesity.

2.3.2.7 Cardioprotective Properties

Cardiovascular disease (CVD) is one of the main causes of death worldwide. Hypertension is a leading cause of cardiovascular diseases such as arteriosclerosis, stroke and myocardial infection which is the world's leading cause of death each year. The incidence of cardiovascular disease is positively correlated with blood lipid concentration and the association between an increased risk of cardiovascular mortality and increased concentrations of triacylglycerols, total cholesterols and low-density lipoprotein (LDL) and low concentrations of high-density lipoprotein (HDL) has been demonstrated in several studies. In addition, cardiovascular risk has been related to specific serum enzymes such as glutamic oxaloacetic transaminase (GOT) and glutamic pyruvic transaminase (GPT) for causes of death worldwide.

In recent years, there has been considerable interest in the potential for using natural food components as functional food to treat hypertension especially with patients with borderline to mild high blood pressure that does not warrant the prescription of anti-hypersensitive drugs. Bamboo shoot has been regarded as a kind of ideal vegetable and medicinal material for the prevention of hypertension. Angiotensin converting enzyme (ACE) is an important factor in the pathogenesis of hypertension as it is involved in different blood pressure regulating mechanisms. Liu et al. (2012) evaluated cardiovascular protective functions of bamboo shoot by evaluating the inhibitory peptide (BSP) from bamboo shoot on angiotensin converting enzyme (ACE) including anti-hypertensive effect on spontaneously hypersensitive rats (SHRS) and anti-hyperlipidemic effect on high-fat-induced rats. BSP decreased total cholesterol (TC), triglyceride (TG) and low-density lipoprotein cholesterol (LDL-C) content and malondialdehyde (MDA) level of hyperlipidemic rats, which might contribute to the ACE inhibitory capacity of Asparagine-Tyrosine and the fatty acid synthase inhibitory activity of phenolic compounds (Liu et al 2012). Aqueous extract fractions from by-products of the processing of canned bamboo shoots showed both anti-hypertensive and anti-oxidant activity. Asp-Tyr was isolated and identified as the key active component in bamboo shoot ACE inhibitory peptide (Liu et al. 2013). These findings suggest that BSP exerting both ACE inhibitory and anti-oxidant activity could be a good source of multifunctional food for the prevention of hypertension and attenuation of oxidative stress.

Prevention of cardiovascular diseases has also focused on LDL cholesterol-lowering therapies to recommended levels. Dietary fibres are demonstrated to have beneficial effects in lowering serum cholesterol and the prevention of cardiovascular diseases. Bamboo shoots contain large quantities of dietary fibres consisting of approximately 8% soluble fibre and 92% insoluble fibre. Most dietary fibre in bamboo shoots consists of hemicellulose, cellulose, pectin and lignin. Park and Jhon (2009) studied the effects of bamboo shoot consumption as a dietary fibre source on blood glucose, lipid profiles, hepatic function and constipation symptoms in healthy women receiving a bamboo shoot diet for six days. At the end of each diet, blood biochemical parameters such as glucose, triglycerol, total cholesterol, LDL, HDL, GOT, GPT and atherogenic index were measured. At the end of six days, bamboo shoot diet, total cholesterol and LDL cholesterol decreased by 9.6% and 15.3%, respectively, compared with the control diet but HDL cholesterol levels were not affected. It has been proposed that dietary fibre decreases the serum triacylglycerol by preventing the direct absorption of lipids. Serum-total cholesterol LDL and the atherogenic index were decreased with the bamboo shoot feeding diet compared with the dietary fibre-free diet. Faecal volume and bowel movement frequency in subjects fed with bamboo shoot diet were significantly increased. It is well known that a major role of dietary fibre is to provide a substrate for fermentation of intestinal bacteria. Intestinal micro-organisms comprise up to 50% faecal solids and increased fibre intake generally promotes bacterial proliferation. Results of our study are also in agreement with these outcomes as when Balb/c mice were administered with aqueous extract of fresh shoots of *D. hamiltonii*, a significant decrease was observed in the level of total cholesterol (TC) and low-density lipoprotein (LDL) and, increase in the level of high-density lipoproteins (HDL) when compared with the control group. It has been reported that cholesterol-lowering effects of bamboo shoots have been attributed to inhibition of cholesterol absorption and increase of cholesterol excretion (Lu et al. 2010). Wang et al. (2019) studied the hypolipidemic effect of bamboo shoot soluble fibre obtained by chemical methods in high-fat diet-induced hyperlipidemic mice model. It was observed that the mice had reduced body weight, lowered TC, LDL and increased HDL levels which improved the lipid metabolism of hyperlipidemic mice. Hence, consuming high fibre bamboo shoot may help to prevent CVD.

Lu et al. (2010) investigated the hypolipidemic effect of bamboo shoot oil (BSO) in Sprague-Dawley rats in order to provide insights on how to prevent and cure atherosclerosis. Bamboo shoot oil (BSO) is a novel kind of vegetable oil extracted by supercritical carbon dioxide from bamboo shoots. Hypercholesterolemia was induced in rats by feeding them with high-fat, high-cholesterol diet for six weeks. On administering BSO, a significant decrease was observed in the levels of total cholesterols triglycerol, low-density lipoprotein cholesterol, lipoprotein lipase hepatic lipase and atherogenic index in serum and relative liver weight. It also increases the levels of faecal cholesterol and plasma phytosterol. There was no adverse effect of BSO on the growth and health condition of the rats. The pronounced hypolipidemic effects of BSO might be contributed to its ability to inhibit cholesterol absorption and increase cholesterol excretion. This suggests that consuming BSO may help to manage hypercholesterolemia and could be a useful dietary supplement in lowering cholesterol levels. Cardioprotective activity of *B. blumeana* leaf crude extract was studied by Rosales et al. (2013) on Sprague-Dawley rats against isoproterenol induced myocardial infection. The mice were pre-treated with different doses of leaf extract orally and then myocardial infection was induced by injecting isopropanol intraperitoneally. Investigation of cardioprotective activity showed dose-dependent effect on serum aminotransferase, LDH, creatine kinase. Histopathological studies also revealed damage in bamboo extract treated animals.

2.3.2.8 Hepatoprotective Activity

Liver is one of the most important and complex organs in the human body whose primary function is to filter and detoxify the blood and xenobiotics coming from the digestive tract before it is distributed to the rest of the body. Liver diseases are the main cause of mortality and morbidity worldwide and its damage typically results in leakage of aspartate aminotransferase (AST), alanine aminotransferase (ALT) into the bloodstream. Herbal medicines or plant-derived medicines are used for its treatment for a long time. Hoywegan et al. (2014) explored the hepatoprotective activity of ethanolic leaf extract of *Phyllostachys nigra* in PCM-induced rats and reported a significant reduction in the TBARS level generated during oxidative stress and bilirubin level in serum. This hepatoprotective activity is via decreasing inducible nitric oxide synthase expression through the inhibition of NF-κB.

Various hepatoprotective ability of bamboo has been reported in carbon tetrachloride CCl_4 induced hepatotoxicity in animal models. Methanolic extracts of young shoots of *B. bambos* showed a reduction in AST, ALT, ALP and total bilirubin (Patil et al. 2018). Bamboo salt which is traditionally famous for its medicinal properties mainly in Korea have also shown to decrease serum AST, ALT, LDH and pro-inflammatory cytokine such as TNF-α, IL-6 and IFN-γ (Zhao et al. 2013). Zhang et al. (2014) reported that bamboo leaf flavonoids increase the SOD and GSH-Px activity along with liver glycogen that leads to improved activity of liver enzymes, prevention of liver injury to a high degree, ultimately protecting against chemical injury. Suppression of acetaminophen by *Sasa veitchii* leaf extract shows the hepatoprotective activity by increasing the total anti-oxidant capacity in liver (Yoshioka et al. 2017a). Significant increase in glutathione level in the liver tissues, when treated with different processed (fermented, brine preserved and boiled), shoots of *D. hamiltonii* was reported by Bajwa et al. (2019b). Further, Chauhan et al. (2017) studied the *in-vitro* and *in-vivo* hepatoprotective activity of methanolic leaf extract of *B. arundinacea*. The *in-vitro* study was carried out by monitoring cell viability in Hep G2, Hep 3b tumour cell lines and primary hepatocytes by inducing cytotoxicity by acetamide. The hepatoprotective effect of bamboo is mainly due to the presence of high amount of anti-oxidants.

2.3.2.9 Immunomodulatory Activity

The immune system is one of our most important and complex biological systems in the body and its dysfunction is responsible for various diseases like allergy, asthma, arthritis, cancer and other infectious diseases. Scientific documentations have revealed that modulation of immune responses can control various types of diseases. Many therapeutic effects of plant extracts have been studied and it has been suggested that this is due to their wide array of immunomodulatory effects and influence on the immune system of the human body. Phytochemicals such as flavonoids, polysaccharides, lactones, alkaloids, diterpenoids and glycosides, present in several plants, have been reported to be responsible for the plant's immunomodulating properties. Most of immunostimulants and immunosuppressants in clinical use are the cytotoxic drugs which possess serious side effects. Thus, the search for natural products of plant origin as new leads for development of potent and safe immunosuppressant and immunostimulant agents is gaining much research interest and bamboo is a potential source.

Beta glucans extracted from bamboo (*Sasa sensanensis*) leaves are known to have an immune-modulatory effect in animals (Ohtsuka et al. 2014). These glucans have been used for the treatment of diseases such as viral infections, inflammation and cancer. The immunomodulatory effect of SanSTAGE (TM) which is a pure compound obtained from bamboo leaves (25% of bamboo leaf extract and 75% of dextrin) was studied on peripheral blood leukocyte population and mRNA expression of immune related molecules of dairy cows. Cows supplemented with SanSTAGE (TM) showed an increased number of CD8(+) T cells and expression of perforin (cytotoxicity factor to virally infected cells) and MX-2 (anti-virus factor). The study describes for the first time that oral administration of supplement extracted from Kumaizasa bamboo leaves affects the cellular immune function of dairy cows and can be recommended as part of a diet for the prevention of infectious diseases.

2.3.2.10 Bamboo as a Prebiotic

There is an increasing trend of consumer awareness towards the demand for functional foods as they enhance the health of the consumer. Apart from other food ingredients prebiotics are among those which have attracted much attention. A prebiotic is a non-digestible and selectively fermented ingredient that allows specific changes, both in the composition and/or activity in the gastrointestinal microbiota that confers benefits upon host well-being and health. In general, 'prebiotics' can be considered as 'food' for probiotics. Probiotics can be defined as live microbial food supplements which benefit the health of consumer by maintaining or improving their intestinal microbial balance. Many studies have confirmed that the prebiotics incorporated in the diet is a valid approach to the dietary manipulation of the colonic microbiota leading to the increase in demand for prebiotics. Extensive studies are now focused on the prebiotic potential of polysaccharides extracted from natural sources instead of commercially available prebiotics. Azmi et al. (2012) extracted bamboo shoot crude polysaccharides (BSCP) from *Gigantochloa* sp. leaves and elucidated the function of extract in supporting the growth of *Bifidobacterium animalis, B. longum, Lactobacillus acidophilus* and also its ability to suppress the growth of *Salmonella* spp. Fourier Transform Infra-Red (FTIR) spectroscopy of BSCP revealed that the extract contains β-glucan which is a valuable compound for the medical and food industries. These relate to the resistance of BSCP towards artificial human gastric juice which is more than 99%. Prebiotic activity tested using BSCP as a carbon source showed a significant increase in the growth of *B. animalis, B. longum* and *L. acidophilus* as compared to the use of fructo-oligosaccharides (FOS), whereas survivability of *Salmonella choleraesuis* was found to be slower. This indicated that BSCP could be a promising source of natural prebiotic as not all carbohydrates could exert similar beneficial effects as commercial prebiotics.

3 Nutrients in Bamboo Shoots

Bamboo shoot is one of the most highly nutritious health promoting vegetables, and it is projected globally to be a future health food. The nutritional value of edible shoots of different bamboo species has been worked out by several workers (Giri and Janmejoy 1992, Shi and Yang 1992, Tripathi 1998, Chen et al. 1999, Sharma et al. 2004, Xu et al. 2005, Kumbhare and Bhargava 2007, Chongtham et al. 2007, 2008). Bamboo shoots are low in calories, high in dietary fibre and rich in nutrients. The main nutrients in bamboo shoots are protein, carbohydrates, amino acids, minerals, fat, sugar, fibre and inorganic salts. The shoots have a good profile of minerals, consisting mainly of potassium, calcium, manganese, zinc, chromium, copper, iron, plus lower amounts of phosphorus and selenium (Shi and Yang 1992, Chongtham et al. 2007, Saini et al. 2017, Bajwa et al. 2019b). Fresh shoots are a good source of thiamine, niacin, vitamin A, vitamin B6 and vitamin E (Visuphaka 1985, Xia 1989, Shi and Yang 1992). They are rich in protein, containing between 1.49 to 4.04 g (average 2.65 g) per 100 g of fresh shoots. They contain 17 to 19 amino acids, 8 of which are essential for the human body (Qiu 1992, Ferreira et al. 1995, Rawat 2017). Tyrosine amounts to 57–67% of the total amino acid content of the shoots (Kozukue et al. 1999). Fat content is comparatively low (0.26–0.94%) which can be estimated by Soxhlet extraction method and the shoots contain important essential fatty acids.

The total sugar content, 2.5% on average, is lower than that of other vegetables. The water content is 90% or more. Major advances have been made in fresh shoot production and processing and in the analysis of nutrient components of edible shoots. Based on nutritional analyses, it has been determined that bamboo shoots are a good source of food energy and are being projected as a new health food (Chongtham et al. 2011). This is because bamboo shoots are endowed with these health-enhancing properties:

i) Rich in nutrients: Shoots have a high content of protein and essential amino acids, carbohydrates, minerals and several vitamins.
ii) Rich in bioactive compounds: Bamboo shoots contain phytosterols and phenols which have cholesterol-lowering and anti-oxidant properties and can thus be considered as nutraceuticals.
iii) High fibre content: Bamboo shoots are a good source of dietary fibre, which helps in lowering blood cholesterol, ease constipation, normalize blood sugar levels and prevent obesity and cardiovascular diseases.
iv) Low fat content: Fat content is extremely low in bamboo shoots which are, therefore, very good for weight-conscious and dieting people.
v) Functions as appetizer: The high cellulosic content of bamboo shoots stimulates appetite. Being crisp, crunchy and tender with a sweet flavor, shoots have a unique and delicious taste that function as an appetizer.
vi) Organic: Bamboo grows naturally without the application of fertilizers and pesticides. Hence, the shoots are organic and free from residual toxicity.

Our group has analyzed shoots of 30 bamboo species, 11 species from *Dendrocalamus* (*D. asper, D. brandisii, D. giganteus, D. hamiltonii, D. hookeri, D. latiflorus, D. longispathus, D. manipureanus, D. membranaceus, D. sikkimensis* and *D. strictus*), 10 from *Bambusa* (*B. balcooa, B. bambos, B. cacharensis, B. kingiana, B. manipureana, B. mizorameana, B. nutans, B. polymorpha, B. tulda* and *B. vulgaris*), 2 each from *Gigantochloa* (*G. albociliata* and *G. rostrata*) and *Thyrsostachys* (*T. oliveri* and *T. siamensis*) and one each from *Cephalostachyum* (*C. capitatum*), *Chimonobambusa* (*C. callosa*), *Schizostachyum* (*S. dullooa*), *Melocanna* (*M. baccifera*) and *Phyllostachys* (*P. mannii*). The shoots of the different species can be recognized due to their unique physical appearance and shape.

3.1 MACRO-NUTRIENTS

Macro-nutrients present in the shoots include amino acids, proteins, carbohydrates, fibre and fat (Table 3.1). Some of the nutrient components in bamboo shoots are higher than those contained in commonly consumed vegetables (Chongtham et al. 2011). However, significant nutritional changes occur during processing and so appropriate processing methods need to be adopted to ensure that maximum nutrients are retained (Figure 3.1).

3.1.1 Protein

Protein is vital for building and repairing body tissues; formation of bones, muscles, teeth, hair, nails, skin, cartilage and blood as well as for the synthesis of enzymes, hormones and antibodies. Protein content in the freshly harvested shoots of 24 bamboo species was estimated which showed a range from 1.27 to 5.87 g/100 g f.w., highest being in *Bambusa bambos* followed by *Chimonobambusa callosa* (4.57 mg/100 g f.w.) and lowest in *B. tulda* (Table 3.1). *B. kingiana, B. polymorpha, B. vulgaris, D. giganteus* and *D. membranaceus* had more or less similar protein content (Sundriyal and Sundriyal 2001, Sharma et al. 2004, Bhatt et al. 2005). With harvesting age of shoots, protein content was reported to reduce in 10-day-old shoots of four bamboo species and 16-day-old shoots of three bamboo species when compared to freshly harvested juvenile shoots (Chongtham et al. 2007, Pandey and Ojha 2013) (Figure 3.2).

To remove cyanogenic glycosides and reduce acridity, young shoots are subjected to processing like soaking, drying, boiling and fermentation, which reduces the protein content (Tabet et al. 2004, Zhang et al. 2011, Park and Jhon 2013, Badwaik et al. 2014, 2015, Pandey and Ojha 2014). Variation in protein content has also been reported at different stages of shoot growth. Chongtham et al. (2008) revealed that canned shoots have the lowest (1.93%) protein content followed by fermented (2.57%) and raw shoots (3.11%) in *D. giganteus* species. Protein content in seven species (*Phyllostachys aurea, P. aureosulcata, P. bissetii, P. glauca, P. nuda, P. rubromarginata* and *Pseudosasa japonica*) at three stages of growth (< 60, 90–150 and > 180 cm) revealed a range from 5.1 to 25.80% (Christian et al. 2015). The apical portions of *D. giganteus* shoots were reported to have higher protein (46.1%) content compared to lower portion (40.4%) (Ferreira et al. 1992); however, no significant variation in the protein content in the upper (33.4%) and lower (33%) part of oven-dried shoots of *Yushania alpina* was reported by Karanja et al. (2016).

TABLE 3.1

Comparative Account on the Macro-Nutrients (g/100 g f.w.) and Vitamins (mg/100 g f.w.) Content in Fresh Juvenile Bamboo Shoots and Some Common Vegetables

Name of Species	Carbohydrate	Amino Acid	Starch	Protein	Fat	Vitamin C	Vitamin E	Ash	Moisture
B. balcooa	3.22 ± 0.13	2.13 ± 0.03	1.21 ± 0.02	3.70 ± 0.09	0.47 ± 0.01	2.63 ± 0.02	0.42 ± 0.03	0.86 ± 0.02	90.68 ± 0.09
B. bambos	1.72 ± 0.08	2.31 ± 0.01	1.24 ± 0.08	5.87 ± 0.39	0.53 ± 0.04	1.63 ± 0.03	0.60 ± 0.04	0.88 ± 0.04	90.09 ± 0.08
B. cacharensis	2.40 ± 0.04	2.42 ± 0.03	0.72 ± 0.03	3.19 ± 0.04	0.46 ± 0.04	2.10 ± 0.03	0.47 ± 0.04	0.65 ± 0.00	92.60 ± 0.06
B. kingiana	5.44 ± 0.11	3.71 ± 0.95	0.34 ± 0.03	3.57 ± 0.09	0.35 ± 0.03	2.10 ± 0.12	0.50 ± 0.10	1.38 ± 0.23	90.00 ± 1.02
B. mizorameanea	1.98 ± 0.11	1.94 ± 0.01	1.02 ± 0.10	3.17 ± 0.12	0.38 ± 0.02	1.67 ± 0.13	0.27 ± 0.07	0.98 ± 0.02	89.21 ± 1.16
B. manipureana	2.81 ± 0.02	2.80 ± 0.02	0.82 ± 0.02	3.45 ± 0.04	0.41 ± 0.01	2.50 ± 0.03	0.55 ± 0.03	0.69 ± 0.00	91.68 ± 0.08
B. nutans	2.76 ± 0.10	2.21 ± 0.02	1.36 ± 0.08	3.47 ± 0.23	0.70 ± 0.05	1.52 ± 0.03	0.49 ± 0.02	0.82 ± 0.05	91.21 ± 0.21
B. polymorpha	5.44 ± 0.04	3.42 ± 0.02	0.38 ± 0.04	3.64 ± 0.02	0.46 ± 0.00	2.60 ± 0.13	0.49 ± 0.12	0.76 ± 0.22	90.26 ± 1.67
B. tulda	1.09 ± 0.04	1.65 ± 0.03	0.89 ± 0.12	1.27 ± 0.02	0.48 ± 0.06	1.42 ± 0.06	0.61 ± 0.14	0.85 ± 0.13	83.60 ± 1.26
B. vulgaris	6.51 ± 0.04	3.57 ± 0.04	0.27 ± 0.05	3.64 ± 0.02	0.50 ± 0.01	4.80 ± 0.10	0.52 ± 0.09	1.01 ± 0.21	90.60 ± 0.82
C. capitatum	2.53 ± 0.02	3.14 ± 0.02	0.83 ± 0.03	3.70 ± 0.04	0.39 ± 0.03	2.43 ± 0.05	0.71 ± 0.04	0.65 ± 0.02	92.70 ± 0.24
C. callosa	1.26 ± 0.01	4.61 ± 0.02	0.71 ± 0.02	4.57 ± 0.03	0.43 ± 0.02	2.59 ± 0.03	0.81 ± 0.02	0.75 ± 0.02	91.23 ± 0.10
D. asper	4.90 ± 0.11	3.11 ± 0.06	0.36 ± 0.08	3.59 ± 0.06	0.40 ± 0.06	3.20 ± 0.05	0.91 ± 0.13	0.95 ± 0.02	89.40 ± 0.98
D. brandisii	4.90 ± 0.104	3.01 ± 0.10	0.49 ± 0.04	2.31 ± 0.12	0.24 ± 0.09	1.59 ± 0.09	0.42 ± 0.09	0.60 ± 0.11	89.80 ± 0.15
D. giganteus	5.65 ± 0.06	2.26 ± 0.04	2.38 ± 0.04	3.64 ± 0.05	0.49 ± 0.02	2.21 ± 0.02	0.56 ± 0.03	1.03 ± 0.00	89.02 ± 0.03
D. hamiltonii	3.33 ± 0.04	2.33 ± 0.02	1.74 ± 0.02	3.37 ± 0.03	0.42 ± 0.02	2.48 ± 0.07	0.68 ± 0.03	0.76 ± 0.02	91.33 ± 0.18
D. hookeri	2.15 ± 0.06	1.93 ± 0.01	1.62 ± 0.09	2.53 ± 0.01	0.41 ± 0.02	1.35 ± 0.00	0.29 ± 0.01	0.82 ± 0.03	91.13 ± 1.11
D. latiflorus	2.50 ± 0.08	1.85 ± 0.05	0.98 ± 0.02	3.13 ± 0.07	0.38 ± 0.00	2.38 ± 0.05	0.52 ± 0.03	0.94 ± 0.01	90.14 ± 0.04
D. longispathus	2.62 ± 0.01	2.96 ± 0.03	1.02 ± 0.02	3.08 ± 0.01	0.47 ± 0.01	3.08 ± 0.02	0.78 ± 0.06	0.78 ± 0.07	91.36 ± 0.75
D. manipureanus	2.46 ± 0.05	2.23 ± 0.03	1.11 ± 0.08	2.81 ± 0.06	0.39 ± 0.02	2.43 ± 0.04	0.51 ± 0.04	0.78 ± 0.06	90.24 ± 0.14

(Continued)

TABLE 3.1 (CONTINUED)
Comparative Account on the Macro-Nutrients (g/100 g f.w.) and Vitamins (mg/100 g f.w.) Content in Fresh Juvenile Bamboo Shoots and Some Common Vegetables

Name of Species	Carbohydrate	Amino Acid	Starch	Protein	Fat	Vitamin C	Vitamin E	Ash	Moisture
D. membranaceus	3.48 ± 0.03	3.20 ± 0.02	1.49 ± 0.04	3.65 ± 0.09	0.44 ± 0.05	1.83 ± 0.04	0.65 ± 0.03	1.00 ± 0.04	89.02 ± 0.33
D. sikkimensis	2.99 ± 0.03	1.87 ± 0.02	1.31 ± 0.08	3.03 ± 0.13	0.51 ± 0.01	2.43 ± 0.03	0.59 ± 0.04	0.76 ± 0.02	91.24 ± 0.04
D. strictus	6.17 ± 0.02	3.07 ± 0.02	0.31 ± 0.05	2.60 ± 0.07	0.32 ± 0.04	2.43 ± 0.12	0.58 ± 0.03	0.71 ± 0.09	90.10 ± 0.93
G. albociliata	4.59 ± 0.09	3.52 ± 0.11	0.31 ± 0.04	3.05 ± 0.11	0.51 ± 0.09	1.00 ± 0.08	0.60 ± 0.04	0.73 ± 0.04	89.23 ± 0.30
G. rostrata	4.32 ± 0.11	3.16 ± 0.08	0.21 ± 0.03	3.56 ± 0.11	0.56 ± 0.12	3.20 ± 0.09	0.49 ± 0.05	0.68 ± 0.05	90.56 ± 1.02
M. baccifera	2.22 ± 0.01	2.43 ± 0.05	0.85 ± 0.02	3.22 ± 0.02	0.34 ± 0.02	1.44 ± 0.04	0.40 ± 0.07	0.55 ± 0.09	93.42 ± 0.84
P. mannii	2.73 ± 0.02	2.36 ± 0.06	1.09 ± 0.02	3.24 ± 0.03	0.44 ± 0.01	3.23 ± 0.05	0.53 ± 0.04	0.86 ± 0.03	90.34 ± 0.12
S. dullooa	0.82 ± 0.03	3.20 ± 0.02	0.45 ± 0.01	0.95 ± 0.02	0.40 ± 0.01	0.71 ± 0.04	0.60 ± 0.02	0.53 ± 0.03	93.77 ± 0.04
T. oliveri	4.09 ± 0.08	2.84 ± 0.12	0.56 ± 0.04	3.23 ± 0.08	0.35 ± 0.09	2.50 ± 0.08	0.38 ± 0.07	1.01 ± 0.01	88.56 ± 1.56
T. siamensis	5.07 ± 0.12	2.90 ± 0.10	1.01 ± 0.02	3.35 ± 0.12	0.41 ± 0.10	2.80 ± 0.10	0.37 ± 0.06	1.38 ± 0.05	86.83 ± 1.50
Values reported are measurement replication means ± standard deviation (n = 3 replicates).									
				Some common vegetables*					
Amaranthus gangeticus (Amaranth)	6.1	1.3	–	4.0	0.5	1.0	43.3	1.5	85.7
Abelmoschus esculantus (Ladies finger)	6.4	0.3	–	1.9	0.2	1.2	13.0	1.1	88.3
Brassica oleracea var. *capitata* (Cabbage)	5.6	0.3	–	1.8	0.1	2.6	32.2	0.7	91.9
Cucumis sativus (Cucumber)	2.5	0.1	0.1	0.6	0.1	0.7	3.2	0.4	96.3

(Continued)

TABLE 3.1 (CONTINUED)

Comparative Account on the Macro-Nutrients (g/100 g f.w.) and Vitamins (mg/100 g f.w.) Content in Fresh Juvenile Bamboo Shoots and Some Common Vegetables

Name of Species	Carbohydrate	Amino Acid	Starch	Protein	Fat	Vitamin C	Vitamin E	Ash	Moisture
Cucurbita maxima (Pumpkin)	6.5	0.2	–	1.4	0.4	0.7	9.0	0.8	92.6
Daucus carota (Carrot)	10.6	0.2	–	0.9	0.2	1.2	3.0	1.1	86.0
Lagenaria siceraria (Bottle gourd)	3.4	0.4	–	0.6	0.1	0.6	12.0	0.4	92.4
Phaseolus vulgaris (French bean)	20.1	0.3	–	18.8	2.0	4.6	–	4.3	10.8
Raphanus sativus (Radish)	3.4	0.1	–	0.7	0.1	1.6	15.0	0.6	94.4
Spinacea oleracea (Spinach)	2.9	0.3	–	2.0	0.7	0.6	28.1	1.7	92.1
Solanum melongena (Brinjal)	4.0	0.2	–	1.4	0.3	1.3	12.0	0.8	92.7
Solanum tuberosum (Potato)	22.6	0.2	15.4	1.6	0.1	0.4	19.7	1.1	74.7

*Source: Chongtham et al. 2011.

Note: '–' indicates data not available,

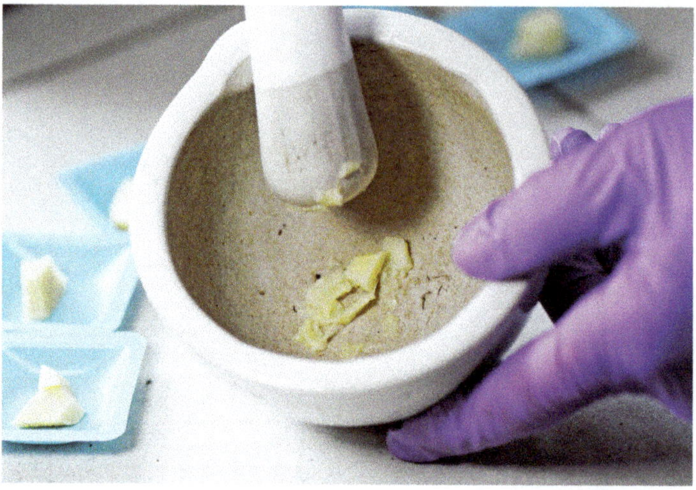

FIGURE 3.1 Crushing of bamboo shoot for extraction and estimation of macro-nutrients.

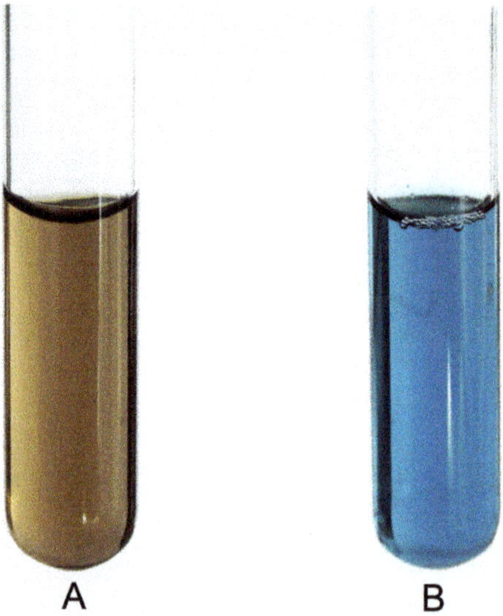

FIGURE 3.2 Colorimetric analysis of protein using Bradford reagent. The colour changes from (A) brown to (B) blue, indicating the presence of protein in bamboo shoot.

3.1.2 Amino Acids

Amino acids are essential macro-nutrients in diets, which are prerequisites not only for the synthesis of protein but as precursors for the formation of secondary metabolites that participate in the regulation of signaling pathways and multiple cellular processes in the body. More than 300 amino acids are known in nature but merely 20 are required for protein synthesis. Functional amino acids hold boundless potential in the prevention and treatment of metabolic diseases (e.g. obesity, diabetes and cardiovascular disorders), lactation failure, fetal and postnatal growth restriction, male and female infertility, organ (e.g. intestinal, neurological and renal) dysfunction and infectious disease. Unlike nonessential amino acids that are synthesized by the body itself, essential amino acids are obtained from the diet; and have numerous imperative functions in human health.

Twelve to nineteen amino acids have been reported from bamboo shoots (Figure 3.3). Of the 30 species investigated, the amino acid content ranged from 1.65 to 4.61 mg/100 g f.w. (Table 3.1). An in-depth analysis of only limited bamboo species has been investigated by few researchers (Zhang et al. 2011, Park and Jhon 2013, Zheng et al. 2013, Sun et al. 2015, Xu et al. 2015, Rawat 2017). Whereas Zhang et al. (2011) reported twelve free amino acids in the shoots of *Phyllostachys praecox*, Rawat (2017) reported 19 amino acids detected by HPLC in five bamboo species viz. *B. balcooa*, *D. giganteus*, *D. hamiltonii*, *D. membranaceus* and *P. mannii*, out of which eight are essential. All essential amino acids (viz. histidine, isoleucine, leucine, lysine, methionine, phenylalanine, threonine and valine) except tryptophan were detected in the shoots of the four species (Figure 3.4) and their concentrations ranged from 0.46-21.11μg/mg d.w. They were in the descending order as valine (2.51-21.11) > leucine (1.59-12.84) > methionine (4.58-9.02) > threonine (0.46–8.91) > isoleucine (1.6–7.80) > phenylalanine (1.98–7.54) > histidine (1.63–4.21) > lysine (1.05–3.96). Out of all the detected amino acids, asparagine and tyrosine showed the highest concentration while ornithine and glycine had the lowest. Overall, shoots were dominant in asparagine, tyrosine and essential amino acids, that is valine, leucine and isoleucine. Prevalence of asparagine and tyrosine has also been observed by Park and Jhon (2013) in the shoots of *P. pubescens*. Cooking, pickling and other processing methods reduce the amino acid content in bamboo shoots (Zhang et al. 2011, 2013).

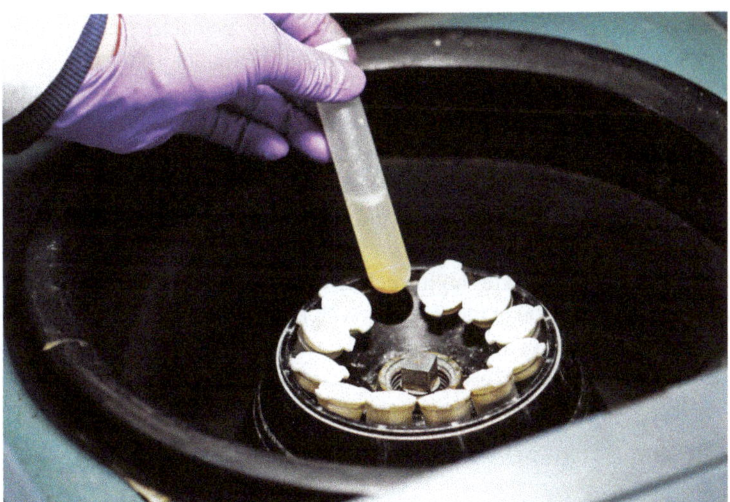

FIGURE 3.3 Extraction of amino acids from bamboo shoot through centrifugation at 10,000 rpm for 15 mins.

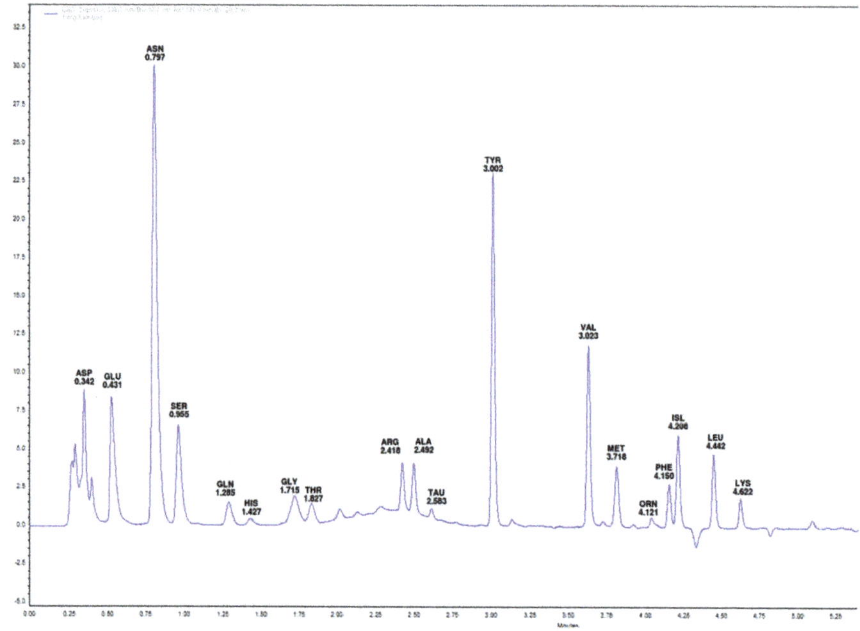

FIGURE 3.4 HPLC chromatogram of fresh shoots of *Phyllostachys mannii* showing peaks of different amino acids with retention time in minutes.

3.1.3 Carbohydrates

Carbohydrates are an important source of energy in human diets, comprising 40–80% of total energy intake. In addition to providing easily available energy for oxidative metabolism, carbohydrate-containing foods are vehicles for important micronutrients and phytochemicals. Dietary carbohydrate is important to maintain glycaemic homeostasis and for gastrointestinal integrity and function. As examined by different researchers, the carbohydrate content ranged from 2.0 to 9.94% in the freshly harvested shoots and is affected by harvesting age and processing methods of various bamboo species (Chongtham et al. 2008, Pandey and Ojha 2013). Sugar content in the fresh and boiled shoots of *P. pubescens* and *P. nigra* has been reported by Park and Jhon (2013). They detected three sugars with high fructose content followed by glucose and galactose and showed a reduction in these sugars with boiling except galactose in the shoots of *P. pubescens*. Karanja et al. (2016) investigated upper and lower parts of *Yushania alpina* shoots and reported 23.6% and 17.3% carbohydrate content, respectively.

3.2 MICRONUTRIENTS

Micronutrients have a pivotal role in human nutrition by regulating several metabolic processes, maintaining tissue functions and their satisfactory intake has a significant influence on public health and well-being. Deficiency in micronutrients can retard growth and cognitive development, impair immunological functioning and increase the risks of non-communicable diseases including skeletal, cardiovascular and metabolic disorders. Any food that we consume is generally subjected to some form of processing and the latter generally causes changes in the food matrix and the integral constituents of foods as well. In addition to, improving the digestibility of macronutrients by softening and loosing of food matrix, processing is known to enhance the bioavailability of minerals by altering and inhibiting certain inherent factors like phytate and soluble dietary fibre (Figure 3.5).

3.2.1 Minerals

Minerals, the major group of micronutrients are indispensable for normal body growth and development due to their functionalities and potentials in body metabolism and homeostasis that include maintenance of hormonal and regulatory functions of our body and building of muscles and bones. One of the most important challenges for agriculture, besides enhancing food production, is to provide almost all the essential minerals and organic nutrients to humans for maintenance of health and proper organ function. Dietary minerals are of great interest to health specialists and consumers, due to the number of processes they are involved in and there is continuous research highlighting the benefits of their adequate and balanced intake. Minerals in the food are critical for metabolism and normal functioning of muscles, heart, nerves, bones, serve as cofactors and coenzymes for various enzyme systems and therefore are crucial for maintaining human health and well-being (Awuchi et al. 2020). Macro-mineral elements (potassium, phosphorus, magnesium, calcium, sodium) are required in large amount (>100 mg/day) and present in large quantities in the body, whereas micro-mineral or trace elements (Iron, zinc, copper, nickel, manganese) are required in small quantity (<100 mg/day) and also present

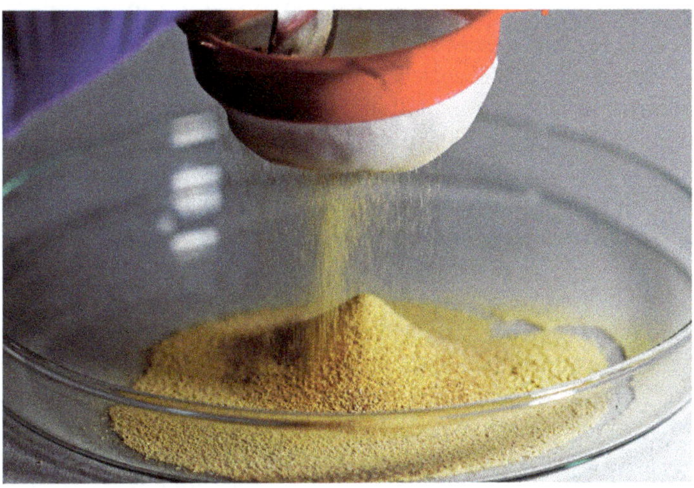

FIGURE 3.5 Bamboo shoot sample preparation for mineral estimation; oven-dried powder sieved to attain 0.25 mm-sized particles.

in small amounts in tissues and body fluids. It is estimated that approximately 60% of the world's population is iron (Fe)-deficient and approximately 30% is zinc (Zn)-deficient in addition to other essential nutrient elements including calcium (Ca), magnesium (Mg) and copper (Cu) deficiencies.

The role of trace metals in enzyme functions has been studied extensively in nutrition and biochemistry. Selenium, copper, zinc, iron and manganese are indispensable metals, for the activities of various anti-oxidant enzymes. Bamboo shoots are endowed with rich quantities of useful minerals such as selenium, iron, phosphorus, sodium, calcium, magnesium, zinc and iron.

Many researchers have evaluated the mineral content in leaves, shoots and bamboo shoot fortified food products using different methods such as an atomic absorption spectrophotometer flame photometer, wavelength dispersive X-ray fluorescence (WDXRF) spectrometry, plasma spectrometer and ICP-AES optical emission spectrometer methods. The mineral content may vary depending upon the species, age, plant part, harvesting season, growing locations and methods used for sample preparation and estimation (Table 3.2, Figure 3.6).

3.2.2 Macro-Minerals

3.2.2.1 Potassium

The shoots are labeled as a heart-protective vegetable because of its high content of potassium (K) that helps to maintain normal blood pressure and a steady heartbeat and is a vital electrolyte for sustaining fluid equilibrium in cells. High K intake has also other beneficial effects such as reducing the risk of stroke, preventing the development of renal vascular, glomerular and tubular damage, decreasing urinary calcium excretion, reducing the formation of kidney stones and demineralization of bones. Severe K deficiency or hypokalemia occurs when a person's K levels fall below 3.6 mmol/L (Weiner et al. 2018). The K content in bamboo shoots ranges from 4190 to 6660 mg/100 g of f.w. (Table 3.2). Waikhom et al. (2013) explored 10 elements in 30-day-old shoots of 12 bamboo species and found that all bamboo shoots are rich in K and poor in sodium content. The K content ranged from 1310 to 3533 mg/100 g dry weight (d.w.), maximum in *D. manipureanus* and minimum in *Schizostachyum dullooa*. A higher range (2670–9630 mg/100 g d.w.) of K was recorded by Christian et al. (2015) in six species of *Phyllostachys* and *Pseudosasa japonica* whereas Karanja et al. (2016) observed higher K content in upper portions of *Yushania alpina* shoots (35,900 μg/g d.w.) compared to lower portions (27,600 μg/g d.w.).

3.2.2.2 Calcium

It is required for strong bone and teeth and plays a major role in muscle contraction and relaxation, blood clotting, proper nerve function and body immune defenses. Analysis of 19 bamboo species was carried out and Ca content ranged from 100 to 220 mg/100 g dry weight (Table 3.2). In subsequent reports, Ca content in different bamboos species exhibited a range from 15 to 80 mg/100 g f.w. in the fresh shoots (Park and Jhon 2013, Sood et al. 2013, Pandey and Ojha 2014, Hailu and Addis 2016) and 10 to 267 mg/100g d.w. in the dried shoots (Mainka et al. 1989, Tabet et al. 2004, Waikhom et al. 2013, Christian et al. 2015, Karanja et al. 2016). The Ca content is

TABLE 3.2

Macro- and Micro-Mineral Elements in Different Bamboo Species Estimated by Wavelength Dispersive X-Ray Fluorescence Spectrometry

	Macro-Mineral Elements (mg/100 g d.w.)							
Species	**K**	**P**	**Mg**	**Ca**	**S**	**Na**	**Cl**	**Si**
Bambusa balcooa	4230	560	210	180	230	20	1220	150
B. bambos	5980	750	230	190	260	20	1530	130
B. cacharensis	4480	550	180	110	250	10	1150	120
B. manipureana	6480	670	210	100	260	20	1410	110
B. nutans	5230	580	200	180	250	20	1230	160
B. tulda	5210	640	190	100	280	20	1680	120
B. vulgaris	4190	460	130	110	200	10	1660	140
Cephalostachyum capitatum	5630	610	170	180	270	20	1200	80
C. callosa	6570	750	220	220	280	20	680	100
Dendrocalamus giganteus	4590	540	190	210	270	40	590	120
D. hamiltonii	5230	560	200	150	220	40	870	190
D. hookeri	5740	680	220	150	290	30	1460	170
D. latiflorus	4390	480	160	120	230	20	910	170
D. longispathus	5610	580	200	130	240	10	950	140
D. manipureanus	6200	630	240	140	320	20	1270	140
D. membranaceus	6120	620	200	160	240	90	930	150
D. sikkimensis	5200	530	240	180	270	30	880	160
Melocanna baccifera	6480	620	300	210	340	30	1350	120
Phyllostachys mannii	6660	930	230	130	330	60	850	70

	Micro-mineral elements (mg/100g d.w.)				
	Fe	**Zn**	**Cu**	**Mn**	**Ni**
Bambusa balcooa	8.2	6.8	2.6	2.5	0.9
B. bambos	8.0	10	2.5	3.6	0.7
B. cacharensis	5.8	7.2	2.4	2.3	0.7
B. manipureana	5.9	8.5	1.6	1.3	0.9
B. nutans	8.8	9.5	1.9	9.7	0.8
B. tulda	7.0	7.7	2.4	2.5	0.7
B. vulgaris	6.7	6.0	2.2	2.5	0.8
Cephalostachyum capitatum	6.8	9.0	2.6	6.0	1.2
C. callosa	6.5	8.0	3.4	3.5	0.9
Dendrocalamus giganteus	6.9	6.1	5.1	1.3	0.8
D. hamiltonii	7.4	6.8	2.6	1.2	0.7
D. hookerii	6.0	8.4	2.9	2.4	0.7
D. latiflorus	4.7	7.9	1.9	3.6	1.2
D. longispathus	6.8	8.2	2.1	2.3	0.7
D. manipureanus	7.9	9.0	2.1	3.2	0.8
D. membranaceus	6.8	8.5	2.2	1.5	0.9
D. sikkimensis	10	8.3	2.5	4.3	1.1
Melocanna baccifera	7.2	10	2.8	5.5	1.0
Phyllostachys mannii	9.1	10	2.6	9.0	0.8

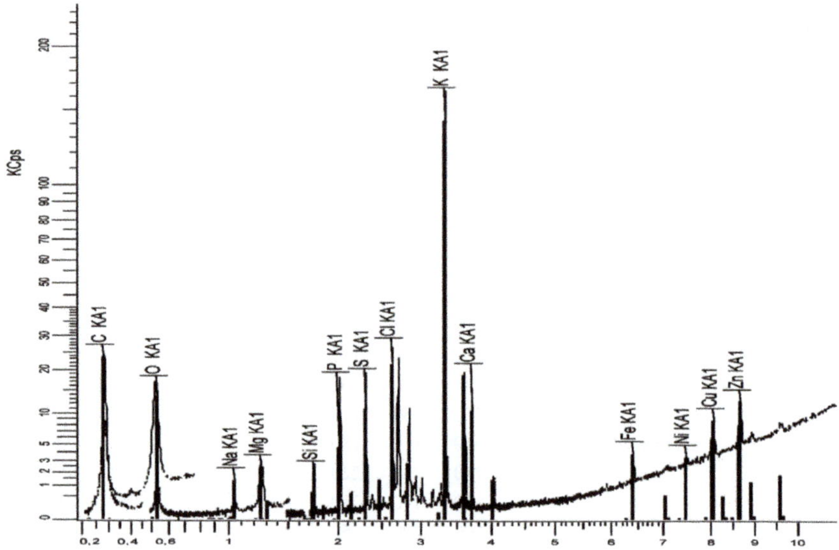

FIGURE 3.6 Wavelength dispersive X-ray fluorescence spectra of *Dendrocalamus giganteus* shoot depicting different peaks of macro- and micro-mineral elements.

quite unstable and a drastic decrease was observed while cooking and other processing methods (Chongtham et al. 2008, Pandey and Ojha 2014, Hailu and Addis 2016). However, Ca content increased after boiling by 22.5% and 31.5% in *Sinoarundinaria nigra* and *P. pubescens*, respectively (Park and Jhon 2013).

3.2.2.3 Phosphorus

This mineral is required for the growth and renewal of tissues. Phosphorus (P) compounds carry, store and release energy and they assist many enzymes and vitamins in extracting the energy from nutrients. The P content was quantified in the fresh shoots of different bamboo species which varied from 50 to 90 mg/100 g (Gopalan et al. 1978, Yamaguchi 1983, Duke and Atchley 1986, Park and Jhon 2013, Sood et al. 2013, Pandey and Ojha 2014). Dried shoots have a higher phosphorous content ranging from 70 to 1049 mg/100 g (Bhargava et al. 1996, Bhatt et al. 2003, Kumbhare 2003, Waikhom et al. 2013, Karanja et al. 2016), whereas other processing methods like boiling and cooking have reduced its content in shoots of various species of bamboo (Park and Jhon 2013, Pandey and Ojha 2014, Hailu and Addis 2016).

3.2.2.4 Sodium

Sodium (Na) is an important extracellular electrolyte and plays an important role in maintaining water balance and the functioning of the nerves and muscles. Only a few researchers in recent years examined the Na content of bamboo shoots and indicated lower values compared to other macro-minerals. Na content ranged from 0.19 to 7.34 mg in the fresh shoots (Chongtham et al. 2008, Park and Jhon 2013, Sood et al. 2013, Hailu and Addis 2016). Like K content, Na content was also observed in the higher range in dried shoots, that is from 10 to 70 mg (Waikhom et al. 2013, Christian et al. 2015). However, the content remained unchanged in 10 days old, canned and fermented shoots of *D. giganteus* (Chongtham et al. 2008), showed increase by 36–136% when boiled in water and further increased drastically, that is by 4- to 20-fold when boiled in 1–10% NaCl concentration (Park and Jhon, 2013, Pandey and Ojha 2014). In cooking as well, Na content increased by 41% in *Oxytenanthera abyssinica* shoots (Hailu and Addis 2016).

3.2.2.5 Magnesium

It is essential when trying to keep the normal fluid balance of body, contraction and relaxation of muscles and functioning of several enzymes. As investigated by various researchers, Magnesium (Mg) content in various bamboo species ranged from 5.38 to 170 mg in the fresh shoots (Bhargava et al. 1996, Bhatt et al. 2003, 2005, Chongtham et al. 2007, Park and Jhon 2013, Sood et al. 2013, Pandey and Ojha 2014) and 69–390 mg in dried shoots (Waikhom et al. 2013, Awol 2015). Whereas upon various other processing methods, the changes in Mg content was inconsistent, it was reduced by 34–45% boiling in salt in few species (Park and Jhon 2013, Pandey and Ojha 2014), but did not get altered significantly after canning and fermentation (Chongtham et al. 2008).

3.2.2.6 Sulphur

Sulphur (S) is the third most abundant mineral in our body, found in muscle, skin and bones and plays an important role in various physiological processes. It is basically ignored in nutritional circles, although it is a critical nutrient necessary for vibrant health and prevention of chronic diseases. Sulphur is a part of some of the amino acids in our body and is involved in protein synthesis, as well as several enzyme reactions. It helps in the production of collagen, which is a substance that forms connective tissues, cell structure and artery walls. Additionally, it is a part of keratin, giving strength to hair, skin and nails. Sulphur can help ease the effects of several skin disorders, including acne, psoriasis, warts, dandruff, eczema and folliculitis, which cause inflamed hair follicles. Without adequate sulphur, glucose metabolism becomes defective that leads to muscle and fat cell damage as the result of becoming glucose intolerant. Impaired glucose metabolism resulting from insufficient sulphur is also implicated as a factor in obesity and the dangerous condition known as Metabolic Syndrome. Sulphur is reported to be anti-cancerous, lowers blood cholesterol and skin infirmities. Sulphur content in 19 bamboo species ranged from 200 mg/100 g d.w. to 340 mg/100 g d.w. (Table 3.2). In three species *D. manipureanus, Phyllostachys manii* and *Melocanna baccifera*, the sulphur content was 320, 330 and 340 mg/100 g d.w., respectively whereas in all the other species, the value was below 300 mg/100 g d.w. Saini et al. (2017) reported the sulphur content in *B. bambos* (260 mg/100g) and *B. balcooa* (230 mg/100g) fresh shoots which increased significantly by 9–11% after soaking and 8–13% after storage in water for six months.

3.2.2.7 Silicon

Silicon (Si) is a non-metallic element and the second most abundant element in the Earth's crust with a great affinity for oxygen, forming 92% silica and silicates. It is also the most abundantly available trace element after iron and zinc. Chemically, silica is an oxide of silicon, viz. silicon dioxide and is generally colourless to white and insoluble in water. When associated with metals or minerals the family of silicates is formed. Humans are exposed to numerous sources of silica/silicon including dust, food, pharmaceuticals, cosmetics and medical implants and devices. As a metalloid, silicon has been used in many industrial applications including use as an additive in the food and beverage industry. As a result, humans are exposed to silicon through both environmental exposures and also as a dietary component. Bamboo extract is the richest known source of natural silica, containing over 70% organic silica. This is more than 10 times the level found in the widely used Horsetail plant (*Equisetum*) that contains 5% to 7% silica.

Tabasheer or *Banslochan* mainly obtained from bamboo internodes consists of pure silica and is a part of the pharmacology of traditional *Ayurvedic* and *Unani* medicine in the Indian subcontinent (Rawat et al. 2018). It acts as stimulant, astringent, febrifuge, tonic with anti-spasmodic and aphrodisiac properties and is the main ingredient in *Sitopaladi* ayurveda medicine (Chongtham and Bisht 2017). Menghao et al. (2012) investigated the effect of silica extract of *Phyllostachys edulis* on bone loss in ovariectomized rats and observed that Si supplementation increased significantly the femoral and lumbar bone mass density. Si content is highest in *D. hamiltonii* (190mg/100g d.w.) followed by *D. hookeri* and *D. latiflorus* (170mg/100g d.w.) as indicated in Table 3.2. Minimum content was detected in *P. mannii* (70mg/100g d.w.). Thus, bamboo shoot is a Si rich vegetable that has significant prospects for dietary supplementation (Rawat et al. 2018). Moreover, the abundance of Si in bamboo shoot offers the opportunities to be used in the nutraceutical and cosmetics industry.

3.2.3 Micro-Mineral Elements

3.2.3.1 Iron

It is a prerequisite for haemoglobin formation, normal functioning of the central nervous system, oxidation of carbohydrates, protein and fats. Iron acts as a carrier for oxygen from the lungs to the body's tissues. Iron deficiency ultimately leads to anemia, a condition in which the blood lacks healthy red blood cells required to carry oxygen, resulting in morbidity and death. It is estimated that about 29% of non-pregnant women, 38% of pregnant women and 43% of preschool children are affected by anemia; which is due to iron deficiency (WHO 2015). Examination on fresh shoots of different bamboo species depicted a range of Fe content from 0.1 to 3.37 mg (Gopalan et al. 1978, Yamaguchi 1983, Chongtham et al. 2007, NMBA 2009, Park and Jhon 2013) while in dried shoots it varied from 1.03-25.8 mg (Rajyalakshmi and Geervani 1994, Waikhom et al. 2013, Christian et al. 2015). Of 19 species analyzed (Table 3.2) *D. sikkimensis* had the highest Fe content (10mg/100g d.w.) followed by *P. mannii* (9.1mg/100g d.w.) and *B. nutans* (8.8mg/100gg d.w.). All of the other species had Fe content in the range of 4.7–8.2 mg/100 g d.w. Very few studies are available on the iron content of processed bamboo shoots. Significant reduction in iron content with an increase in harvesting age (10 days old) and growth (>60 cm) of shoots was noted by Chongtham et al. (2007) and Christian et al. (2015).

With boiling, increase in iron content by 13.5% in *P. pubescens* while a decrease in *Sinoarundinaria nigra* and *Oxytenanthera abyssinica* species by 25.46% and 6.25%, respectively, have been observed (Park and Jhon 2013, Hailu and Addis 2016).

3.2.3.2 Zinc

Zinc (Zn) content in fresh and processed shoots have been determined by many researchers. Zn plays an important role in lowering oxidative damage to cellular DNAs and thus shows anti-oxidant property while enhancing the function of the immune system and is an essential component of a large number of Zn-dependent enzymes, particularly in the synthesis and degradation of carbohydrates, lipids, proteins and nucleic acids (Rukaguer et al. 2001, Kaur et al. 2014). After iron, Zn is the major cause of micronutrient deficiency (Bailey et al. 2015; Table 3.2). Zn content in 19 bamboo species were determined and it ranges from 6.1 to 10 mg/100 g d.w. with highest recorded in *B. bambos*, *M. baccifera* and *P. manni*. Other studies indicate that the Zn content ranged from 0.57 to 1.01 mg in the fresh shoots of bamboo species (Chongtham et al. 2007, Park and Jhon 2013, Hailu and Addis, 2016) while it varied from 1.15 to 12.8 mg in the dried shoots (Waikhom et al. 2013, Christian et al. 2015, Karanja et al. 2016). Rui and Liangru (2008) have also analyzed Zn concentration in 80 bamboo species and reported the highest Zn content in *Phyllostachys* spp. viz. *P. atrovaginata*, *P. bambusoides*, *P. rivalis* and *P. aureosuleata*. The decrease in Zn content during the growth of shoots of different bamboo species was examined by Christian et al. (2015). With boiling, Zn content decreased by 13.75% to 39% in some bamboo species (Park and Jhon 2013, Hailu and Addis 2016).

3.2.3.3 Copper

Copper (Cu) is an essential trace element in mammalian nutrition as a component of metalloenzymes in which it acts as an electron donor or acceptor. It also acts as a co-factor of many redox enzymes. Beyond its role in iron metabolism, the need for Cu also derives from its involvement in a myriad of biological processes, including anti-oxidant defense, neuropeptide synthesis and immune function. Analysis of Cu content in the bamboo shoots has been worked out by few researchers and indicated a range from 0.07 to 6.12 mg at different stages of shoot growth of various bamboo species (Sood et al. 2013, Waikhom et al. 2013, Christian et al. 2015). In 19 species (Table 3.2) Cu content ranged from 1.6 to 5.1 mg/100g d.w. Cu content after cooking and boiling of shoots has been reported to reduce by 12.5 and 36% in *Sinoarundinaria nigra* and *Oxytenanthera abyssinica* species, respectively (Park and Jhon 2013, Hailu and Addis 2016).

3.2.3.4 Manganese

Manganese (Mn), an essential trace mineral indispensable for bone formation and bone health in general, is found in all tissues and is required for normal amino acid, lipid, protein and carbohydrate metabolism. It is also involved in the function of numerous organ systems and is needed for normal immune function, regulation of blood sugar and cellular energy, reproduction, digestion, bone growth and it aids in defense mechanisms against free radicals. Mn is vital as a co-factor in enzymes that facilitate metabolism of carbohydrates, proteins and fats. The uptake of manganese by humans mainly takes place through food, such as spinach, tea and herbs. The foodstuffs that contain the highest concentrations are grains and rice, soya beans, eggs, nuts, olive oil, green beans and oysters. After absorption in the human body, manganese will be transported through the blood to the liver, the kidneys, the pancreas and the endocrine glands. Shoots of bamboo species *B. nutans* (9.7 mg/100 g d.w.) and *P. mannii* (9.0 mg/100 g d.w.) showed high Mn content as indicated in Table 3.2. Saini et al. (2017) estimated the manganese content in the fresh shoots of *Bambusa balcooa* (2.5 mg/100 g) and *B. bambos* (3.6mg/100 g) which depletes up to 50% after boiling, soaking and fermentation.

3.2.3.5 Selenium

Selenium (Se) is an essential trace element and is of fundamental importance to human health. Being a constituent of selenoproteins, Se has structural and enzymatic roles. It is a co-factor for an enzyme, glutathione peroxidase and has anti-oxidant properties. Dietary deficiency of selenium markedly decreases tissue glutathione peroxidase activity by 90% and results in peroxidative damage and mitochondrial dysfunction (Xia et al. 1985). The essential role of selenium in the removal of free radicals and the maintenance of normal human health is epitomized by the etiology of Keshen disease in China. This disease was discovered by Chinese scientists and results from a severe deficiency of dietary selenium (Yang et al. 1983).

Selenium content in 16 bamboo species have been evaluated (Elangbam 2006). Selenium content in the shoots ranged from 0.1 μg/100 g to 1 μg/100 g f.w., in which *B. nutans* had the minimum and *D. asper* had the maximum.

3.3 VITAMIN C (ASCORBIC ACID)

Vitamin C is known to have many biological functions such as in collagen formation, absorption of inorganic iron, reduction of plasma cholesterol level and enhancement of the immune system. It is also required for the prevention of scurvy and maintenance of healthy skin, gums and blood vessels. Being water-soluble, it is found in the aqueous fractions of the cell and in body fluids. Vitamin C, as an anti-oxidant, reportedly reduces the risk of arteriosclerosis, cardiovascular diseases and some forms of cancer. Many investigators have worked on different bamboo species to determine vitamin C content. The vitamin C content as determined by Chongtham et al. (2011) in the raw shoots of various bamboo species, ranged from 0.71 mg to 4.80 mg/100 g f.w. (Table 3.1). Bhatt et al. (2005) also reported vitamin C content for a number of bamboo species ranging from 3.0% to 12.9%, highest being in *D. hamiltonii* and lowest being in *D. sikkimensis*. According to Bhargava et al. (1996), vitamin C content ranged from 8% to 23% in shoots of various bamboo species. The shoots of three bamboo species (*Dendrocalamus giganteus, D. latiflorus, D. sikkimensis*) when evaluated for their vitamin C content, revealed that *D. sikkimensis* (2.43 mg/100 g f.w.) has higher vitamin C content followed by *D. latiflorus* (2.38 mg/100 g f.w.) and *D. giganteus* (2.21 mg/100 g f.w.) (Rawat et al. 2016). Vitamin C content was analyzed in 30 bamboo species (Table 3.1). *B. vulgaris* had highest content (4.8 mg/100 g d.w.) The cause of variations in vitamin C content might be related to the differences in genotype, climatic conditions, maturity at harvest, growing condition, soil state and condition of post-harvest processing and preservation. Vitamin C content of some bamboo species such as *Dendrocalamus longispathus* (23.0 mg/100 g f.w.), *Pleioblastus amarus* (15.4 mg/100 g f.w.) and *Phyllostachys praecox* (12 mg/100 g f.w.) is even higher than some commonly used vegetables like tomatoes (10.6 mg/100 g f.w.), carrot (9.28 mg/100 g f.w.), potatoes (11.45 mg/100 g f.w.), cucumber (6.99 mg/100 g f.w.) and ginger (11.50 mg/100 g f.w.) (Ogunlesi et al. 2010).

3.4 VITAMIN E (TOCOPHEROLS)

The term ‘vitamin E’ refers to a family of eight naturally occurring homologues that are synthesized by plants from homogentisic acid. As an anti-oxidant, vitamin E plays a protective role in many organs and systems. Other functions include enzymatic activities, gene expression and neurological functions. Out of eight possible isomers of vitamin E, α-tocopherol is the most biologically important anti-oxidant. Vitamin E shows protective effects against coronary heart disease due to the inhibition of LDL oxidation. It is considered as the ‘standard anti-oxidant’ to which other compounds with anti-oxidant activities are compared, especially in terms of its biological activity and clinical relevance. Fresh bamboo shoots are a good source of vitamin E (Visuphaka 1985, Xia1989, Shi and Yang 1992, Chongtham et al. 2008). Vitamin E content of shoots ranged from 0.27 mg/100 g f.w. to 0.91 mg/100 g f.w. in different bamboo species (Table 3.1) and is comparatively higher than reported in some commonly used vegetables such as cabbage (0.08 mg/100 g f.w.), cauliflower (0.15 mg/100 g f.w.) and broccoli (0.49 mg/100 g f.w.). Vitamin E may work synergistically with vitamin C in enhancing immune function. Recent research evidence indicates that the combined use of vitamin E and vitamin C helps to prevent Alzheimer disease. It is also needed for the development of the retina in the eyes and protects against cataracts and macular degeneration. Bamboo shoot is not only rich in vitamin C and E, but it is a good multivitamin food that can act as a foundation of good health.

4 Bioactive Compounds in Bamboo Shoots

Food is no longer considered to be just a means by which to curb hunger and/or satisfy the appetite. Modern scientific research has highlighted the active role played by food in the prevention and cure of several chronic diseases such as cardiovascular diseases, cancers, metabolic disorders and so on, as well as the role food plays in improving physical and mental well-being. Scientific studies have attributed the positive impact of foods to their phytochemical constituents or bioactive compounds. Bioactive compounds are extra-nutrient, secondary metabolites with potent health promoting effects. These compounds though not essential for fundamental plant physiological processes, play some important biological functions such as defense against herbivores, the attraction of pollinators and cell signalling. Many epidemiological studies suggest that large consumption of fruit and vegetables can counteract the development of several chronic and degenerative diseases because of the presence of bioactive molecules in these foods (Mattioli et al. 2018). Several groups of bioactive compounds are known to exist naturally in a wide variety of plant foods and food products, for example polyphenols, carotenoids, anthocyanins, phytosterols, dietary fibres, alkaloids, glycosides and so on, and impart specific health benefits upon consumption of such plant foods and food products (Bernhoft et al. 2010, Singh et al. 2016). Hence, a lot of research is being carried out focusing on new bioactive molecules in plants and on the effects that these molecules have on human health. Foods particularly rich in bioactive compounds play an active role in the prevention and cure of chronic diseases and are often termed as functional foods.

Because of the associated health benefits backed by strong scientific evidence, consumption of bioactive compound rich foods especially fruits and vegetables have gone upscale in recent times, driven by increased health consciousness among people. Globally, the health sector continues to expand faster than the rest of the economy (Figure 4.1). The use of bamboo shoots in the traditional medicinal system has been known for centuries across Asia, but it is only recently that the presence of several bioactive compounds such as phytosterols, phenolic compounds and dietary fibres has been confirmed scientifically. These bioactive compounds have been proven to impart bamboo shoots with several health benefits such as improvement of bowel function and digestion, reducing serum cholesterol, neuroprotective, anti-inflammatory, anti-microbial and anti-oxidant properties, prevention of diabetes, obesity, metabolic disorders, cardiovascular diseases and even certain types of cancer.

4.1 PHENOLIC COMPOUNDS

Phenolic compounds constitute a large and diverse class of natural secondary metabolites widespread in plants produced mostly via shikimate, phenylpropanoid, flavonoid, anthocyanin and lignin pathways and have attracted both public and

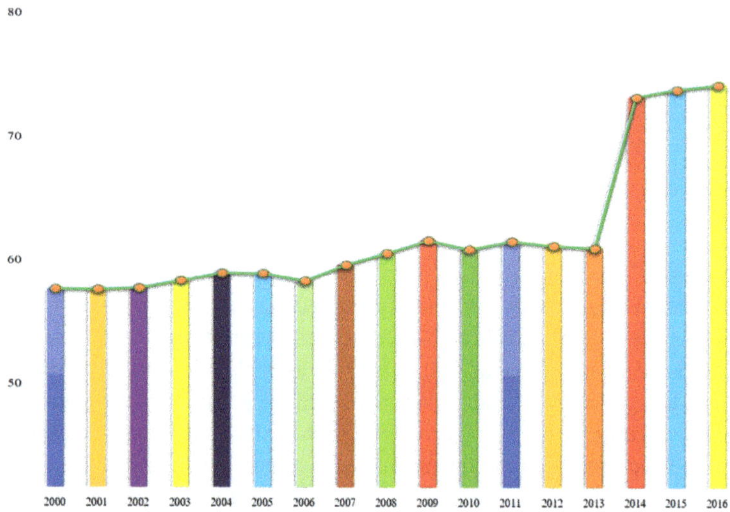

FIGURE 4.1 Increasing domestic health expenditure of the world, 2000–2016 as a percent of government expenditure (WHO 2019).

scientific interest because of their health promoting effects and potential applications. Structurally, phenols are simple aromatic hydrocarbons having either one (phenol) or more than one hydroxyl group substitution (polyphenols). Based on their molecular structure, more than 8,000 different phenolic compounds have been identified (Ribas-Agusti et al. 2018). A major group of plant phenolic compounds includes flavonoids (flavones, flavonols, anthocyanidins, isoflavones, etc.), tannins, chalcones, coumarins and phenolic acids (Giada 2013). Phenolic compounds signify the largest groups of natural anti-oxidants mainly because of the strong hydrogen-donating properties of their hydroxyl groups. They prevent the oxidative damage of various biomolecules such as DNA, lipids and proteins by scavenging various reactive species such as super-oxide radicals, hydroxyl radical, peroxyl radicals, hypochlorous acid and peroxynitrous acid, and also by chelating metal ions thus playing an important role in prevention of various chronic diseases such as cardiovascular diseases, gastric ulcers, cancer or hepatic encephalopathy and so on. Other health benefits of phenols include anti-diabetes, anti-hypertension, anti-inflammatory, anti-allergic, anti-microbial and cardioprotective properties (Puupponen-Pimiä et al. 2001, González-Gallego et al. 2007, Landete 2012, Saliu et al. 2012). These health beneficial effects of phenols have been ascribed to their strong anti-oxidant property. The major anti-oxidants and other nutrients which play an important role in the anti-oxidant defense system of bamboo shoots are vitamins C and E, phenolic compounds and minerals such as selenium, copper, manganese, iron and zinc (Chongtham et al. 2018). All of these anti-oxidants may act together to reduce reactive oxygen levels more effectively than single dietary anti-oxidants because they can function as synergists. Apart from their strong anti-oxidant nature, preventive action of phenolic compounds against non-transmissible chronic diseases can also be linked to their regulatory roles on several metabolic processes such as enzyme inhibition, protein phosphorylation, modification of gene expression and so on (Laura et al. 2019). Phenolic acids present in the tender bamboo shoots have mild anti-inflammatory properties and are potent anti-oxidants that prevent cancer and blood vessel injury that can lead to atherosclerosis. It has also been confirmed that there is a significant correlation between total phenolic content and anti-oxidant activity in bamboo shoots (Velioglu et al. 1998, Nemenyi et al. 2015). The phenolic compounds in bamboo consist mainly of caffeic acid, catechin, chlorogenic acid, ferulic acid, p-coumaric acid p-hydroxybenzoic acid, protocatechuic acid and syringic acid Figure 4.2 and Figure 4.3.

In our studies conducted on 20 bamboo species, total phenol content ranged from 362 mg/100 g to 907 mg/100 g f.w. with the least in *Bambusa balcooa* and the highest in *Dendrocalamus latiflorus* (Table 4.1). Nemenyi et al. (2015) analyzed total phenolic content and its relationship with total anti-oxidant capacity in shoots of 14 species of *Phyllostachys* viz. *P. aureosulcata*, *P. aureosulcata* f. *aureocaulis*, *P. aureosulcata* f. *spectabilis*, *P. bissetii*, *P. flexuosa*, *P. humilis*, *P. iridescens*, *P. nigra* var. *nigra*, *P. nigra* var. *henonis*, *P. mannii*, *P. sulphurea* var. *sulphurea*, *P. violascens*, *P. viridiglaucescens* and *P. vivax* f. *aureocaulis*, collected on four harvest dates. The highest values of total phenols were measured in the case of *P. aureosulcata* (1321.95 µg GAE/ml) and lowest was in the case of *P. vivax* f. *aureocaulis* (826.22 µg GAE/ml), while the highest anti-oxidant capacity values were obtained in the case of *P. iridescens* (184.24 µg GAE/ml) and the lowest in the case of *P. humilis* (89.63 µg GAE/ml). Table 4.1

Kozukue et al. (1998) studied the changes in phenolic compounds in bamboo shoots during storage at 20°C. They found that the content of crude phenolic

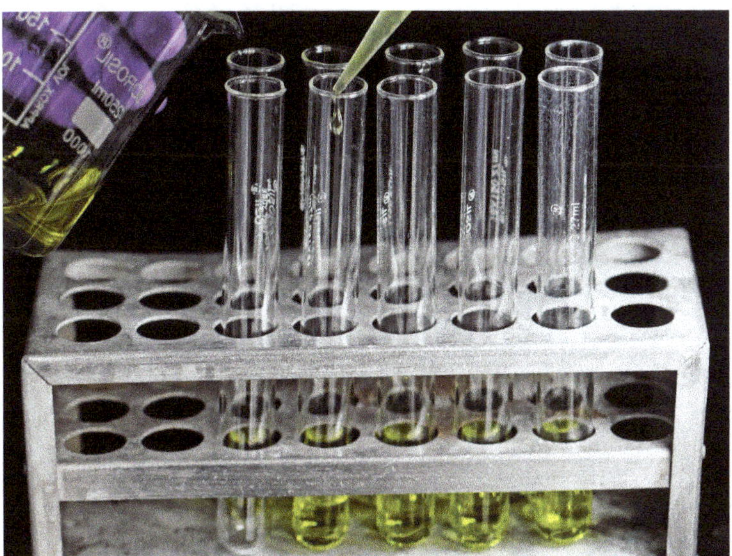

FIGURE 4.2 Total phenol estimation from bamboo shoot extract using Folin-Ciocalteu reagent.

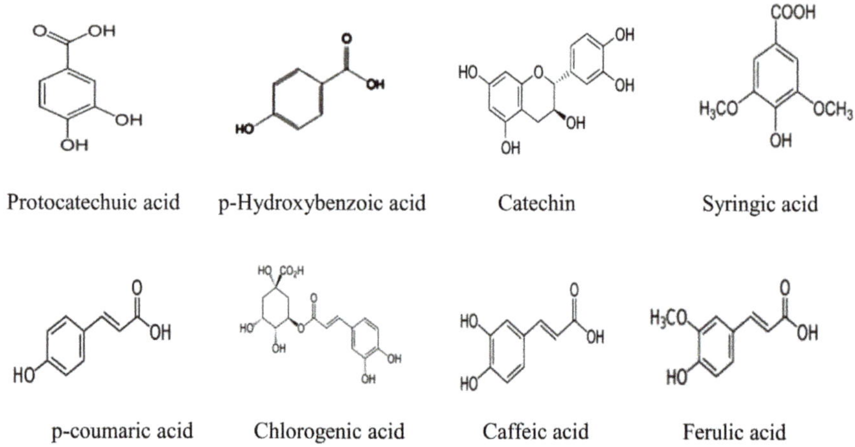

FIGURE 4.3 Some phenolic compounds in bamboo shoots. (Modified from Chongtham et al 2011.)

TABLE 4.1
Phenol and Phytosterol Content in Some Species of Bamboo Shoots

Sr. No.	Species	Phenol (mg/100g f.w.)	Phytosterol (mg/100g d.w.)
1.	*Bambusa balcooa*	362.36 ± 4.80	127.24 ± 2.86
2.	*B. bambos*	721.24 ± 6.80	198.69 ± 7.92
3.	*B. cacharensis*	375.84 ± 4.40	149.41 ± 4.34
4.	*B. manipureana*	383.60 ± 8.22	162.34 ± 1.79
5.	*B. mizorameana*	776.79 ± 5.21	262.48 ± 1.22
6.	*B. nutans*	558.96 ± 2.32	91.37 ± 2.44
7.	*B. tulda*	561.70 ± 2.17	99.13 ± 1.66
8.	*B. vulgaris*	395.47 ± 5.70	133.04 ± 3.03
9.	*Cephalostachyum capitatum*	357.11 ± 6.90	159.18 ± 3.03
10.	*Chimonobambusa callosa*	532.25 ± 3.67	137.35 ± 1.00
11.	*Dendrocalamus giganteus*	616.50 ± 4.80	196.14 ± 1.23
12.	*D. hamiltonii*	678.56 ± 2.34	131.73 ± 1.68
13.	*D. hookeri*	539.10 ± 6.11	150.28 ± 2.17
14.	*D. longispathus*	420.59 ± 3.62	91.37 ± 3.45
15.	*D. manipureanus*	720.62 ± 4.35	157.46 ± 2.63
16.	*D. membranaceus*	471.73 ± 7.56	178.07 ± 12.35
17.	*D. latiflorus*	907.39 ± 3.54	89.90 ± 0.02
18.	*D. sikkimensis*	450.29 ± 5.00	122.08 ± 4.27
19.	*Melocanna baccifera*	426.07 ± 5.48	144.53 ± 4.34
20.	*Phyllostachys mannii*	382.23 ± 2.08	265.49 ± 3.16

Values reported are measurement replication means ± standard deviation (n = 3 replicates).

compounds soon after the harvest was 165 mg and 106 mg per 100 g f.w., in the apical and basal portions of the shoots, respectively, and these levels decreased during storage. They also identified 25 individual phenolic compounds in the shoots using GC-MS analysis, including 5-dehydroshikimic acid, shikimic acid, p-hydroxyphenylethanol, p-hydroxyphenylpropionic acid, ferulic acid, 5-Dihydroshikimic acid and shikimic acid, caffeic acid and chlorogenic acid. Lu and Xu (2004) studied the polyphenolic content of the different portions of shoots of *Phyllostachys heterocycla* var. *pubescens* and found that polyphenol content was maximum in the apical region (around 60 mg/g f.w.) and it decreased towards the middle and basal portions. Shen et al. (2006) studied the total polyphenol content of the *Phyllostachys praecox* shoots which was around 1.6 mg/g f.w. Ito et al. (2007) also studied the effect of lig-8, a lignophenol derivative from bamboo, on the protection from neurodegenerative disorders.

The functional properties of edible shoots of *Phyllostachys pubescens* and *Phyllostachys nigra* were evaluated from shoot extracts for their anti-oxidant capacity, anti-microbial activity, angiotensin converting enzyme inhibition activity, ascorbic acid and phenolic compound content (Park and Jhon 2010). Using high performance liquid chromatography, eight phenolic acids (protocatechuic acid, p-hydroxybenzoic acid, catechin, caffeic acid, chlorogenic acid, syringic acid, p-coumaric acid and ferulic acid) were identified amongst which protocatechuic acid, p-hydroxybenzoic acid and syringic acid were the most abundant. Comparison of anti-oxidant capacities between extracts of bamboo shoots was performed and anti-microbial test of phenolic compounds on some bacterial and fungal strains was conducted. Of the two species tested, *P. nigra* showed higher extraction yield, anti-oxidant capacity and ascorbic acid and phenolic compound content than *P. pubescens* (Park and Jhon 2010). Two anti-microbial peptides designated Pp-AMP-1 and Pp-AMP-2 which have anti-microbial activity against pathogenic bacteria and fungi, were purified from the shoot of *Phyllostachys pubescens* using chitin affinity chromatography (Fujimura et al. 2005). The presence of tannins, steroids, phenols and flavonoids were reported from methanol and ethyl acetate extracts of fermented shoots (Singh et al. 2012). Their therapeutic potential was confirmed by the anti-microbial property of the methanolic extract against four bacterial strains, *Staphylococcus aureus*, *Bacillus subtilis*, *Pseudomonas aeruginosa* and *Escherichia coli*, and three fungal strains, viz. *Aspergillus niger*, *Candida albicans* and *Fusarum oxyporum*. Dichloromethane extracts prepared from bamboo shoot skins of Moso bamboo *Phyllostachys pubescens* have been reported to have anti-bacterial activity against *Staphylococcus aureus* (Tanaka et al. 2011). Moso bamboo shoot skins have been traditionally used as a preservative to maintain the taste of tea in China and as a packaging material for rice balls and meat in Japan.

Yang et al. (2010), while investigating the effect of nitric oxide on browning and lignification of peeled bamboo shoots of *Phyllostachys violascens*, determined the total phenols of the shoot samples which was 23.5 mg/g of f.w. which decreased upon storage. Pandey et al. (2012) analyzed the total phenol content in the fresh shoots of four species, that is *Bambusa bambos*, *B. tulda*, *Dendrocalamus asper* and *D. strictus* and reported maximum total phenol content in *D. strictus* (1.25 g/100 g). The total by-products of canned bamboo shoots were analyzed by Liu et al. (2013), who showed that the ethyl extract fraction exhibited high anti-oxidant capacity that was attributed to flavonoid and phenolic acid content and could thereby be used for the prevention of hypertension and attenuation of oxidative stress. Pandey and Ojha (2013) analyzed the effect of harvesting age on the total phenolic content in shoots of three species, that is *Bambusa tulda*, *Dendrocalamus asper* and *D. strictus*, with *D. strictus* having maximum phenol content (2.26%) at optimum harvesting age. Furthermore, they isolated four different phenolic acids in the shoots namely gallic acid, vanillic acid, chlorogenic acid and caffeic acid. The total phenol content and anti-oxidant activity in the fresh shoots of *Bambusa balcooa* were determined by Badwaik et al. (2014). The total phenol content was 97.5 mg/100 g, whereas the anti-oxidant activity was found to be 26.62 % of DPPH radical scavenging activity. Furthermore, Badwaik et al. (2015) studied the total phenol content and anti-oxidant activity in fresh shoots of four species, that is *Bambusa balcooa*, *B. pallida*, *B. tulda* and *Dendrocalamus hamiltonii*. Total phenol of four species ranged from 79.85 mg/100 g to 101.65 mg/100 g, and total anti-oxidant activity ranged from 19.17% to 27.12% of DPPH radical scavenging activity. Thomas et al. (2016) studied the total phenol content of shoot extracts of *Bambusa polymorpha* and found it to be 246 mg GAE/100 g. They also reported that the addition of bamboo shoot extracts significantly lowered the levels of lipid oxidation in pork nuggets thus confirming the strong anti-oxidant property of phenols present in bamboo shoot extract.

Rawat et al. (2016) estimated the total phenol content of the young shoots of *Dendrocalamus giganteus*, *D. latiflorus* and *D. sikkimensis* which ranged from 450.29 to 627.39 mg/100 g f.w. Total phenol content of leaves and culm extract of five native species viz. *Aulonemia aristulata*, *Chusquea bambusoides*, *C. capituliflora*, *C. meyeriana* and *Merostachys pluriflora* were estimated by Wróblewska et al. (2019) and the content ranged from 43.64 mg GAE/g to 87.81 mg GAE/g. Chauhan et al. (2017a) analyzed the total phenol content, total flavonoid content, anti-oxidant activity and anti-lipid peroxidation activity of different fractions of methanolic extracts of *Bambusa arundinacea* shoots. They found that total phenol content and total flavonoid content was highest in n-butanol fraction 56.6 mg GAE/g d.w. and ethyl acetate fraction 47 mg QUE/g d.w., respectively. Anti-oxidant activity and anti-lipid peroxidation activity, on the other hand, was found to be highest in the case of ethyl acetate fractions, 40.33 IC_{50} of DPPH and 61.89, respectively. Chauhan et al. (2017a) revealed that bamboo shoots are viable sources of natural anti-oxidants being particularly rich in phenolic and flavonoid content and can thus be further exploited for their applications in functional foods and nutraceuticals. Chauhan et al. (2017b) analyzed the hepatoprotective activity of *Bambusa arundinacea* shoot extracts against thioacetamide induced cytotoxicity in HepG2 and Hep3b tumor cell lines (*in-vitro*) and against liver injury in Wistar rats (in-vivo). They reported that methanolic extracts of bamboo shoot were able to significantly reduce thioacetamide induced decrease in cell viability *in-vitro* and showed a protective effect against liver injury in rats *in-vivo* in a dose dependent manner and authors attributed these properties to the presence of high phenolic and flavonoid content in shoots. Wani et al. (2019) while screening shoots of *Bambusa balcooa* for the presence of phytochemicals to be used against bovine reproductive disorders, found that total phenol content ranged from 1.01 to 3.17 mg GAE/g while the total flavonoid content was between

0.88 to 12.24 mg CNE/g. Shoots of *D. hamiltonii* in paste form were used for fortifying cookies as reported by Santosh et al. (2018) who reported that the addition of shoot paste increased the total phenol content of the cookies by 40 to 60%, indicating a strong potential of bamboo shoots for food fortification.

4.2 PHYTOSTEROLS

Plant sterols or phytosterols, the structural and functional counterpart of cholesterol in plant kingdom have gained lots of acclaim in recent times due to their potential implications for human health. They are the major parts of the non-saponifiable fraction of lipids. Scientific evidences supporting their beneficial action on reducing serum cholesterol and low-density lipoprotein (LDL) cholesterol levels, reducing blood cholesterol levels, anti-microbial, anti-inflammatory and anti-cancerous properties as well as their other beneficial health effects have resulted in promotion of phytosterol-rich plant-based diets (Jones et al. 1997, Plat and Mensink 2005, Jones and AbuMweis 2009, Woyengo et al. 2009, Moreau et al. 2018, Vilahur et al. 2019). Sitosterol, campesterol and stigmasterol are the major plant sterols and constitute about 65%, 30% and 3%, respectively.

Phytosterols are present in both fresh and fermented bamboo shoots. In shoots of 20 species (Table 4.1) phytosterol ranged from 89.90 to 265.49 mg/100 g d.w. Srivastava (1990) estimated the phytosterol content in the fresh shoots of two species *Bambusa tulda* and *Dendrocalamus giganteus* and it was found to be 0.21% and 0.39%, respectively, on a dry weight basis. Major phytosterols including β-sitosterol, campesterol and stigmasterol are reported from shoots of several bamboo species (Figure 4.4) including *Bambusa oldhamii*, *B. edulis*, *Dendrocalamus latiflorus*, *Phyllostachys edulis*, *P. pubescens* and *P. makinoi*. They proposed a hypocholesterolemic formulation with potent cholesterol lowering properties and suggested that these phytosterols act by inhibiting or reducing the cholesterol absorption and cholesterol synthesis and/or by faecal extraction of neutral and acid sterols (He and Lachance 1998, Lachance and He 1998).

Sarangthem et al. (2003) estimated the total phytosterol content of seven different bamboo species, that is *Arundinaria callosa*, *Bambusa balcooa*, *B. pallida*, *B. khasiana*, *Cephalostachyum pergracile*, *Dendrocalamus hamiltonii* and *D. strictus* which ranged from 0.12% to 0.19 % with highest being in *B. pallida* and *D. hamiltonii* while the lowest content was reported from *B. khasiana*. Sarangthem and Singh (2003) reported the total phytosterol content of *B. balcooa* and *D. strictus* to be 0.18% and 0.14%, respectively, on dry weight basis.

Effect of genetic variability, parts and seasons on phytosterol content and composition in shoots of four species namely *Dendrocalamus latiflorus*, *Phyllostachys praecox*, *Pleioblastus amarus* and *Phyllostachys pubescens* were analyzed by Lu et al. (2009b). They found that the total phytosterol content in bamboo shoots ranged from 112.4 to 279.6 mg/100 g d.w. in four species with the highest being in *P. pubescens* and lowest being in *D. latiflorus* while the phytosterol composition included β-sitosterol, campesterol, stigmasterol, ergosterol, cholesterol and stigmastanol. Furthermore, they also found out that shoot shells contain much higher phytosterol as compared to shoot body itself (321.8 mg/100 g d.w. in *P. pubescens*) and can be

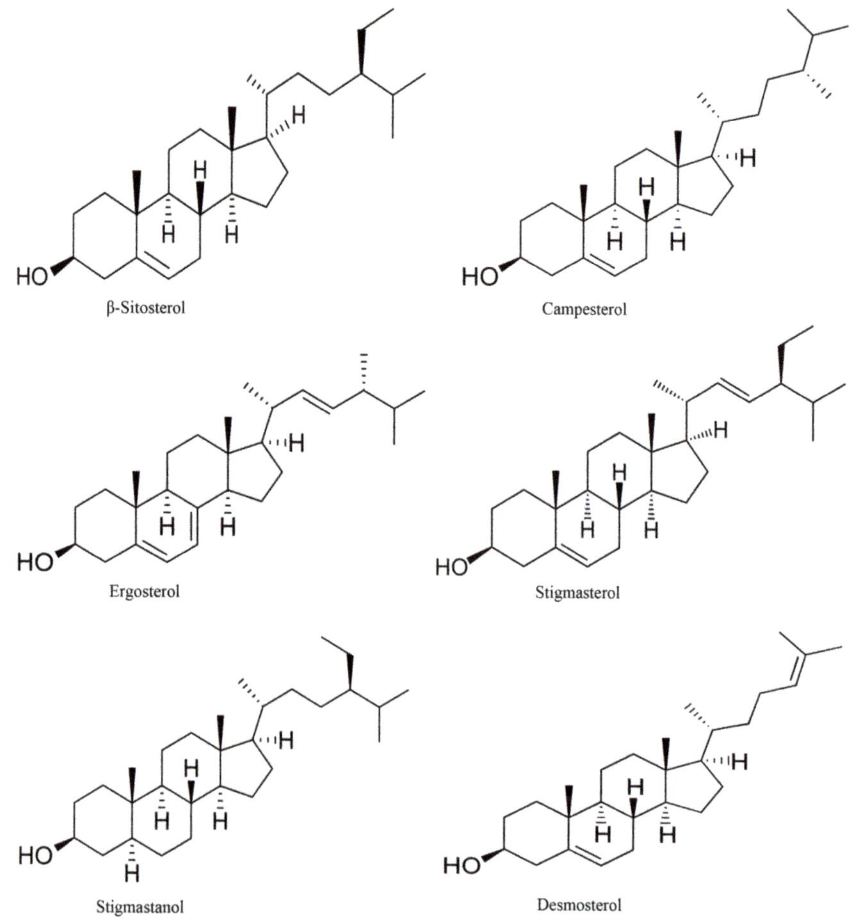

FIGURE 4.4 Chemical structures of some phytosterols in bamboo shoots. (Modified from Chongtham et al. 2011.)

more effective in lowering cholesterol levels. The effect of the harvest seasons on the sterol content and composition in bamboo shoots was investigated using shoots of *P. pubescens* harvested in winter (226.2 mg/100 g), spring (279.6 mg/100 g) and summer (195.3 mg/100 g). The shoot harvested in spring contained the highest level of β-sitosterol (83.33%), those harvested in winter contained the highest level of cholesterol (3.4%) and the shoot harvested in summer contained the highest level of ergosterol (0.86%). These findings suggest that the spring shoot shell of *P. pubescens* is a potential source of dietary sterol which can be generated from industrial waste in the course of processing of bamboo shoots. Phytosterols are precursors of many pharmaceutically important steroid products such as corticosteroids, oral contraceptives and anti-inflammatories, synthetic anabolic steroids and estrogenic hormones. Thus, succulent bamboo shoots which are easily available in large quantities can be used as a source of phytosterols.

Shoots of *Phyllostachys pubescens* were subjected to supercritical CO_2 extraction method to extract bamboo shoot oil (BSO) and several phytosterols and their derivatives such as β-sitosterol, campesterol, stigmasterol, ergosterol, cholesterol, stigmastanol were identified in it using GC-MS analysis. Maximum concentration of 26% is that of β-sitosterol (Lu et al. 2009a,b). Furthermore, Lu et al. (2010) studied the hypolipidemic effect of BSO extracted from *P. pubescens* in rats and proved that BSO with its relatively higher phytosterol content compared to other vegetable oil, can be an ideal dietary supplement for lowering serum cholesterol levels. In another study, Lu et al. (2011) analyzed the effect of this phytosterol-rich BSO on non-bacterial prostatitis (NBS). Their result showed that BSO was able to inhibit prostate inflammation by altering the expression pattern of inflammatory cytokines, their receptors and other genes related to inflammation mechanism. Therefore, it was proposed that BSO can be a useful raw ingredient in future medicinal formulations aimed at treating chronic non-bacterial prostatitis. Tanaka et al. (2013) studied the anti-microbial activity of bamboo shoot skins of *P. pubescens* and found that the dichloromethane-soluble methanol extract from the shoot skins was able to inhibit the growth of bacteria *Staphylococcus aureus*. They further isolated the active constituents responsible for anti-microbial activity and identified phytosterols namely stigmasterol and dihydrobrassicasterol by NMR and mass spectrometry. These studies, therefore, support the fact that bamboo shoot contains very high quantities of major phytosterols and have potential health benefits to human populations.

Bajwa et al. (2015) evaluated the total phytosterol content of four bamboo species, that is *Bambusa nutans, Dendrocalamus giganteus, D. hamiltonii and D. latiflorus* which ranged from 136.23 to 198.2 mg/100 g f.w. The total phytosterol content of bamboo shoots of 12 species *Dendrocalamus brandisii, D. strictus, D. giganteus, D. flagellifer, D. hamiltonii, D. sericeus, Bambusa tulda, B. balcooa, B. nutans, B. kingiana, B. khasiana* and *Cephalostachyum pergracile* was determined by Ingudam and Sarangthem (2016). Total phytosterol content of shoots ranged from 40.5 mg/100 g (*B. kingiana*) to 293.8 mg/100 g (*D. hamiltonii*) on a dry weight basis. Phytosterol content in all the investigated species was highest in the top apex portion of the shoots followed by the middle and basal part. Furthermore, outer culm sheaths of shoots which were generally discarded during the processing of shoots also contained significant phytosterol content ranging from 35.5 mg/100 g to 119.7 mg/100 g d.w.. Rawat et al. (2016) reported that young shoots of *Dendrocalamus giganteus, D. latiflorus and D. sikkimensis* contain significantly high quantities of total phytosterol, which ranged from 89.90 to 196.14 mg/100g f.w. These studies, therefore, support the fact that bamboo shoot contains very high quantities of major phytosterols and has potential health benefits to human populations.

Saini (2019) used gas chromatography combined with mass spectrometry (GC-MS) to analyze phytosterols of shoots of *B. bambos*, *B. nutans* and *D. sikkimensis*. The GC-MS chromatography showed various peaks of multiple compounds which on reckoning with NIST library affirmed the presence of three main phytosterols, β-sitosterol, stigmasterol and campesterol (Figure 4.5). β-sitosterol was the dominant sterol with maximum concentration in the fermented shoots in all the three species (Table 4.2) The fermented shoots in all three species also had the highest content of campesterol. The stigmasterol content was quite variable in the different processed forms.

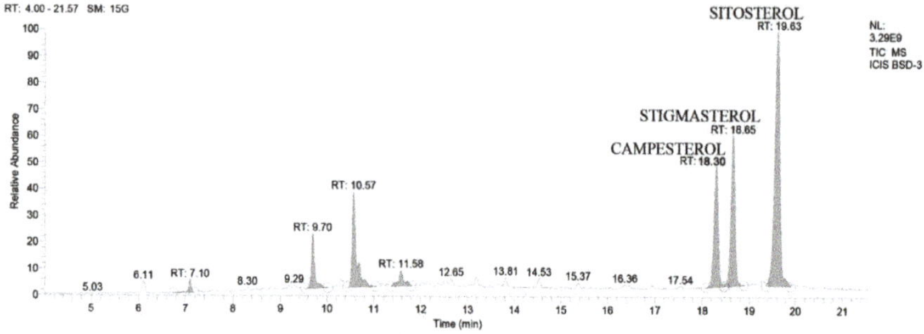

Component Name	RT	Calculated Amount	Area
CAMPESTEROL	18.30	137.363	281209910.08
STIGMASTEROL	18.65	282.308	276634552.94
SITOSTEROL	19.64	710.713	805061478.64

FIGURE 4.5 GC-MS chromatogram showing phytosterols in oven-dried shoots of *B. bambos*.

The phytosterol content in bamboo shoots is higher than the quantity present in commonly consumed vegetables, fruits and vegetables (Table. 4.3). Amongst vegetables, beet root had the highest phytosterol content (171 mg/100 g f.w.) whereas, in legumes, chickpea had the highest content (121 mg/100 g f.w.). This is quite less as compared to bamboo shoots wherein, the phytosterol content ranged from 131.4 to 196 mg/100 g f.w. (See Table 4.2, Table. 4.3 and Figure 4.6.)

4.3 DIETARY FIBRES

Dietary fibre is defined as edible parts of plants or analogous carbohydrates that are resistant to digestion and absorption in the small human intestine with complete or partial fermentation in the large intestine. Based on water solubility, dietary fibre is divided into two forms: (i) insoluble dietary fibre (IDF), which includes celluloses, some hemicelluloses, galactomannans, xylans, xyloglucans and lignin; and (ii) soluble dietary fibre (SDF), which includes β-glucans, pectins, gums mucilages and some hemicelluloses (Căpriţă et al. 2010). Consumption of food or food products rich in dietary fibre content has been shown to be beneficial in improving digestive function, reducing serum cholesterol levels, normalizing blood sugar levels, easing constipation, prevention of diabetes, obesity and cardiovascular diseases (Fernandez 2001, Merchant et al. 2003, Anderson 2008, Delzenne et al. 2019). Dietary fibre has not only health benefits, but also imparts some functional properties to foods, for example increase water holding capacity, oil holding capacity, emulsification and/or gel formation. Dietary fibre incorporated into food such as bakery and dairy products, jams, meats and soups can modify textural properties, avoid synaeresis, stabilize high fat food and emulsions and improve shelf-life (Elleuch et al. 2011).

Bamboo shoots contain a significant amount of dietary fibre, classified as neutral detergent fibre (NDF), which determines the indigestible component of the plant material consisting of hemicelluloses, cellulose and lignin and acid detergent fibre (ADF) primarily representing cellulose and lignin (Chongtham et al. 2009). Chen

TABLE 4.2

Major Phytosterols β-Sitosterol, Stigmasterol and Campesterol (ppm on a Dry Weight Basis) in Shoots of Three Bamboo Species

		Treatment					
Species		**Freeze-Dried**	**Oven-Dried**	**Sun-Dried**	**Boiled**	**Soaked**	**Fermented**
B. bambos	**β-Sitosterol**	865.14	710.71	1015.32	1118.98	1155.75	1412.52
B. nutans		810.14	741.25	1035.63	850.63	912.12	1290.83
D. sikkimensis		433.40	428.71	527.94	560.90	683.04	744.27
B. bambos	**Stigmasterol**	130.80	282.30	212.02	146.32	164.38	302.11
B. nutans		131.51	162.27	150.47	237.95	256.53	240.91
D. sikkimensis		72.97	82.07	76.47	66.55	185.18	126.88
B. bambos	**Campesterol**	171.96	137.36	216.21	216.15	254.47	288.13
B. nutans		137.80	133.28	192.28	133.44	172.78	270.81
D. sikkimensis		83.72	68.65	96.49	104.26	105.84	144.83

TABLE 4.3

A Comparative Account of Total Phenolic (mg/100 g f.w.) and Phytosterol Content (mg/100 g d.w.) of Bamboo Shoots and Some Common Food Items

Species	Phenols	Phytosterols	References
	Bamboo Species		
Bambusa nutans	558.96 ± 23.24	181.59 ± 3.88	Saini 2019
Dendrocalamus latiflorus	659.11 ± 0.84	160.76 ± 1.29	Devi 2018
D. hamiltonii	678.56 ± 2.34	131.73 ± 1.68	Rawat 2017
D. giganteus	609.32 ± 1.2	196.14 ± 1.23	Sharma 2018
Phyllostachys mannii	382.23 ± 2.08	265.49 ± 3.16	Rawat 2017
	Vegetables		
Broccoli (*Brassica oleracea* var. *italica*)	87.50 ± 8.10	18.3± 1.30	Kaur and Kapoor 2002, Jimenez-Escrig et al. 2006
Beet root (*Beta vulgaris*)	323.0 ± 11.70	171.00 ± 70	Kaur and Kapoor 2002, Piironen et al. 2003
Carrot (*Daucus carota*)	55.0 ± 0.90	18.6 ± 1.5	Kaur and Kapoor 2002, Jimenez-Escrig et al. 2006
Cauliflower (*Brassica oleracea* var. *botrytis*)	96.0 ± 0.90	44.3 ± 1.2	Kaur and Kapoor 2002, Jimenez-Escrig et al. 2006
Cabbage (*Brassica oleracea* var. *capitata*)	92.5 ± 2.40	27.4 ± 1.9	Kaur and Kapoor 2002, Jimenez-Escrig et al. 2006
Beans (*Phaseolus vulgaris*)	97.0 ± 1.10	18.8 ± 0.8	Weihrauch and Gardner 1978, Jimenez-Escrig et al. 2006
	Fruits		
Apple (*Pyrus malus*)	296.3 ± 6.40	16.0 ± 0.9	Sun et al. 2002a, Jimenez-Escrig et al. 2006
Banana (*Musa paradisiaca*)	90.4 ± 3.20	20.1 ± 1.2	Sun et al. 2002a, Jimenez-Escrig et al. 2006
Cherry (*Prunus avium*)	105.4 ± 27.0	20.1 ± 1.4	Karakaya et al. 2001, Jimenez-Escrig et al. 2006
	Legumes		
Chickpea (*Cicer arietinum*)	2.20	121.2 ± 4.7	Jimenez-Escrig et al. 2006, Han and Baik 2008
Lentils (*Lens culinaris*)	12.00	117.3 ± 5.6	Jimenez-Escrig et al. 2006, Han and Baik 2008
	Nuts		
Almond (*Prunus amygdalus*)	239	148.6 ± 4.5	Jimenez-Escrig et al. 2006, Kornsteiner et al. 2006
Peanut (*Arachis hypogaea*)	420	143.6 ± 4.1	Jimenez-Escrig et al. 2006, Kornsteiner et al. 2006
	Beverages		
Coffee (Instant)	146–151		Schulz et al. 1999
Black Tea	80.5–134.9		Khokhar and Magnusdottir 2002
Green Tea	65.8–106.2		Khokhar and Magnusdottir 2002
Red wine	242		Baroni et al. 2012

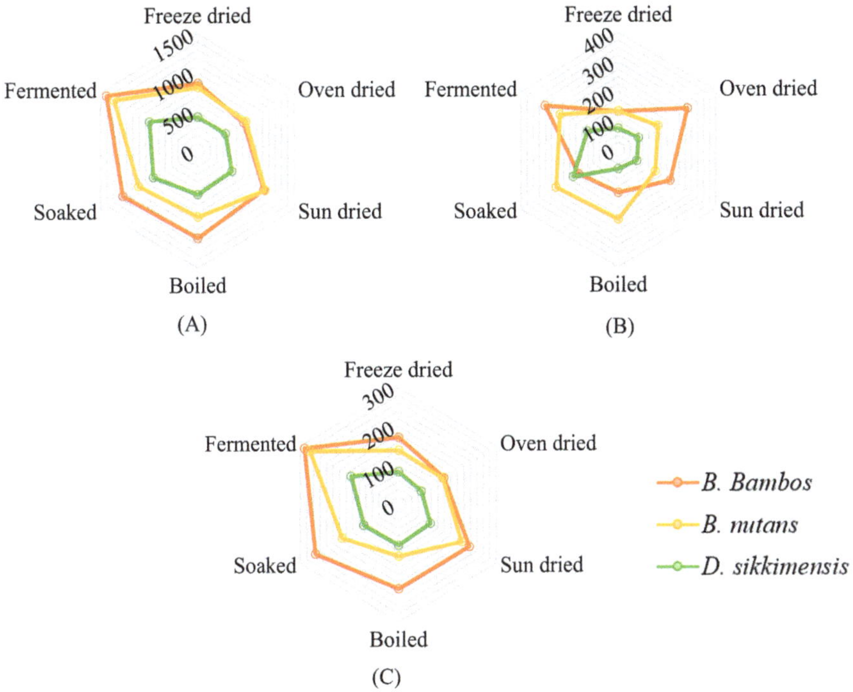

FIGURE 4.6 Radar chart showing (A) β-Sitosterol, (B) Stigmasterol, (C) Campesterol contents in the shoots of different processed forms of three bamboo species (ppm on dry weight basis).

et al. (1985) reported a high content of hemicelluloses, a major component of dietary fibre, in ten bamboo species that exists in the form of polyxylose. The crude fibre content of an apical and basal portion of *Dendrocalamus giganteus* shoots was reported by Ferreira et al. (1992) to be 0.96% and 0.97%, respectively, on a fresh weight basis. Rajyalakshmi and Geervani (1994) while analyzing the nutritive value of common foods consumed by tribals of South India, reported the crude fibre content in the shoots of *Bambusa arundinacea* (*Bambusa bambos*) to be 6.90% on a dry weight basis. Muchtadi and Adawiyah (1996) while studying the effect of drying on the nutritional characteristic of *Dendrocalamus asper* shoots reported the crude fibre content to be 5.2 g/100 g. Qiu et al. (1999) studied the nutritional constituents of *Phyllostachys heteroclada* shoots and reported that the crude fibre in the shoots ranged from 0.63% to 0.71%. The crude fibre content in the shoots of 11 bamboo species, that is *Bambusa balcooa*, *B. nutans*, *B. tulda*, *Dendrocalamus giganteus*, *D. hamiltonii*, *D. hookeri*, *D. longispathus*, *D. sikkimensis*, *Melocanna baccifera*, *Phyllostachys bambusoides*, *Teinostachyum wightii* was reported by Bhatt et al. (2005) to be in the range of 23.1 to 35.5%, with the highest being in the shoots of *M. baccifera*. Kumbhare and Bhargava (2007) while investigating the effect of processing on the nutritional values in the shoots of four central Indian bamboo species, that is *Bambusa nutans*, *B. vulgaris*, *Dendrocalamus asper*, *D. strictus* found out the crude fibre content in fresh shoots in the range of 0.71 % to 0.98%, which was significantly lesser as compared to previous reports on bamboo shoots. Chongtham et al. (2007) in a study to determine the nutrient changes in emerging juvenile shoots of five commercially important bamboos, that is *Bambusa bambos*, *B. tulda*, *D. asper*, *D. giganteus* and *D. hamiltonii* found that crude fibre in freshly emerged shoots ranged from 2.64 to 3.97% whereas in ten-day-old shoots, there was an increase in the fibre content ranging from 8.20% to 13.84%. Thirty bamboo species were analyzed for their fibre content by our team and it was found that the NDF content ranged from 2.25 to 7.4 g/100 g f.w. (Table 4.4). The fibre content was estimated by heat digestion using ADF and NDF reagent (Figure 4.7). The residue obtained was subjected to 500⁰C in a muffle furnace (Figure 4.8) and further analyzed for different fibre components. The fibre content of bamboo shoots is higher than most of the commonly consumed vegetables (Chongtham et al. 2011). Studies have been conducted to compare the nutrient and fibre content in fresh, fermented and canned shoots in a commercially important bamboo *Dendrocalamus giganteus* (Chongtham et al. 2008). The study revealed that freshly harvested shoots are richer in nutrient components as compared to canned and fermented shoots. There is an overall decrease in the nutrient components except for dietary fibre content during fermentation and canning.

Pandey et al. (2012) determined the crude fibre content in the fresh shoot samples of four species, that is *Bambusa bambos* (0.82 g/100 g), *B. tulda* (0.75 g/100 g), *Dendrocalamus asper* (0.76 g/100 g) and *D. strictus* (0.96 g/100 g). Moreover, they studied the effect of harvesting age on the dietary fibre content of the shoots of *Bambusa tulda*, *Dendrocalamus asper* and *D. strictus* (Pandey and Ojha 2013) and reported that dietary fibre content of the shoots increased with the harvesting age with optimum age of harvesting for the extraction of dietary fibre in case of *B. tulda* was 20 days (5.20%), for *D. asper* it was 18 days (3.86%) and for *D. strictus* it was 16 days (5.46%). Sood et al. (2013) analyzed the dietary fibre content in the shoots of *Dendrocalamus hamiltonii*. Their results showed crude fibre at 1.50%, NDF at 2.54%, ADF at 2.08% and Lignin at 0.49%. Shoots grown in Masha area of Ethiopia were studied by Awol (2015) who reported the fibre content to be 18.81%. Badwaik et al. (2015) reported fibre content ranging from 3.16 g/100 g to 3.92 g/100 g in fresh shoots of four species, that is *Bambusa balcooa*, *B. pallida*, *B. tulda* and *Dendrocalamus hamiltonii* which ranged from 3.16 g/100g to 3.92 g/100g. Thomas et al. (2016) determined the crude fibre content of shoot extracts of *Bambusa polymorpha* to be 5.8%. Figure 4.7 and Table 4.4.

Health benefits of dietary fibre from the bamboo shoot have been studied intensively. Naito et al. (1980) patented a methodology to make bamboo shoot powder under pressure and heat from the shoots of *Phyllostachys* species and their study confirmed the therapeutic effect of bamboo shoot powder administration against the acquired intestinal diverticulum mainly because of the high water-swellable fibrous material of the bamboo shoot. They suggested the use of bamboo shoot powder as a food additive for the prevention of intestinal diverticulum and hyperlipemia. Shi and Yang (1992) proposed that high cellulose content bamboo shoots may be helpful in improving gut microbial flora, reduce the fat products and improve the peristalsis of the intestine which could prevent intestine cancers. Shimizu et al. (1996) investigated the effect of bamboo shoot dietary fibre on the faecal steroidal profiles of rats and found an increase in faecal wet weight suggesting an improvement in bowel movement. The role of bamboo shoot dietary fibre in regulating intestinal microbial

TABLE 4.4
Dietary Fibre and Its Components in the Juvenile Shoots of Some Species (g/100 g f.w.)

Name of species	NDF	ADF	Lignin	Cellulose	Hemicellulose
Bambusa balcooa	6.07 ± 0.04	0.51 ± 0.02	0.30 ± 0.02	0.21 ± 0.01	5.56 ± 0.06
B. bambos	3.95 ± 0.12	0.48 ± 0.01	0.30 ± 0.02	0.18 ± 0.00	3.47 ± 0.06
B. cacharensis	4.78 ± 0.15	0.69 ± 0.02	0.35 ± 0.01	0.34 ± 0.02	4.09 ± 0.15
B. kingiana	4.49 ± 0.06	3.19 ± 0.04	2.01 ± 0.02	1.18 ± 0.02	1.30 ± 0.03
B. manipureana	4.30 ± 0.20	0.65 ± 0.02	0.33 ± 0.01	0.31 ± 0.02	3.65 ± 0.22
B. mizorameana	4.67 ± 0.02	1.68 ± 0.03	0.18 ± 0.01	1.49 ± 0.01	2.99 ± 0.09
B. nutans	5.34 ± 0.14	1.17 ± 0.05	0.78 ± 0.01	0.40 ± 0.02	4.17 ± 0.08
B. polymorpha	3.81 ± 0.05	2.29 ± 0.01	1.30 ± 0.01	0.99 ± 0.03	1.51 ± 0.04
B. tulda	4.62 ± 0.02	0.80 ± 0.03	0.54 ± 0.04	0.26 ± 0.04	3.82 ± 0.09
B. vulgaris	4.24 ± 0.01	3.28 ± 0.02	2.40 ± 0.01	0.78 ± 0.01	0.96 ± 0.09
Cephalostachyum capitatum	4.40 ± 0.09	0.65 ± 0.03	0.22 ± 0.03	0.43 ± 0.06	3.75 ± 0.12
Chimonobambusa callosa	4.68 ± 0.06	0.82 ± 0.02	0.32 ± 0.02	0.50 ± 0.02	3.86 ± 0.01
Dendrocalamus asper	3.54 ± 0.06	3.00 ± 0.01	1.26 ± 0.01	1.74 ± 0.00	0.47 ± 0.05
D. brandisii	4.02 ± 0.08	3.06 ± 0.06	2.01 ± 0.01	1.05 ± 0.05	0.96 ± 0.02
D. giganteus	5.60 ± 0.02	0.83 ± 0.01	0.49 ± 0.04	0.34 ± 0.02	4.77 ± 0.14
D. hamiltonii	4.78 ± 0.06	0.94 ± 0.02	0.68 ± 0.05	0.26 ± 0.02	3.84 ± 0.09
D. hookeri	5.01 ± 0.05	1.03 ± 0.02	0.11 ± 0.03	0.92 ± 0.06	3.97 ± 0.03
D. latiflorus	5.88 ± 0.01	0.87 ± 0.03	0.44 ± 0.02	0.43 ± 0.02	5.01 ± 0.04
D. longispathus	4.42 ± 0.12	0.68 ± 0.01	0.36 ± 0.04	0.32 ± 0.04	3.74 ± 0.13
D. manipureanus	7.40 ± 0.02	0.63 ± 0.02	0.21 ± 0.04	0.42 ± 0.03	6.77 ± 0.02
D. membranaceus	5.33 ± 0.12	1.93 ± 0.07	0.37 ± 0.03	1.56 ± 0.06	3.40 ± 0.04
D. sikkimensis	4.66 ± 0.04	0.93 ± 0.00	0.51 ± 0.04	0.42 ± 0.01	3.73 ± 0.05
D. strictus	2.25 ± 0.00	1.38 ± 0.02	0.64 ± 0.02	0.93 ± 0.09	0.84 ± 0.09
Gigantochloa albociliata	4.15 ± 0.10	3.75 ± 0.05	2.70 ± 0.05	1.05 ± 0.00	0.40 ± 0.02
G. rostrata	4.20 ± 0.09	3.32 ± 0.02	1.82 ± 0.02	1.50 ± 0.02	0.93 ± 0.06
Melocanna baccifera	4.32 ± 0.14	0.61 ± 0.03	0.16 ± 0.03	0.45 ± 0.04	3.71 ± 0.12
Phyllostachys mannii	5.72 ± 0.03	1.41 ± 0.05	0.17 ± 0.01	1.24 ± 0.01	4.31 ± 0.03
Schizostachyum dullooa	5.40 ± 0.08	0.53 ± 0.04	0.22 ± 0.04	0.31 ± 0.02	4.87 ± 0.03
Thyrsostachys oliveri	3.91 ± 0.02	2.84 ± 0.04	1.28 ± 0.01	1.56 ± 0.03	1.06 ± 0.09
T. siamensis	3.71 ± 0.05	2.15 ± 0.01	1.20 ± 0.01	1.25 ± 0.00	1.56 ± 0.04

Values reported are measurement replication means ± standard deviation (n = 3 replicates).

flora in mice model was studied by Anping (2005), who concluded that bamboo shoot dietary fibre can be useful in relieving constipation.

Park and Jhon (2009) compared the effect of a high-fibre bamboo shoot diet with a fibre-free control on eight women in the age group 21–23 years. Blood biochemical parameters such as glucose, triacylglycerols, total cholesterol, high-density

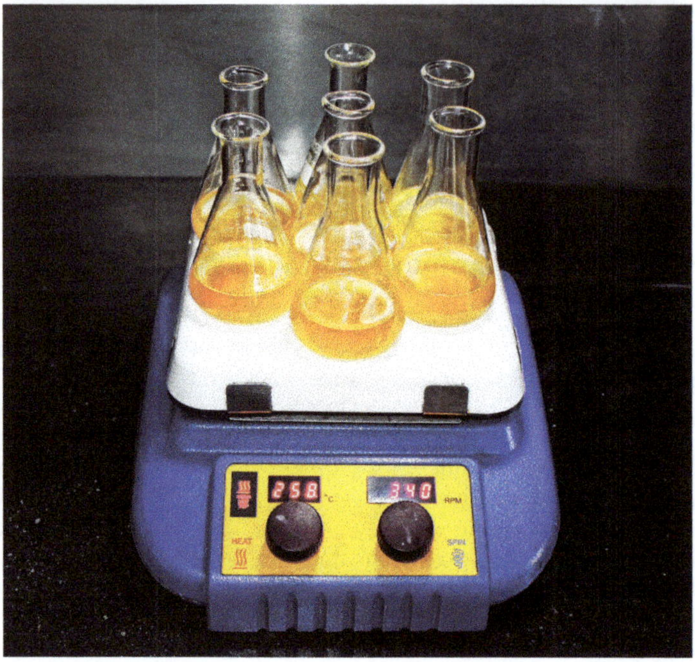

FIGURE 4.7 Heat digestion for estimation of acid detergent fibre (ADF) from bamboo.

lipoprotein cholesterol, low-density lipoprotein cholesterol, glutamic pyruvic transaminase, glutamic oxaloacetic transaminase and atherogenic index were measured. Serum total cholesterol, low-density lipoprotein cholesterol and the atherogenic index were decreased with the bamboo shoot diet feeding compared with the dietary fibre-free diet. Faecal volume and bowel movement frequency in the subjects fed with bamboo shoot diet were significantly increased. These results indicated that bamboo shoots included in the diet as a fibre source has a beneficial effect on lipid profile and bowel function.

Peng et al. (2012) studied the hemicellulosic fractions from *Phyllostachys pubescens* stem to promote its potential uses in the food industry. Hemicelluloses are characterized as complex heteropolysaccharides consisting of xylose, glucose, arabinose, galactose mannose and uronic acid (Sun et al. 2002b). Water-soluble hemicelluloses H_1 and four alkali-soluble hemicellulosic fractions H_2, H_3, H_4 and H_5 have been obtained which constituted a total yield of 59.6% based on the original hemicelluloses (Peng et al. 2012). Sugar composition analysis showed that the hemicelluloses were mainly composed of xylose (44.39–72.71%), arabinose (26.36–51.87%), ribose (0.93–2.72%) and uronic acid (0.29–5.27%). In addition to utilization in papermaking, hemicelluloses could be utilized in the food industry and energy industry to produce xylitol (Prakash et al. 2011), xylose and functional xylooligosaccharides (Yoon et al. 2006) and bioethanol (Velmurugan and Muthukumar 2011).

Mahayotpanya and Phoungchandang (2016) analyzed the crude fibre content of different portions (lower, middle and upper) of *Dendrocalamus asper* shoots and found that fibre content in different portions of fresh shoots ranged from 8.61 to 13.93% d.w.

with the highest content present in the lower portion of the shoots. Content of NDF and ADF components of dietary fibre in the young shoots of three *Dendrocalamus* species, that is *D. giganteus*, *D. latiflorus* and *D. sikkimensis* were determined by Rawat et al. (2016). In their study they found that NDF content ranged from 4.66 g/100 g f.w. to 5.88 g/100 g f.w. while the ADF content ranged from 0.83 g/100 g f.w. to 0.93 g/100g f.w. Sharma and Barooah (2017) analyzed the fibre content of a traditional fermented bamboo shoot product known as *khorisa* and prepared to utilize shoots of three different bamboo species separately, namely *Bambusa balcooa*, *Dendrocalamus giganteus* and *D. hamiltonii*. Their results showed that *khorisa* contains a high amount of crude fibre ranging from 8.965 to 11.138 g/100 g. Sood et al. (2017) also reported the fibre content of young shoots of four bamboo species viz. *Bambusa bambos*, *Dendrocalamus asper*, *D. hamiltonii* and *Phyllostachys pubescens* with fibre content ranging from 1.20 to 1.50%. Various components of dietary fibre from the shoot powder of *Phyllostachys praecox* were characterized by Wang et al. (2017) which included rhamnose, arabinose, xylose, mannose, glucose and galactose. The total dietary fibre content of bamboo shoot powder was 20.18%, of which 18.27% was insoluble dietary fibre, while 1.9% was soluble dietary fibre.

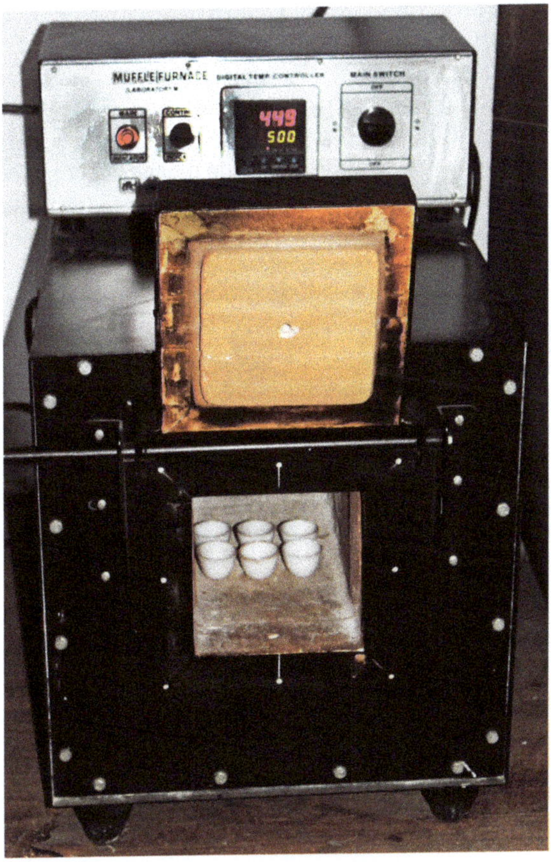

FIGURE 4.8 Ignition of neutral detergent fibre (NDF) residue in muffle furnace at 500°C.

Other bioactive compounds with health benefits have been isolated from bamboo shoots. Hartayanie et al. (2016) isolated and successfully tested the anti-microbial activity of lactic acid bacteria (LAB) extracted from pickle prepared from fermented *Dendrocalamus asper* shoots against pathogenic *Escherichia coli*. He et al. (2016) analyzed the prebiotic activity of water-soluble heteropolysaccharide fractions isolated and characterized from *Phyllostachys praecox* shoots, that is WBP1 and WBP2. Results showed that both these heteropolysaccharides were able to improve the growth of *Bifidobacterium adolescentis* and *B. bifidum* bacterial species showing the potential application of these heteropolysaccharides in functional food industries. Sukmaningsih et al. (2017) evaluated the potential aphrodisiac activity of *Gigantochloa nigrociliata* shoot extracts in the male mice. Their results revealed that in the case of mice fed with bamboo shoot extract, testosterone serum levels, sperm count, sperm viability and sperm motility enhanced significantly thereby improving the sexual behaviour of male mice. These findings suggest that bamboo shoots have potential aphrodisiac activity and can be utilized in various health products in this regard. Tanabe et al. (2017) isolated PCT N-glycan rich glycoproteins from bamboo shoots suggesting that bamboo shoots could serve as an excellent source for the plant antigenic glycans to synthesize immune-active neo-glycopolymers which have potent immunoactive properties.

Bioactive compounds obtained from natural plant resources have now gained prominence for their use as prophylactic agents in the prevention and treatment of several chronic human diseases. These secondary metabolites or phytochemicals have shown to exert a wide range of biological activities. In general, these bioactive compounds have low potency in comparison to pharmaceutical drugs, but since they are ingested regularly and in significant amounts as part of the diet, they may have a noticeable long-term physiological effect. Bamboo represents a hugely versatile natural resource that possesses tremendous potential for fighting global food insecurity. Bamboo shoots are not only rich in basic nutrient components but also contain an array of infused bioactive compounds bestowing them with several health benefits. With the backing of sound scientific evidence, the establishment of bamboo shoots as one of the most sought after ingredients for the functional food industry is inevitable thus making them one of the prominent contributors towards securing a healthy future for mankind.

5 Anti-Nutrients in Bamboo Shoots

Bamboo shoots, apart from being highly nutritious and endowed with several health benefits, contain some anti-nutrients which raise concerns over their biosafety. Anti-nutrients are mainly defence-related secondary metabolites produced by plants with specific biological functions as governed by the structure and functional nature of these compounds which range from simple carbohydrates to complex proteins. Although essential components of natural plant defence mechanisms against herbivore and pest attacks, they tend to affect the bioavailability and metabolisms of various essential nutrient components of plant foods if consumed in higher quantities. Moreover, few anti-nutrient compounds may also cause some serious health complications. Therefore, along with the identification and characterization of various nutritional facets of plants, it is also necessary to screen the presence of anti-nutrients so that the biosafety aspects of such food material can be validated appropriately and strategies for their removal can be developed. Some of these compounds are not harmful to the plant and also to the consumer directly but, they combine with nutrient elements and compounds and render them unavailable in the consumer's system thus indirectly acting as an anti-nutrient. Due to an increase in scientific awareness about the potentially harmful health effects of these anti-nutrient compounds, there is a recent surge in the scientific inquiries pertaining to the identification and removal of anti-nutrient contents of plants and plant-based food products. It is essential to remove these compounds also from bamboo shoots to make them fit for consumption. Anti-nutrients found in bamboo include cyanogenic glucosides, saponins, glucosinolates, tannins, oxalates and phytates. For centuries, people in east and south-east Asia have developed various methods and techniques to remove these anti-nutrients from the shoots and make them palatable through processing. Processing of bamboo shoots is also done for increasing the shelf life of highly perishable young juvenile shoots, proper handling and long-distance transportation. However, all shoots do not require rigorous processing as shoots of some species have a negligible amount of anti-nutrient, especially cyanogenic glucosides.

5.1 CYANOGENIC GLYCOSIDES

Cyanogenic glycosides are amino acid–derived constituents of plants produced as secondary metabolites that release hydrogen cyanide when chewed or digested. Plants synthesize cyanogenic glycosides as a defence mechanism against the attack of herbivores, insects and pathogens. They occur in at least 2,500 plant species, represented within most plant families of which a number of species are used as food. There are approximately 25 known cyanogenic glycosides and these are generally found in the edible parts of plants, such as apples, apricots, cherries, peaches, plums, almonds, cassava, bamboo shoots, linseed/flaxseed, lima beans, chickpeas, cashews, etc. The toxicity of cyanogenic glycosides and their derivatives is dependent on the release of hydrogen cyanide. The act of chewing or digestion leads to the hydrolysis of the substances, causing cyanide to be released. Symptoms of cyanide toxicity in humans have been reported to include rapid respiration, low blood pressure, headache, dizziness, vomiting, stomachache, diarrhea, convulsion and in severe cases death.

Young juvenile bamboo shoots are sweet or bitter in taste. Shoots of *Phyllostachys, Melocanna* and *Chimonobambusa* have a sweet taste and do not require much processing, whereas shoots of *Bambusa* and *Dendrocalamus* are mostly bitter in taste and require vigorous processing. The acridity and bitterness of bamboo shoots along with peculiar smell is due to a compound called cyanogenic glycoside which is one of the strongest deterrents in bamboo shoots that keep away many insects, microbes and animals from it. If not removed properly, cyanogenic glycosides are also toxic to humans. Since the potential toxicity of hydrogen cyanide from ingested cyanogenic glycosides depends on a number of nutritional factors that are involved in detoxification mechanisms, there is still insufficient quantitative data to estimate the accurate safe exposure level of cyanogenic glycosides (FAO/WHO 2012). The cyanogenic glycoside in bamboo shoots is known as taxiphyllin which is structurally p-hydroxylated mandelonitrile triglochin (Jones 1998, Moller and Seigler 1998, FSANZ 2004). Taxiphyllin is unusually least stable among other similar anti-nutrient compounds and also thermolabile, hence it can be decomposed readily by the action of heat. However, the cyanogen content varies according to the species, age, parts of the plant, harvesting time as well as environmental factors. There are only a few animals like the giant panda, golden lemur and mountain gorilla which can digest the high amount of cyanogenic glycoside present in some bamboos. There are also many known incidents of accidents and fatalities due to the consumption of the shoots without removing this anti-nutrient compound. A folk tale from north-east India says, 'a long time ago, people died due to eating fresh raw bamboo shoots in the forest during hunting'. Since then the descendants of some clans in north-east India, for example, *Nongsiej* and *Jerwa* from Meghalaya, do not eat bamboo shoots.

In intact cells, cyanogenic glucosides are stored in vacuoles and protected from degrading enzymes. But, when physical processes, such as chewing by herbivores or when cell integrity is destroyed by physical processes such as by freezing or maceration, the two components come into contact and in this process, cyanogenic glucoside is hydrolyzed in two steps (Figure 5.1 and Figure 5.2). First, a β-glycosidase enzyme converts the cyanogens into cyanohydrins which are further converted into aldehyde or ketone and hydrogen cyanide by hydroxynitrilelyase enzyme. Hydrogen cyanide is readily absorbed and rapidly distributed in the body through blood. In humans, cyanide is chiefly detoxified by a mitochondrial enzyme rhodanase which converts cyanide to thiocyanate which is then excreted via urine. Cyanide inhibits the mitochondrial enzyme, cytochrome oxidase through combination with their copper and iron ions, respectively which result in inhibition of respiration. The detoxification of cyanide needs amino acids rich in sulphur like cysteine and methionine in the diet.

The cyanogen content varies in different bamboo species. In some species, like *Phyllostachys* and *Chimonobambusa,* the cyanogens content is minimum

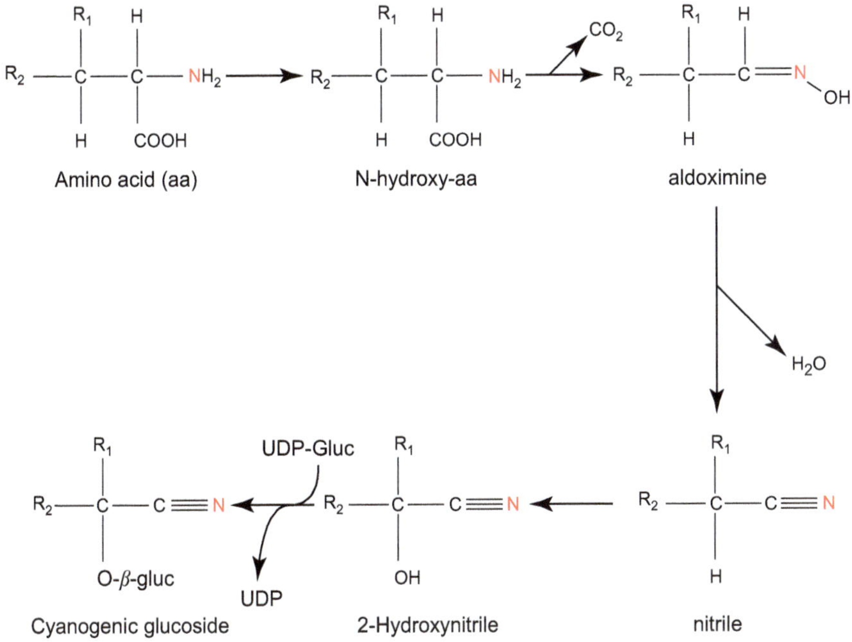

FIGURE 5.1 Biosynthetic pathways of cyanogenic glycoside. (Source: Rawat et al 2015.)

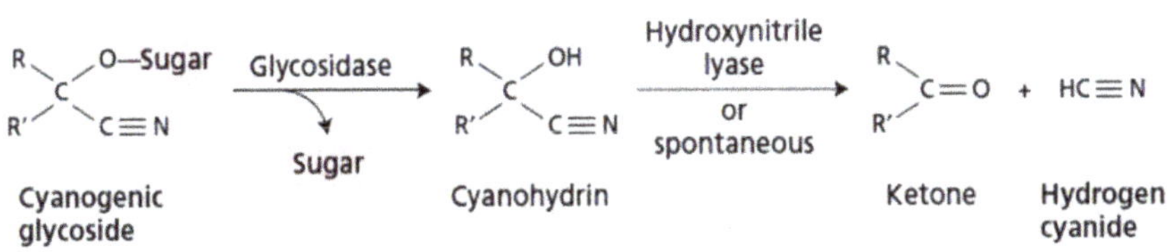

FIGURE 5.2 Enzymatic breakdown pathways of cyanogenic glycoside. (Source Rawat et al 2015.)

(36.32 mg/kg f.w. and 55.97 mg/kg f.w., respectively), whereas in some species of *Dendrocalamus* and *Bambusa*, the cyanogen content exceeds 1,000.0 mg/kg or more of fresh weight of shoots (Table 5.1). The amount of cyanogenic glycoside in the shoot varies with age as well as in different parts of the shoot. The cyanogen content in bamboo shoot is determined by using picrate paper (Figures 5.3 and 5.4) as given by Haque and Bradbury (2002). In fresh shoots, Waikhom et al. (2013) reported that total cyanogenic glycoside varies from 300–2604 ppm (tip portion), 210–2243 ppm (middle portion) and 199–920 ppm (basal portion). It has been observed that as the young shoot matures, the amount of cyanogenic glycosides content increases for the protection of shoots from pathogens, other animals and insects (Haque and Bradbury 2002, Haorongbam et al. 2009). Cyanogenic content in the fresh shoots also varies according to genotype, geographic location and age of the shoots (Haque and Bradbury 2002, Haorongbam et al. 2009, Pandey and

TABLE 5.1
Total Cyanogenic Glucoside Content in Fresh Bamboo Shoots

Sr.No.	Species	Amount (mg/kg)	References
1.	*Bambusa arundinacea*	1060.00	Haque and Bradbury 2002
2.	*B. balcooa*	1108.32	Rawat et al. 2015
3.	*B. bambos*	678.39	Rawat et al. 2015
4.	*B. cacharensis*	1155.26	Devi 2018
5.	*B. jaintiana*	434.02	Rawat et al. 2015
6.	*B. manipureana*	642.05	Devi 2018
7.	*B. nutans*	1224.43	Devi 2018
8.	*B. tulda*	867.24	Devi 2018
9.	*B. vulgaris*	523.25	Devi 2018
10.	*Cephalostachyum capitatum*	138.60	Devi 2018
11.	*Chimonobambusa callosa*	55.97	Devi 2018
12.	*Dendrocalamus asper*	766.66	Rawat et al. 2015
13.	*D. calostachys*	636.76	Rawat et al. 2015
14.	*D. flagellifer*	1893.67	Rawat et al. 2015
15.	*D. giganteus*	688.17	Rawat et al. 2015
16.	*D. hamiltonii*	733.92	Rawat et al. 2015
17.	*D. hookeri*	767.45	Devi 2018
18.	*D. latiflorus*	1027.22	Devi 2018
19.	*D. longispathus*	952.78	Devi 2018
20.	*D. manipureanus*	1347.98	Devi 2018
21.	*D. membranaceus*	514.80	Rawat et al. 2015
22.	*D. sikkimensis*	1335.31	Devi 2018
23.	*D. strictus*	1717.85	Rawat et al. 2015
24.	*Melocanna baccifera*	315.22	Devi 2018
25.	*Phyllostachys mannii*	36.32	Rawat et al. 2015
26.	*Thyrsostachys oliveri*	1097.71	Rawat et al. 2015

Ojha 2013, Waikhom et al. 2013). Young shoots of bamboo growing at lower altitudes have a high amount of cyanogenic glycoside as compared to the species growing at higher altitudes (Waikhom et al. 2013).

5.2 OXALATES

Oxalates, a dianion with a chemical formula, $C_2O_4^{2-}$, is a salt formed from oxalic acid and are naturally occurring substances found in a wide variety of plants (Figure 5.5). Oxalic acid forms strong bonds with various minerals such as calcium, magnesium, sodium and potassium resulting in the formation of oxalate salts like calcium-oxalate, magnesium oxalate, etc. Some oxalate salts such as sodium and potassium are soluble, whereas calcium-oxalate salts are basically insoluble. The insoluble calcium-oxalate has the tendency to precipitate in the kidneys or urinary tract, thus forming sharp-edged calcium-oxalate crystals that play a role in the formation of kidney stones. When plants rich in oxalates are consumed, they are known

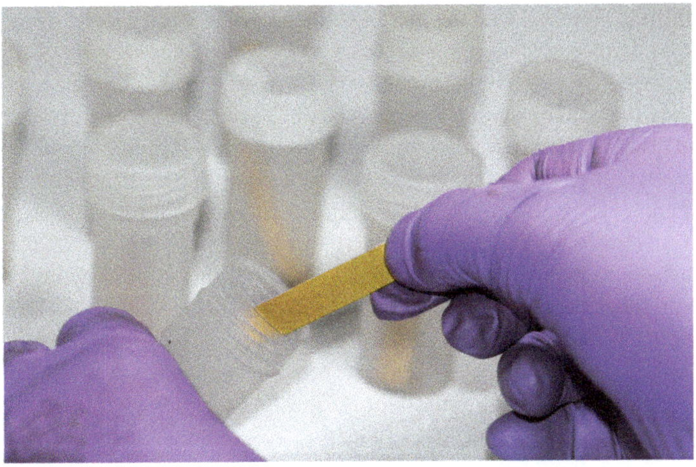

FIGURE 5.3 Cyanogenic glycosides estimation using picrate paper.

FIGURE 5.4 Picrate paper changing colour from light yellow (A) to light brown (B) depending upon the cyanogenic glycoside concentration.

to cause adverse effects on animals as well as human health. After their consumption and release, oxalates combine with Ca^{2+}, $Fe^{2+}$and Mg^{2+} and other minerals rendering them unavailable in the consumer's system. Over-consumption of oxalate-rich foods leads to the occurrence of kidney stones as absorbed oxalates cannot be metabolized by humans and are excreted in the urine. Foodstuff rich in oxalate content has been scientifically linked with the increased incidence of kidney stone formation. No safe limit on oxalate consumption has been formulated so far because of the dietary variations across the populations though some scientific studies have been conducted to determine the relationship between intake of oxalate and risk of developing nephrolithiasis (kidney stones). A study by Taylor and Curhan (2008) found that for men, oxalate consumption up to 214 mg/day did not result in the incidences of kidney stones whereas, for younger and older women, the upper safe limit of oxalate consumption was found to be 183 and 185 mg/day, respectively. High oxalate levels may also disturb the carbohydrate metabolism by inhibiting succinic dehydrogenase.

Bamboo shoots are known to contain oxalates varying from 112.20 mg/100g to 460 mg/100g (Kozukue et al. 1983, Judprasong et al. 2006, Juajun et al. 2012, Ruan et al. 2013). Oxalate content of fresh shoots of four bamboo species (*Bambusa tulda*, *Dendrocalamus giganteus*, *D. latiflorus* and *D. membranaceus*) ranged from 262.59 mg/100g to 277.37 mg/100g (Table 5.2). Even though having high quantities of oxalate content, there has been no clinical study so far linking the oxalate in bamboo shoots with the occurrence of stone diseases. On the contrary, the use of sliced bamboo shoots as herbal treatment of kidney stones by Muslim *Maibas* of Manipur is reported by Ahmed and Singh (2011). Moreover, as shown by various other studies (Jaworska 2005, Ogbadoyi et al. 2006, Catherwood et al. 2007, Juajun et al. 2012) and our own studies, it was found that various processing treatments reduce the oxalate content thereby lowering the chances of potential adverse health effects even further.

5.3 GLUCOSINOLATES

Glucosinolates constitute a large group of sulphur-rich natural phytochemicals which play a role in plant defence mechanism towards herbivore and pest attacks. Chemically, they are thioethers consisting of a sugar entity, β-D-thioglucose which is linked to an organic aglycone via an ester bond (Figure 5.5). These compounds upon hydrolysis yield isothiocyanate, nitrile, thiocyanate and other related compounds that impart a specific bitter and hot taste that is very prominent in cruciferous vegetables. They are natural components of many pungent plants such as mustard, cabbage and horseradish. In plants, these compounds normally remain intact unless brought into contact with the enzymes glucosinolase or thioglucosidase when plant tissue is crushed either by mastication or by pest injury thus releasing its hydrolysis products

TABLE 5.2
Anti-Nutrient Content in Shoots of Four Bamboo Species

Species	Glucosinolates (mg/100g)	Oxalate (mg/100g)	Saponins (mg/100g)	Phytates (mg/100g)	Tannins (mg/100g)
B. tulda	29.11	283.02	228.43	85.41	48.31
D. giganteus	26.33	285.50	232.21	89.63	50.67
D. latiflorus	25.41	262.59	241.39	93.67	39.72
D. membranaceus	26.99	277.37	246.03	95.84	41.60

and providing protection against further damage by herbivores or pests (Chew 1988). So far, around 100 glucosinolates have been identified signifying their importance in the plant kingdom. Upon human consumption, plants rich in glucosinolate compounds are known to be involved in several biological activities which are attributed chiefly to their hydrolysis products. Their hydrolysis products thiocyanate, isothiocyanates and oxazolidine-2-thiones have potent anti-thyroid properties and interfere with the functioning of thyroid hormones by inhibiting iodine uptake by the thyroid, blocking the incorporation of iodine into thyroxine precursors and by suppressing thyroxine secretion from the thyroid. Besides their anti-nutritional effects, hydrolysis products of glucosinolates have been shown to have potent anti-cancerous properties.

In bamboo shoots, glucosinolate content ranged from 25.41 mg/100g to 29.11 mg/100 g on a dry weight basis (Table 5.2). Our studies revealed that total glucosinolate content in fresh shoots of four investigated bamboo species (*Bambusa tulda*, *Dendrocalamus giganteus*, *D. latiflorus* and *D. membranaceus*) ranged from 25.41 mg/100g to 29.11 mg/100g (Table 5.2). Earlier, Chandra et al. (2004) elucidated glucosinolate content in fresh shoots *Bambusa arundinacea* but their result (9.57 mg/kg) is significantly less than the values obtained by Sharma (2018). The presence of glucosinolates and their hydrolysis products in bamboo shoots has been linked with the incidence of thyroid malfunctioning and endemic goitrogenesis (Chandra et al. 2004, Chandra et al. 2012). But there are several other clinical studies conducted on human subjects that did not report any adverse effect on thyroid functioning even after the administration of as high as 174.60 mg/day glucosinolates (Kensler et al. 2005, Shapiro et al. 2006, Clarke et al. 2011). Hence, suggested impact of bamboo shoot glucosinolates on goitrogenesis is not conclusive especially when bamboo shoots are mostly consumed in processed, that is, boiled, soaked or fermented form which tends to reduce the glucosinolate content of the shoots. Therefore, there is a need for more clinical trials in this regard. On the other hand, there is a substantial and growing body of research evidence confirming the chemopreventive actions of glucosinolates and their hydrolysis products against carcinogenesis (Shapiro et al. 2001, Hayes et al. 2008, Fahey et al. 2012). Thus, the presence of glucosinolates in bamboo shoots as reported in the current study and their related anti-cancerous properties adds more weightage to this already valuable health food.

5.4 PHYTATES

Phytate or phytic acid is a saturated cyclic acid with chemical formulae $C_6H_{18}O_{24}P_6$ and is the chief form of phosphorus storage in many plant organs especially seeds and grains (Figure 5.5). It forms complexes with dietary minerals, especially with iron and zinc and causes a mineral-related deficiency in humans. Phytate affects the bioavailability of several minerals especially Zn, Fe and Mn. It also negatively impacts protein and lipid utilization and is a major concern for individuals who depend mainly on plant derivative foods.

Phytate in fresh shoots of *Dendrocalamus hamiltonii* and *Bambusa balcooa* were determined to be 35.95 mg/100g to 30.67 mg/100g which reduced to as low as 22.46 mg/100g upon fermentation (Sarangthem and Singh 2013). In another study, phytate content in the fresh shoots of six bamboo species was found to be between

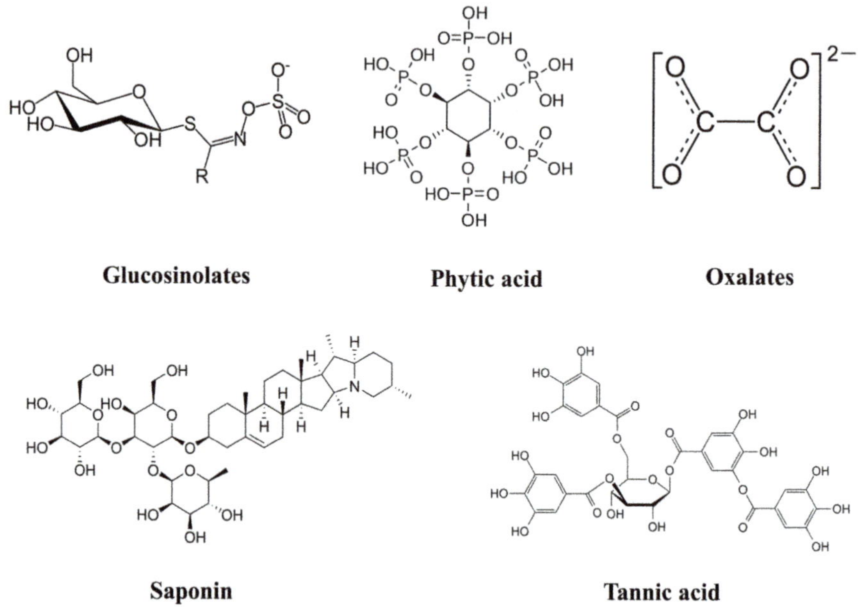

FIGURE 5.5 Chemical structures of anti-nutrients present in bamboo.

19.80 to 66.44 mg/100g (Mina et al. 2014). Our studies in fresh shoots of four investigated species (*B. tulda*, *D. giganteus*, *D. latiflorus* and *D. membranaceus*) revealed phytate content to be between 85.41 mg/100g to 95.84 mg/100g (Table 5.2). Earlier reports have highlighted that processing techniques, such as soaking, cooking and fermentation, result in the reduction of the phytate content of plant-based foods (Svanberg et al. 1993, Greiner and Konietzny 1999).

5.5 SAPONINS

Saponins are glucosides with foaming characteristics and are found in most vegetables, beans and herbs (Figure 5.5). The best-known sources of saponins are peas, soybeans and some herbs with names indicating foaming properties such as soapwort, soaproot, soapbark and soapberry. Commercial saponins are extracted mainly from *Yucca schidigera* and *Quillaja saponaria*. In plants, saponins are involved in plant defence mechanism against microbial attack.

Saponins show a high physiological activity upon consumption which arises primarily because of their strong physiological interaction as surface acting agents with other components of food and their ability to interact with the membranes of the mucosal cells. They have been shown to demonstrate haemolytic action towards red blood cells and can be toxic if given intravenously possibly by affecting the cAMP levels in the plasma, brain, adipocytes and adrenal glands. Saponins are also known to form insoluble saponin-mineral complexes, with Fe, Zn and Ca, thus affecting mineral availability for absorption. Thus, by affecting mineral availability they act as a potent inhibitor of metabolism and growth. However, saponins are also linked with some positive effects on health with anti-oxidant and hypolipidemic properties, suppressive actions against colon cancer and also have the ability to lower cholesterol levels in blood plasma and liver by forming complexes with cholesterol. Saponins have been shown to have potent anti-oxidant and hypolipidemic effects. They also possess anti-bacterial activity and modify ruminal fermentation by suppressing ruminal protozoa and selectively inhibiting some bacteria. They are known to have potent suppressive action against colon cancer.

Saponin content was investigated in the fresh shoots of four species (*Bambusa tulda*, *Dendrocalamus giganteus*, *D. latiflorus* and *D. membranaceus*) and was found to be between 228.43 mg/100 g to 246.03 mg/100 g (Table 5.2). Singh et al. (2012) also reported the presence of saponin content in the fresh shoots of *B. balcooa*. Sarangthem and Singh (2013) quantified the saponin content in the fresh shoots of *D. hamiltonii* and *B. balcooa* which was 95.32 mg/10 g and 103.32 mg/100 g, respectively. Various processing treatments caused a marked reduction in the saponin content of the shoots.

5.6 TANNINS

Tannins are a large group of water-soluble phenolic compounds having a molecular weight between 500 and 3,000 D (Figure 5.5). These polyphenols contain a large number of hydroxyl or other functional groups (1 to 2 per 100 D) and therefore are capable of forming cross-linkages with proteins and other macromolecules. These compounds form complexes with proteins, starch and digestive enzymes to cause a reduction in the nutritional values of foods. They can cause a browning reaction in foods through the action of polyphenol oxidase by darkening reactions. Tannins have been reported to be responsible for decreases in growth rate, net metabolizable energy and protein digestibility. Other deleterious effects of tannins include damages to the mucosal lining of the gastrointestinal tract, alteration of excretion of certain cations and increased excretion of proteins and essential amino acids. Tannins inhibit the enzymatic activities of cellulase, pectinase, amylase, lipases, proteolytic enzymes, β-galactosidase and those microbial enzymes involved in the fermentation of cereal grains thereby severely compromising the metabolism. But some recent studies have shown tannins to have anti-microbial, anti-cancerous and anti-mutagenic properties.

In fresh shoots of bamboo species (*Bambusa tulda, Dendrocalamus giganteus*, and *D. membranaceus*) the tannin content ranged between 39.72 mg/100 g to 48.31 mg/100 g (Table 5.2). In the shoots of some other species of bamboo from north-east India, tannin was estimated 45.49 mg/100 g in *D. hamiltonii* to 31.49 mg/100 g in *B. balcooa* (Sarangthem and Singh 2013). They also reported that fermentation caused an increase in the content of tannin as compared to fresh shoots, which ranged from 52.00 to 68.21 mg/100g f.w. of fermented shoots.

6 Processing of Bamboo Shoots

In recent years, food quality and safety have become a major concern to consumers, producers, food industries and regulatory agencies worldwide. The food industry is an increasingly competitive and dynamic domain, with consumers becoming more cognizant about what they consume. Such recent trends may be due to globalization of the food trade and changes in eating habits and consumer demand for healthy, convenience, diversity, minimally processed, long shelf-life, low-calorie content and ready-to-eat products. In order to meet consumer demands, the processing of food has become very challenging, and techniques have been developed to produce food products with better quality. Food processing is a technique implemented to convert raw food stuff into well-cooked and well-preserved intermediate or finished value-added food products that are safe to eat and targets the removal of biological, chemical and physical hazards so that consumers enjoy safe, nutritious and wholesome foods. The aim of food processing is (i) to extend the period during which food remains wholesome (microbial and biochemical), (ii) to provide nutrients required for health, (iii) to provide variety and convenience in diet and (iv) to add value. However, processing affects the contents, activity and bioavailability of nutrients and bioactive compounds as well as the health-promoting capacity of food products. For health and well-being, environmentally friendly procedures with minimal loss of bioactivities are highly desirable. Processing of food items is also necessary for the purpose of security and availability of food during a lean period or for transporting it to the places where it is required.

Due to the seasonal availability of bamboo shoots and its short shelf-life of three to four days after harvesting, it is necessary to process the young shoots using appropriate methods for long-term usage and storage. Moreover, the processing of young raw shoots is also essential to remove cyanogen toxicity and other anti-nutrients like glucosinolates, oxalates, phytates, saponins and tannins. The content of these anti-nutrients in shoots varies from species to species in bamboos. Species like *Bambusa balcooa*, *B. oldhamii*, *Dendrocalamus hookeri*, *D. giganteus*, *D. latiflorus* and *D. longispathus* have a very high amount of cyanogen content in shoots. Around 50 years ago, the processing of bamboo shoots was localized and it was just a household business. In some countries including China, Taiwan and Thailand, bamboo shoot processing and canning turned into a multibillion-dollar business after the 1980s, supplying shoots around the world. Countries like Korea have well developed processing units (Figure 6.1). In countries such as India, Philippines and Bangladesh shoot processing is still a small-scale household business, fulfilling family or local needs only. There is a growing demand for processed and packaged shoots in the national and international markets.

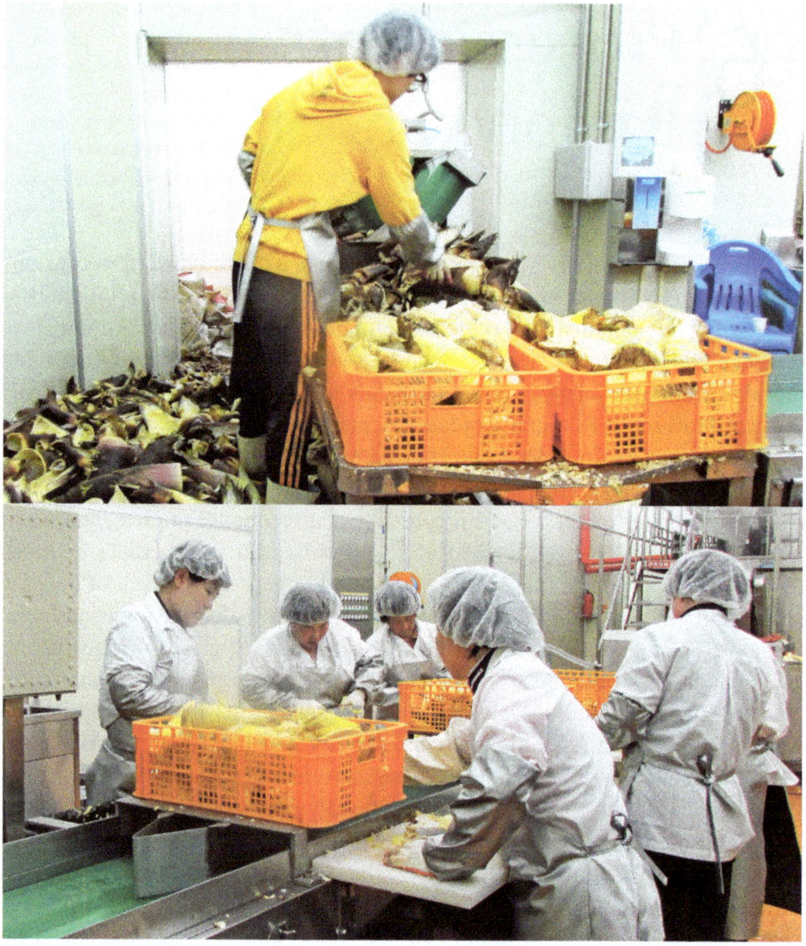

FIGURE 6.1 Bamboo shoot processing unit in Korea.

6.1 HARVESTING OF BAMBOO SHOOTS

Harvesting of shoots is very crucial and needs proper knowledge about the bamboo species and technique for harvesting. Shoots are cut at the time when the maximum soft edible part is available. It is preferable to harvest shoots either early in the morning or late in the evening in order to protect the harvested shoots from the heat of the sun. The juvenile shoots are usually collected at the stage when their tips are just emerging above the ground, that is about 18–20 inches from the ground (Figure 6.2). In most species, this height is attained by the second week of emergence. Harvesting of shoots also requires proper planning and management. Only 20 to 40% of the totally new emerging shoots should be harvested from a particular bamboo grove to maintain the steady supply of shoots year-round. It is essential to allow around 40 to 60% shoots to reach the maturity level to perform photosynthesis and provide the nutrients to the bamboo grove. The extraction of a large number of shoots will

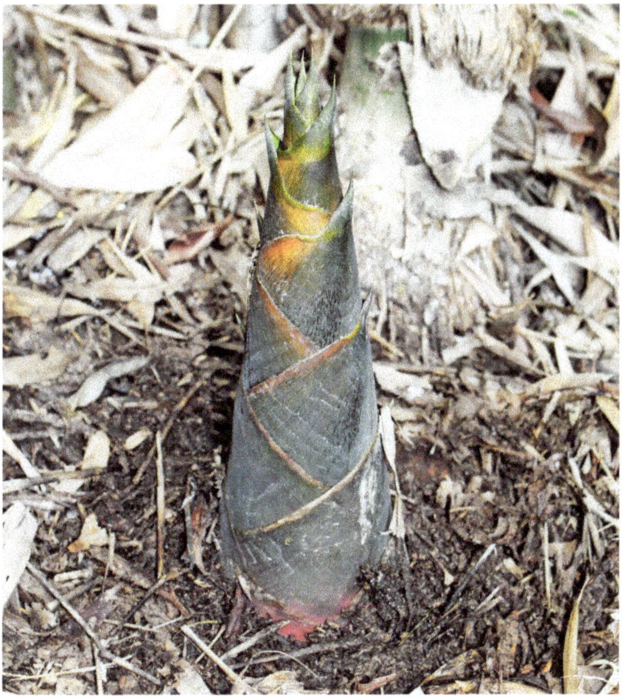

FIGURE 6.2 Young shoot of *Bambusa balcooa*.

certainly affect the future growth and health of the bamboo grove and small shoots will be produced in the following year. Harvesting of shoots from sympodial bamboos like *Dendrocalamus* and *Bambusa* is essential as a way of thinning for the healthy growth of matured and erect culms that are required for timber purpose. In the traditional market system as in north-east India, shoots are generally sold on the roadside along with intact sheaths, unlike in departmental stores where shoots are cleaned, processed and packed in canes, poly packs or glass bottles in a ready to cook form.

While extracting the shoots, care should be taken not to damage the clump, especially the rhizome or other growing culms and shoots. The shoots are harvested by digging around them and carefully severing with a narrow hoe, machete or sharpened narrow-bladed spade (Figure 6.3). After harvesting, they should be processed as soon as possible preferably the same day. The shoots are properly washed and the basal portion of the shoot is discarded as they are generally hard and fibrous. Peeling off and cleaning of shoots is the next important and laborious work after harvesting and transporting shoots at a place that is generally done manually mainly by women, particularly in south-east Asian countries. During peeling off sheaths, the hard portion of the shoot is also discarded. The culm sheaths are removed carefully and the tender edible white/creamy portion of the shoot is extracted. The peeled shoots are immediately put in water to maintain the original colour of the shoots and also to remove the cyanogen content from the shoots. The shoots are then processed as a

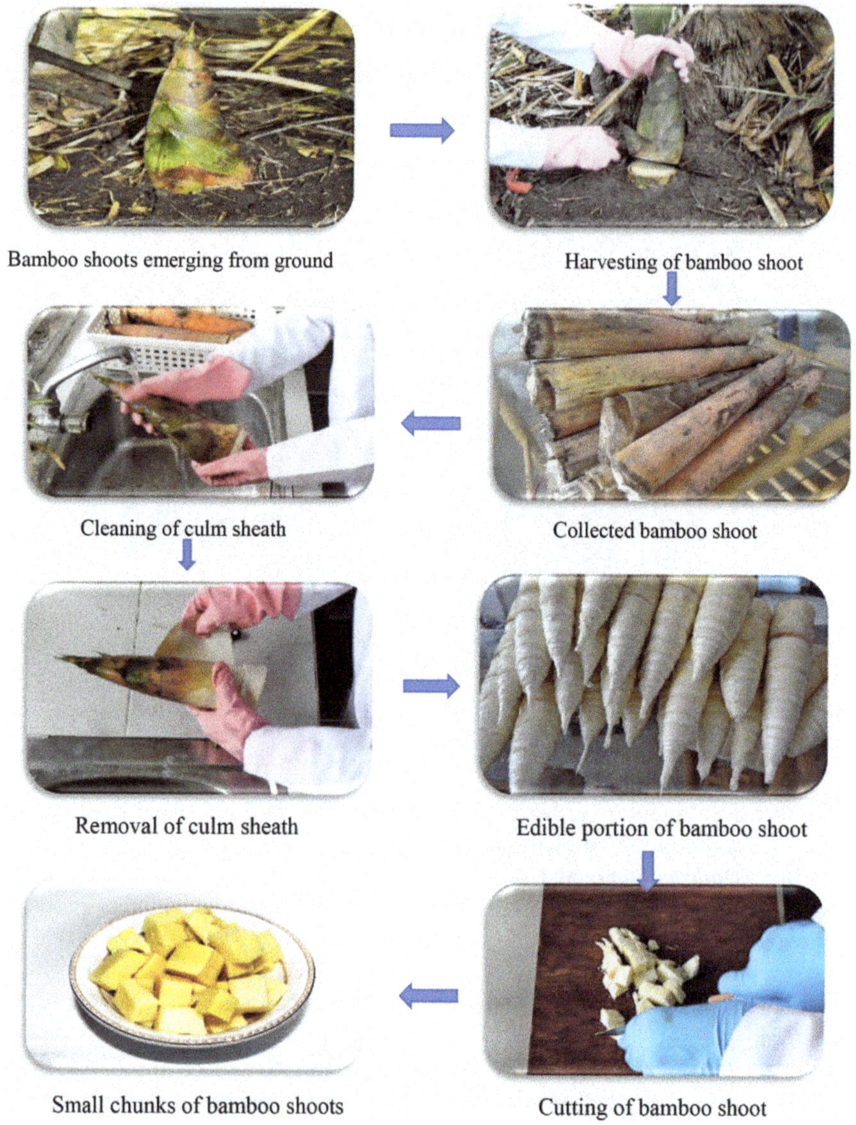

FIGURE 6.3 Bamboo shoot harvesting and processing.

whole or cut in various ways—into halves, thin slices, cubes, big chunks and juliennes (Figure 6.4).

6.2 PRE-COOKING PROCESSING OF SHOOTS

At the time of harvesting, bamboo shoots contain high moisture (up to 90%) and are thus highly perishable and vulnerable to microbial spoilage, mechanical and physical degradation. The harvested shoots need to be processed as soon as possible,

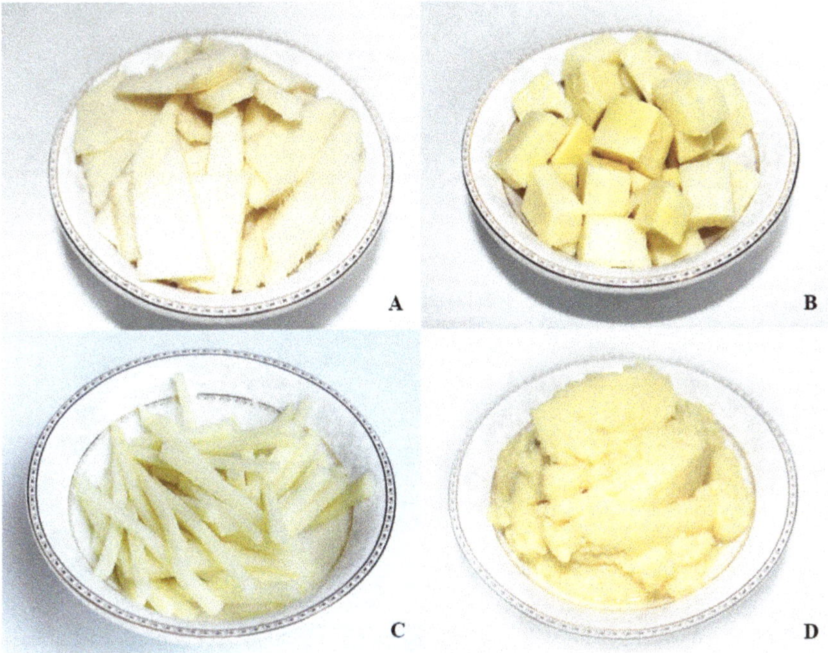

FIGURE 6.4 Different shapes of shoot in pre-cooking: A) slices, B) chunks, C) julienne and D) paste.

preferably the same day. Various processing methods bring changes to the harvested and peeled shoots. In small local markets, people use simple techniques for keeping and maintaining harvested shoots for a short period at ambient temperature or conditions. Most of the shoots are sold with outer sheaths intact but some are sold with the sheaths peeled off (Figure 6.5). But the shelf-life of these shoots is generally not more than two days. The harvested shoots deteriorate rapidly which is one of the main hurdles for the trade of bamboo shoots at the local, national or international markets. For transport from production sites to urban centers or overseas, low temperature and packaging are recommended to reduce transpiration. Liu (1992) attributed the loss of quality to the high respiration rate (4.08 mmol CO_2 $kg^{-1}h^{-1}$) at elevated storage temperature (20°C). Decolouration is a major cause of quality loss in shoots. During storage, shoots quickly undergo browning, lignification and deteriorate rapidly within a few days after harvesting and they need to be preserved to prolong their shelf-life (Zeng et al. 2015). An important factor causing quality deterioration is the development of browning on the shoot surface. Browning reactions are thought to be a consequence of polyphenol oxidase (PPO) and peroxidase (POD) action on phenols to form quinones which ultimately polymerize to produce the browning appearance in fresh-cut fruits and vegetable products.

The deterioration of bamboo shoots is characterized by an unusual increase in firmness and toughness of the flesh from the cut end toward the tip. Lignification may be the cause of this firmness and toughness in the cut shoots and is positively

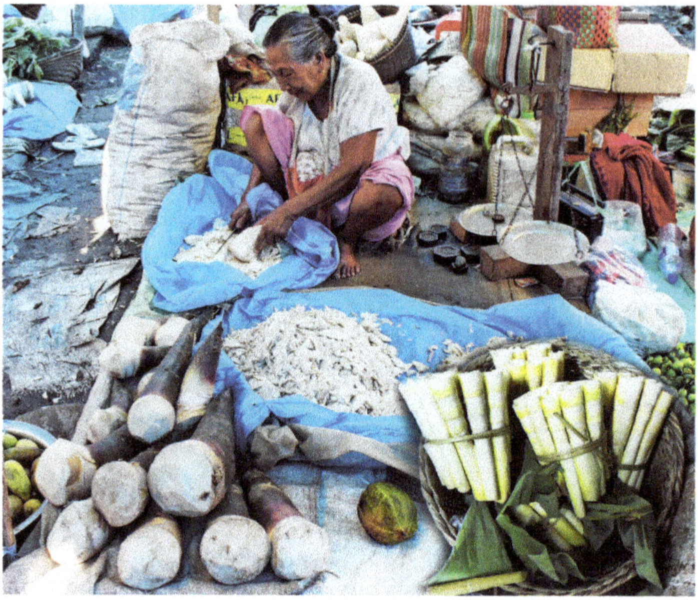

FIGURE 6.5 Woman vendor selling bamboo shoot in a local market of north-east India.

correlated with activities of phenylalanine ammonia-lyase (PAL), cinnamyl alcohol dehydrogenase (CAD) and POD. Hence, delaying or reducing enzymatic browning and lignification could be a way to extend the storage life and maintain the quality of the shoots. The plant hormone ethylene is produced in response to various kinds of environmental stress including wounding and wound-induced ethylene is involved in plant lignifications. Therefore, inhibiting ethylene biosynthesis or its action may play an important role in slowing the lignification process and extend the storage life of bamboo shoots. The effects of 1-methyl cyclopropane (1-MCP) and ethylene on the quality and lignifications of the post-harvest shoot of *Phyllostachys praecox* f. *prevernalis* were examined during storage at 20°C (Luo et al. 2007). An increase in shoot firmness after harvest was positively correlated with the increase of lignin and cellulose contents. Accumulation of lignin in the tissues was also positively correlated with the increased activities of PAL, CAD and POD. Ethylene treatment enhanced firmness, respiration rate and ethylene production, promoted total sugar decrease, but retarded disease incidence. 1-MCP treatment was associated with lower firmness, higher disease incidence and total sugar content, inhibited respiration rate and ethylene production, delayed activities of PAL, CAD and POD and retarded lignin and cellulose accumulation. These results indicated that 1-MCP could be considered for use commercially to maintain post-harvest quality and control lignification disorder in bamboo shoots. Bamboo shoot processing is still done in the traditional way to make them palatable as well as to preserve for longer periods particularly for the lean period and add value and taste to the shoots. However, in modern times with the advent of more scientific and technological knowledge, new techniques have been developed for processing and packaging of bamboo shoots. Detailed biochemical analyses of processed shoots have not been worked out for most of the bamboo species. The majority of the data presented here is from our own research work.

6.3 TRADITIONAL METHODS OF BAMBOO SHOOT PROCESSING

Since ancient times, bamboo shoots have been used for food in countries including China, Korea, Japan, India and many other south-east Asian countries and people have developed their own techniques and methods for processing and consumption of shoots. Processing of shoots is done mainly for two reasons; first, to remove the anti-nutrients from the shoots and secondly for increasing shelf-life. Soaking in water, sun-drying, boiling, blanching, steaming and fermentation are the popular traditional methods of reducing cyanide content leading to the long-term preservation of shoots. During these processes, changes occur in the content of macronutrients, micronutrients, anti-nutrients and bioactive compounds (Tables 6.1–6.9). The processing techniques are region as well as bamboo shoot–specific. In tropical regions of India, Philippines, Thailand and Indonesia, where species like *Dendrocalamus* and *Bambusa* are found which have a very high amount of cyanogen content, shoots need elaborate processing to remove the anti-nutrients. In these regions, removal of this anti-nutrient was the main objective to make the shoots palatable. Bamboos of temperate regions, like *Phyllostachys* do not have much cyanogen content in the shoots and processing are not required. Bamboos like *Melocanna* and *Chimonobambusa* also have very less content of cyanogens and comparatively, need less processing before consumption. Different processing methods for shoots are followed depending on the acridity of the shoots.

6.3.1 SOAKING

Soaking is the simplest method of processing and preservation of bamboo shoots that have been followed from ancient times and the mode varies amongst different communities and tribes. This process washes away the cyanogen and other anti-nutrients. Raw shoots of some species like *Phyllostachys pubescens, P. mannii, Melocanna baccifera* and *Chimonobambusa callosa* are sweet in taste and need little washing before consumption or cooking. Shoots of these species are also eaten raw in a salad without boiling or cooking, whereas raw shoots of some species like *Dendrocalamus sikkimensis, D. hamiltonii, Bambusa bambos* and *B. balcooa* are very bitter and need thorough washing and soaking in water for several hrs. In the *Khasi* tribe of Meghalaya, India, shoots of *D. hamiltonii* are cut into small chunks and stored in plastic bottles or bamboo cylinders filled with water till the brim for more than six months (Figure 6.6). Soaking for 12 to 24 hrs does not change the colour of the shoots as compared to boiling (Figure 6.7). There is also mild fermentation of the shoots in the process. In Arunachal Pradesh, north-east India, the shoots of *D. hamiltonii* and *B. tulda*, due to a very high level of bitterness, are kept overnight in running rivers before using for food. Popular traditional products of Nagaland are *Rhuchak, Voyen, Rhuchu, Ruchan, Rhuyen* and pickle with king chilli, in which different processing methods are employed including slicing of shoots into tiny pieces and soaking in water overnight.

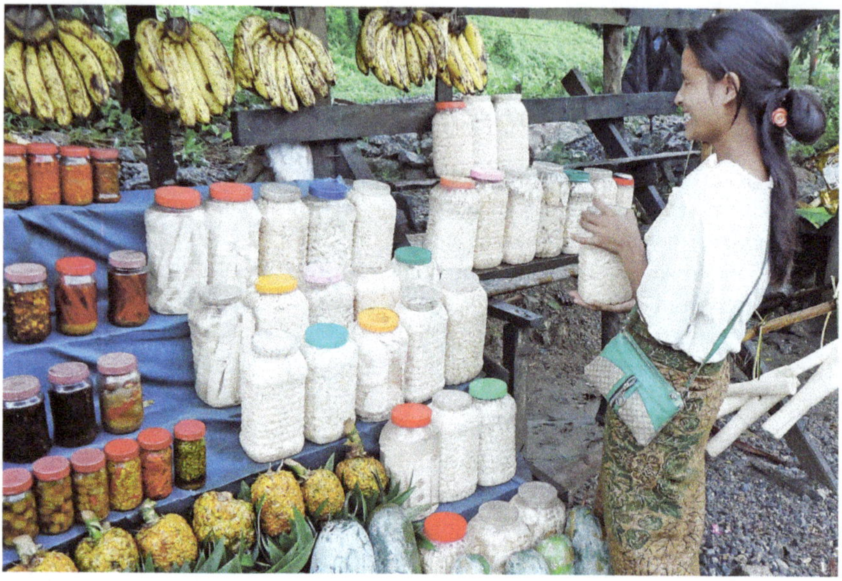

FIGURE 6.6 Females earn a livelihood by selling bamboo shoots in plastic bottles soaked in water.

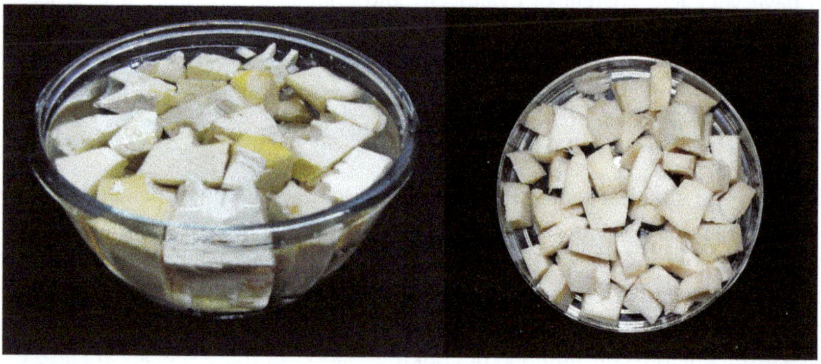

FIGURE 6.7 24 hr soaked shoots of *D. hamiltonii*.

6.3.2 Heat Treatment

Heat treatment is applied to various vegetables to increase the shelf-life and nutritive value of the vegetables and also reduce the anti-nutrient components. It also inhibits disease incidences, respiration, ethylene production and various enzymatic activities of bamboo shoots during storage at 20°C and significantly delays tissue lignifications. Blanching is a heat processing method in which vegetables are put in hot water at 88°C (190°F) for two to five mins or with steam in a conveyor at 100°C (212°F) for one-half to one min. This process inactivates natural enzymes that would cause discolouration and off-flavours and aromas. It also reduces the number of microorganisms, softens tissues for easy packing into containers and shorter cooking time

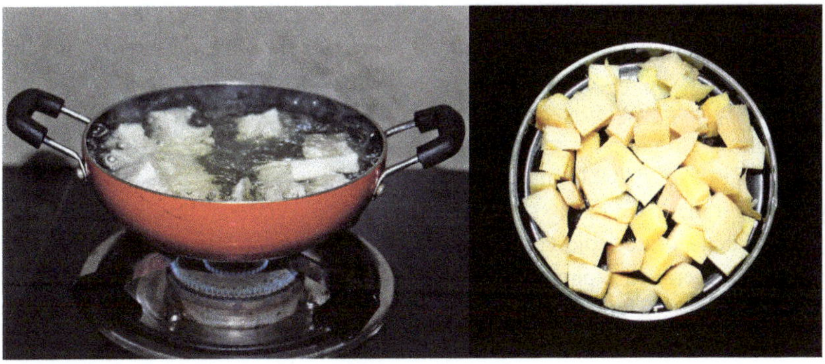

FIGURE 6.8 Boiled shoots of *D. hamiltonii.*

and eliminates intracellular air to prevent oxidation (Ruiz-Ozeda and Penas 2013). The *Sao* community from Thailand preserves the shoots of *Thyrsostachys siamensis* by packing them in plastic bags and steaming by different methods and durations (Chiangthong and Chayawat 2009). For blanching, the fresh bamboo shoots are cut to a uniform size and immersed in a water bath at 75–85°C for 10–20 mins. Effect of blanching on different physical and nutritional quality like total soluble sugars, protein, dietary fibre, fat vitamin, ascorbic acid, phenolic content and radical scavenging capacity was evaluated by Badwaik et al. (2015). Blanching resulted in soft texture and increased yellowness. Loss of nutrients was maximum at 95°C for 20–30 mins and minimum at 75°C for five to ten mins. Loss of anti-oxidant property, total phenolic content and ascorbic content were also noted. A proper combination of time and temperature of blanching is very important to retain the nutrients and quality of the bamboo shoots. In bamboo shoots with high cyanogen content, the shoots are usually boiled for a particular time before consumption. This is mainly done to remove the bitterness of the shoot and the method varies among different tribes and the traditional practices followed. Boiling gives a yellow tinge to the shoots which depend upon the species (Figure 6.8) Rana et al. (2012) optimized the processing conditions by varying NaCl concentration, the thickness of bamboo shoot, amount of NaCl solution and duration of treatment.

6.3.3 Drying

This is probably the most ancient method used by humans to preserve or process their food. The key role of drying is to reduce water activity or moisture content of the food or product, subsequently, decreasing the microbial activity and chemical reactions and improves shelf-life which further makes the commodity available to the consumers throughout the year. This method decreases the bulk and weight and also enables easy handling, storage, packaging and transportation. Although drying is an effective method for long-term preservation, different drying methods may affect the product differently by altering mechanical, physical, biological and chemical properties such as microbial, enzymatic activity, appearance, texture, colour, flavour, hardness rehydration and palatability. Thus, like other processing methods, different drying methods need to be tried to select the best drying method with respect to economical product, functional and physical quality. Many drying methods such as sun-drying, convection oven-drying, freeze-drying, microwave drying and so on are also used to preserve foods.

At the time of harvesting, bamboo shoots contain high moisture (up to 90%) and are thus highly perishable and vulnerable to microbial spoilage, mechanical and physical degradation. During storage, shoots quickly undergo browning and lignification and deteriorate rapidly within a few days after harvesting and they need to be preserved properly to prolong their shelf-life (Zeng et al. 2015). Dehydration is the most common and widely used preservative method, in recent times and a vital facet of food processing. Drying technologies have engrossed major research and development efforts because of the rising demand for better product quality and lower operating cost, as well as lessened environmental impact.

6.3.4 Sun-Drying

Sun-drying is a very simple ancient skill and one of mankind's oldest preservative techniques and reportedly used in ancient Egypt and Mesopotamia. Due to its simplicity, low capital and operating costs and the fact that little expertize is required, it is the most widespread processing technology whose benefits more than compensate for its time-intensive nature - especially when compared to modern mechanical drying methods. However, the main disadvantages of this method are slowness of the process, contamination, no protection from rain or dew that wets the product and encourages mould growth, low and variable quality of products due to over- or under-drying, dependency on weather and the hand labour requirement. While sun-drying is being increasingly adapted in vegetable preservation due to the high cost of other artificial drying methods, conservation of nutrients is important in view of the prevailing micronutrient deficiency problem. In the north-east region of India, sun-drying of bamboo shoots is a common practice. Shoots are cut into shreds or slices, dried in the sun and stored in a dry container or packed in polythene bags (Figure 6.9). It is also a common practice to dry fermented shoots. *Kandha* tribe of Kalahandi, Orissa, India prepare *Handua* which are sun-dried shoots that are pound

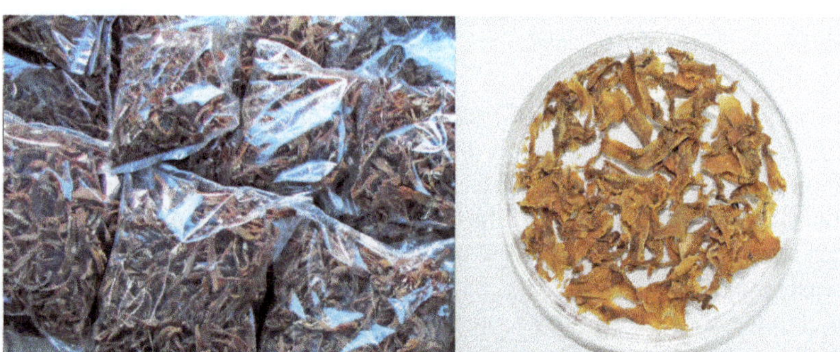

FIGURE 6.9 Sun-dried bamboo shoots sold in the market of Nagaland, India.

before sun-drying (Panda and Padhy 2007). For best sun-drying, humidity below 60% are suitable conditions. The quality of sun-dried shoots depends on the weather (humidity, temperature) and environmental conditions. Shoots after drying in sun for two to three days in suitable conditions are light brown in colour with a pleasant aroma. However, drying more than three days in humid condition with temperature fluctuations makes the shoots soggy and dark brown. A comparison of nutritional composition in the sun-, oven- and freeze-dried shoots reveals that there is not much variation between fat, ash and NDF content but ADF content is highest in sun-dried shoots (Table 6.4).

6.3.5 Oven-Drying

Oven is one of the most common appliances that are used in the culinary world. Oven-drying is the simplest way to dry food and is faster than sun-drying or using a food dryer. It is important to keep the oven temperature at the lowest, that is 140 to 160°F (60 to 70°C) which may possibly be warm enough to dry the shoot. Nutrient content in nine bamboo species was analyzed after oven-drying. Fresh shoots are cut into small cubes and oven-dried at 60°C for 24 hrs. The resultant product was brown in colour and has less volume compared to the fresh sample with woody granular texture (Figure 6.10). Oven-drying is normally not used especially in rural areas due to lack of facility and the cost factor.

6.3.6 Fermentation

Fermentation is one of the ancient methods of food preservation and became widely accepted in many cultures due to its nutritional value and variety of sensory attributes. For centuries, human beings have made fermented food responding to the need to preserve food, prolong shelf-life and improve flavour. Fermented foods which include yogurt, wine, beer, cheese, sauerkraut, kimchi and many more have enhanced nutritional and functional properties due to biotransformation of substrates by bacteria, yeast and/or moulds leading to the formation of bioactive or bioavailable end-products that have unique and diverse flavours important in many foods.

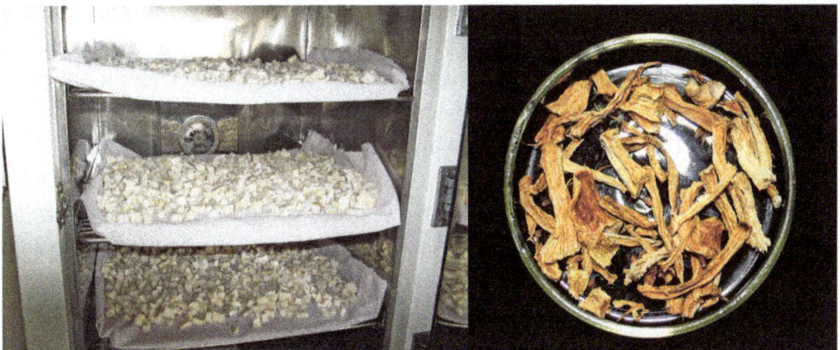

FIGURE 6.10 Oven-dried bamboo shoots of *D. hamiltonii*.

Fermentation is associated with many health benefits due to the micro-organisms associated with the fermentation process and fermented products have recently attracted a lot of scientific interest (Sanlier et al. 2019). Fermented foods are generally associated with a unique group of microflora that synthesizes vitamins and minerals, produces biologically active peptides with enzymes such as proteinase and peptidase and remove some non-nutrients. In addition, they enhance the flavour, increase digestibility, improving nutritional and pharmacological values. Fermentation has the following effects (i) enrichment of the food through development of a wide diversity of flavours, aromas and textures in food; (ii) enrichment of food substrates biologically with vitamins, proteins, essential amino acids and essential fatty acids; (iii) detoxification during the fermentation process; (iv) preservation; and (v) decrease in cooking time and fuel requirements.

6.3.7 Fermented Shoots

For fermenting bamboo shoots, no preservative is used for a storage life of six months to two years. In India, major species used for fermentation include *Dendrocalamus hamiltonii*, *D. hookeri*, *D. giganteus*, *Bambusa manipureana*, *B. tulda* and *Cephalostachyum capitatum*. Except for *C. capitatum*, all of the other species can be used on a commercial scale for the preparation of fermented shoots as they can be preserved up to two to three years, making them available throughout the season. Microbiological analyses of fermented bamboo shoots have shown the presence of lactic acid bacteria (LAB), the predominant strains being *Lactobacillus brevis*, *Lb. curvatus*, *Lb. plantarum*, *Pediococcus pentosaceus*, *Leuconostoc mesenteroides* and *Enterococcus durans* (Tamang et al. 2008). Fermentation involves several steps. Sheaths from the freshly harvested shoot are peeled off, cleaned in water and cut into small slices. Earthen pots or baskets made of bamboo culms are used as a container for fermentation (Figure 6.11). When bamboo baskets are used, the inner surface is layered with banana leaves or perforated polythene sheet to drain off liquid exuded during the fermentation process. The chopped bamboo shoots are put into the container tightly by pressing and covered with banana leaves or polythene. These shoots are subjected to heavy weights like stones or wooden logs to keep the shoots under pressure. If using pots, they are filled tightly with shoots up to the neck and covered. After 10–15 days, fresh chopped shoots are added to the pots. This step is repeated as long as the pots can accommodate the shoots. Sometimes, the pots are perforated at the bottom to allow the exudates to flow out. The shoots become fully fermented after 30–45 days and become ready for consumption and sale in the market (Figure 6.12). Local people, however, prefer much old fermented shoots (four to six months). The principle of bamboo shoot fermentation in all the north-eastern states is similar with slight differences in the processing depending upon the state and ethnic group. The shoots are fermented whole, sliced, crushed-fermented moist and crushed-fermented dry of which the fermented sliced is the most popular.

Fermented bamboo shoots known as *Jiang-sun* is a widely used traditional food in Taiwan. For the fermentation process, shoots of *Dendrocalamus latiflorus* are defoliated, cut and then mixed with salt, sugar and dochi (fermented soybeans) to a final concentration of approximately 20–30 g/kg and layered in a bucket to allow

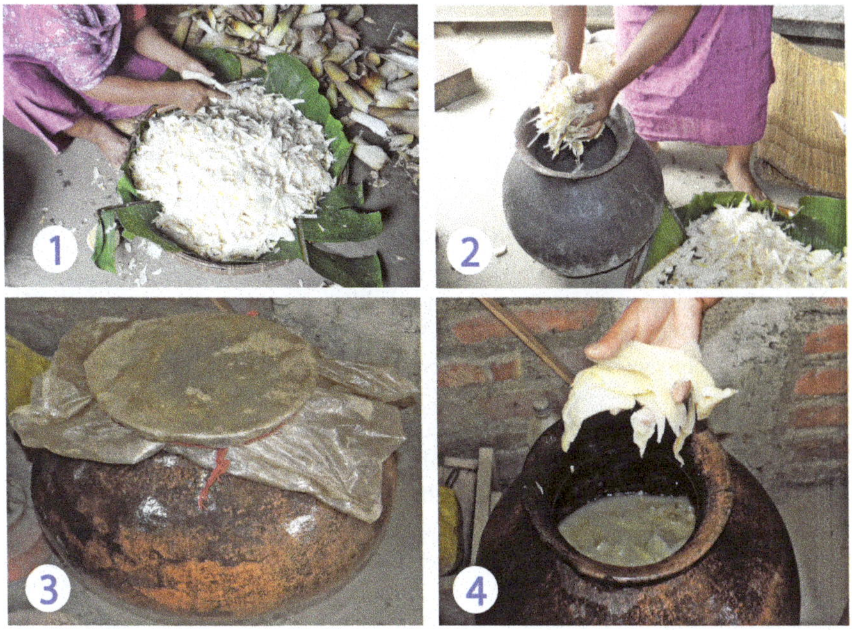

FIGURE 6.11 Traditional methods of bamboo shoot fermentation by the local people of north-east India.

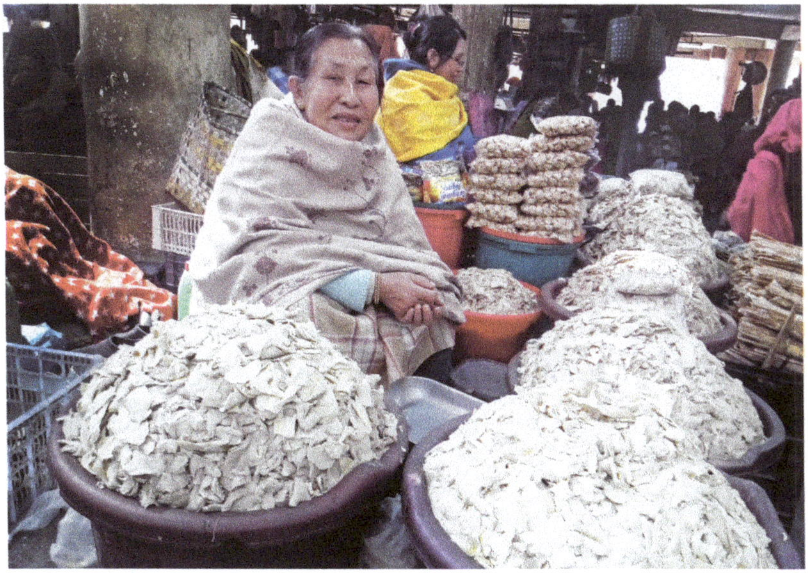

FIGURE 6.12 A woman vendor at Ima Market, Imphal, India, selling fermented bamboo shoot.

fermentation (Chen et al. 2010). *Jiang-sun* is usually used as a seasoning for fish, pork, chicken and various other foods.

6.4 MODERN METHODS OF PROCESSING

6.4.1 Solar-Drying

Banout and Ehl (2010) worked on drying performance and economic aspects of three different drying methods for bamboo shoots in central Vietnam—a double pass solar drier (DPSD), cabinet solar drier (CD) and traditional open sun-drying (OSD). The overall drying efficiency was 23.11%, 15.83% and 9.73% in the case of DPSD, CD and OSD, respectively. DPSD showed a considerable reduction in drying time with maximum drying efficiency as compared to CD and OSD. The construction cost of DPSD was significantly higher than CD but drying cost was found to be lower in the case of DPSD as compared to CD. Overall, DPSD was found to be technically and economically suitable for the drying of bamboo shoots under specific conditions. Piwsaoad and Pusumpao (2015) investigated the performance and artificial neural network (ANN) modeling of the solar dryer for drying bamboo shoot strips. Results showed that drying at a temperature from 31° to 50°C leads to a considerable reduction of drying time as compared to the open-air sun-drying. The product obtained after this dryer was found to be of high quality.

6.4.2 Microwave Drying

Bal et al. (2010) investigated the effect of microwave drying at different power levels (140-350 W) on moisture content, moisture ratio, drying rate, drying time and effective moisture diffusivity in shoots of *Bambusa vulgaris*. Microwave drying reduced the drying time with increased microwave power levels. They further investigated the effect of microwave drying at different power levels (140,210,280 and 350 W) on colour changes kinetics in shoot slices. Colour changes were quantified by tri-stimulus Hunter 'L' (whiteness/darkness), 'a' (redness/greenness) and 'b' (yellowness/blueness) systems. Total colour change, chroma, hue angle and browning index was also calculated by L, a and b values. Hybrid drying system for initial slow drying or by physical and chemical treatment prior to drying of bamboo shoot slices offer the preferred results for colour change which was acceptable to consumers.

6.4.3 Convective Tray-Drying/Hot Air-Drying

Wongsakpairod (2000) compared superheated steam, low-temperature and high-temperature hot air-drying of bamboo shoots in terms of drying kinetics and quality. It was observed that the colour of bamboo shoots was darker by using superheated steam (temperature range 120–160°C) than hot air-drying at the same drying temperature whereas the best colour (lightest) was obtained by low-temperature drying (at 70° C). The bitterness of shoots was reduced after superheated steaming and this data was also in accordance with previous findings that taxiphyllin decomposes at around 116°C. Madamba (2003) found a linear relationship between moisture content and volume change during hot air-drying of bamboo shoots. Bamboo shoots also showed shrinkage parallel to its fibres unlike perpendicular to its fibres.

Kumar et al. (2012) examined the thin layer drying kinetics of bamboo shoot slices of *Dendrocalamus hamiltonii* in a convective tray dryer at three varied temperatures, that is 55, 65 and 75°C. They identified the best-fitted drying model and drying temperature and evaluated its quality by rehydration and sensory features. It was found that the bamboo slices dried at 65° C have superior rehydration as compared to 75° C and 55°C. Furthermore, by using salt solution for rehydration, the rehydration ratio was increased and slices attained more weight irrespective of temperature. It was also noticed that drying of shoots at 65°C yields a product with the highest scores of colour and appearance.

6.4.4 Freeze-Drying

Freeze-drying or lyophilization is a process in which water is frozen, followed by its removal from the sample, initially by sublimation and then by desorption. It is a drying process applicable to the manufacture of certain food products, pharmaceuticals and biologicals that are thermolabile or otherwise unstable in aqueous solutions for prolonged storage periods, but that is stable in the dry state. Coffee was one of the first freeze-dried food products to be created, but now vegetables, fruits, meats, fish, dairy products, herbs and food flavourings are successfully freeze-dried. Freeze-drying maintains the aroma, taste, colour and shape of foods. However, freeze-drying is an expensive practice due to its high operation cost and energy consumption.

Xu et al. (2005) studied the drying methods of (a) hot airflow drying followed by freeze-drying and (b) the reverse of the process. They compared the two processes in terms of cost-effectiveness, energy consumption, rehydration characteristics, physicochemical properties and sensory properties of dried bamboo shoots of *Phyllostachys pubescens*. Dried bamboo shoot slices obtained from the combined freeze and airflow drying were superior to those from single airflow drying concerning sensory, nutrition, cell structure and rehydration ratio features. It was found that 10.5 hr of freeze-drying followed by 4 hr hot air–drying was best in terms of quality and energy consumption which was 21% lower than single freeze-drying.

Cheng (2006) reported that vacuum cooling with hydro cooling and vacuum drying reduces the temperature and water content of the surface and bamboo crust. This process has several advantages including lowering the number of bacteria, prolonged storage time, better quality and appearance whereas some disadvantages include higher equipment cost and lower sugar content. Zheng et al. (2014) evaluated the effect of blanching and drying treatments on the quality of bamboo shoot slices by examining enzyme activity, texture, pectin, microstructure and colour change in shoots of *Dendrocalamus latiflorus*. Microstructure and colour quality of bamboo shoot slices were better maintained after freeze-drying than hot air–drying. The hardness of rehydrated shoot slices decreases more after hot air–drying than freeze-drying. Peroxidase, phenylalanine ammonia-lyase and polyphenol oxidase in shoot slices will become completely inactive at 95°C for 6, 9 and 12 mins blanching treatments, respectively.

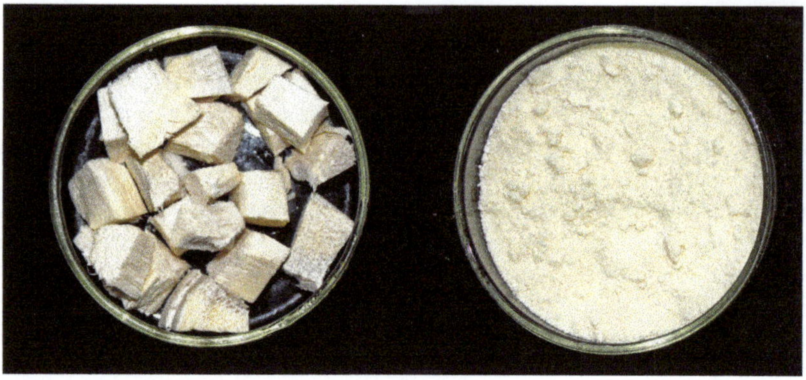

FIGURE 6.13 Freeze-dried shoots and powder of *D. hamiltonii.*

In our experiments conducted on ten species of bamboo, of the different drying methods used, freeze-drying was most efficient in maintaining the colour, aroma and shape of the shoots (Figure 6.13) and retaining the macronutrients (Table 6.4).

6.4.5 Osmotic Dehydration

Osmotic dehydration is the process of partial removal of water from plant tissues by immersion in a hypertonic solution and is considered a valuable tool in minimal processing of foods. Sugar or salt solutions are used to reduce the moisture content of foods before the actual drying process and give the product a quality improvement over the conventional drying process such as reducing the damage of heat to the flavour, colour, inhibiting the browning of enzymes and decrease the energy costs.

Badwaik et al. (2012, 2013, 2014) carried out osmotic dehydration (OD) in shoots of *Bambusa pallida* by using a mixture of sucrose (50 Brix) and varying salt concentrations. Osmotic dehydration, which was used as a pretreatment before the final drying process, was beneficial because it helped in reducing the moisture level to around 71% from an initial moisture content of 93%. Thus, it helped in reducing the drying time to some extent. The shoots were dried by using three drying methods viz. tray drying, vacuum drying and fluidized bed drying at temperatures of 45, 55 and 65°C. The microstructure of bamboo shoots was affected by drying methods. They further evaluated the effect of various processing conditions, that is NaCl concentration (5–15% w/w), process time (30–240 mins) and temperature of the osmotic solution (30–50°C) on water loss, solid gain, rehydration ratio and sensory quality. Experiments were designed according to central composite rotatable design and response surface methodology was used to determine the optimum processing conditions. The optimum conditions for osmotic dehydration were found to be in the range of 8.89–11.08% NaCl in 50 Brix sucrose syrup, 34.09–44.45°C osmotic solution temperature and 72.64–104.48 mins processing duration to achieve quality shoots in terms of maximum water loss, minimum solid gain, better rehydration ratio and sensory quality.

6.4.6 Canning

Canning is a method of preserving food in which the food contents are processed and sealed in an airtight container either metal cans or glass bottles and provides a shelf-life typically ranging from one to five years. In the canning process, vegetables are often cut into pieces, packed in cans and put through severe heat treatment to ensure the destruction of bacterial spores. The containers are sealed while hot so as to create a vacuum inside when they are cooled to room temperature. Properly processed canned vegetables can be stored at room temperature for years. Unfortunately, because of the severe heat treatment, some canned vegetables can have inferior quality and less nutritive value than fresh and frozen products. The nutrient most susceptible to destruction in canning is vitamin C.

Bamboo shoots are also preserved by the canning process which increases its shelf-life. Canned bamboo shoots are normally packed in tin or glass jars containing plain water or brine solution. There are different packs of canned bamboo shoots: bamboo shoot slice, strips, shoot tips, whole, shoot half, cubes or dices. For canning of bamboo shoots, fresh shoots are washed and the outer culm sheaths peeled off. The soft edible portion is extracted and cut into half, slices, cubes and shredded to make strips. This is followed by steaming or boiling in water for 10–20 mins. The processed shoots are then vacuum packed in a tin, glass jars or polypropylene packs containing water or 1–5% brine solution. The amount of water or brine solution should be 50% of the shoots to be packed.

6.5 PROCESSING METHODS FOR REMOVAL OF ANTI-NUTRIENTS

Bamboo shoots need to be processed to remove anti-nutrients especially cyanogenic glucosides to make them safe for consumption. Other anti-nutrients include oxalates, glucosinolates, phytate, tannin and saponin. Appropriate processing methods prior to consumption are needed to remove these anti-nutrients. This can be achieved by several processing methods such as slicing, peeling, soaking, blanching, cooking (boiling, roasting), brine treatment, fermentation, drying and canning.

6.5.1 Cyanogenic Glycoside

Soaking is quite effective in eliminating cyanogens particularly in those species which have low content. The soaking of shoots can be for few hours as in the case of *Chimonobambusa callosa*, *Phyllostachys mannii* and *Melocanna baccifera* all of which have very low cyanogen content in fresh shoots to long-term treatment in closed containers or in running water in rivers and streams in those species which have very high content of cyanogen in the fresh shoots. Shoots of these species are also eaten raw in a salad without boiling or cooking. Whereas raw shoots of some species like *Dendrocalamus asper*, *D. hamiltonii* and *Bambusa bambos* are very bitter and need thorough washing and soaking in water for several hours. The *Khasi* and *Jaintia* tribes of Meghalaya have a unique method of removing the anti-nutrients from the shoots of *D. hamiltonii* which has a high content of cyanogenic glycoside in fresh shoots (Table 6.1). The shoots are chopped in small chips and soaked in plain

TABLE 6.1
Effect of Various Processing Methods On Cyanogenic Glycoside Content (mg/kg HCN f.w.) in Shoots of Different Bamboo Species

Species	Fresh	Boiled (20 mins)	Soaked (12 hrs)	Fermented (3 months)
Bambusa balcooa	1108.32 ± 18.54	133.80 ± 11.64	420.29 ± 9.17	388.24 ± 4.36
B. bambos	1366.50 ± 66.72	170.08 ± 10.08	317.19 ± 11.84	117.82 ± 9.75
B. nutans	1264.82 ± 63.84	210.38 ± 10.08	200.37 ± 9.48	108.50 ± 7.84
B. tulda	1367.76 ± 0.41	83.62 ± 0.70	122.15 ± 0.65	122.02 ± 0.68
Dendrocalamus giganteus	1067.13 ± 0.63	116.60 ± 0.93	258.53 ± 0.61	108.17 ± 0.52
D. hamiltonii	733.91 ± 9.41	95.04 ± 2.39	370.45 ± 3.22	410.27 ± 4.67
D. latiflorus	1171.64 ± 0.92	128.28 ± 0.64	157.43 ± 0.84	34.15 ± 0.50
D. membranaceus	1042.73 ± 0.18	109.43 ± 0.54	246.20 ± 0.55	98.88 ± 1.08
D. sikkimensis	1517.47 ± 14.96	270.28 ± 10.76	357.82 ± 13.64	201.92 ± 20.16
Phyllostachys mannii	36.22 ± 0.11	4.71 ± 0.05	13.49 ± 0.02	21.34 ± 0.07

Values reported are measurement replication means ± standard deviation (n = 3 replicates).

water for more than six months, after which the shoots lose all anti-nutrient elements and become palatable. The decrease in cyanogen also depends on some factors like temperature, time and medium in which the material is soaked. Experimental studies showed that shoots of *D. hamiltonii* and *D. giganteus* showed around 50 and 75% reduction in cyanogenic glycoside when soaked for 12 hrs in plain water and furthermore during fermentation (Table 6.1, Figure 6.14).

Duration of boiling and the amount of water used for boiling greatly affect the reduction of the cyanogenic glycoside. Different processed forms of shoots, that is boiled, soaked and fermented shoots of ten species were analyzed for their cyanogenic content to know the effect of processing methods on cyanogenic content in shoots (Table 6.1). Boiling for 20 mins and soaking for 12 hrs caused a maximum reduction of cyanogenic content in shoots of *Bambusa tulda* (81–93% and 49–91%, respectively). The maximum reduction of cyanogen content (up to 97%) was observed in fermented shoots. Boiling of bamboo shoots in different concentrations of brine has also been reported to reduce the cyanogenic content efficiently. Pandey and Ojha (2014) processed young shoots of *B. bambos*, *B. tulda*, *D. strictus* and *D. asper* by boiling in 1%, 5% and 10% NaCl for different intervals (10, 15, 20, 25 mins). Boiling the shoots in 5% NaCl for 15 mins was found to be the best method for *B.bambos*, ten mins boiling in 1% NaCl for *B. tulda* and *D. asper* and 15 mins boiling in 1% NaCl for *D. strictus*. Rana et al. (2012) optimized NaCl treatment for maximum reduction of cyanide content in *Dendrocalamus strictus* using response surface methodology with four independent variables like the concentration of NaCl, thickness of bamboo shoot, amount of NaCl solution and duration of treatment at three levels of each variable. Cyanide content ranged from 12.8 and 29.6 mg/kg after NaCl treatment. The effect of concentration of NaCl was more effective in reducing the cyanide content

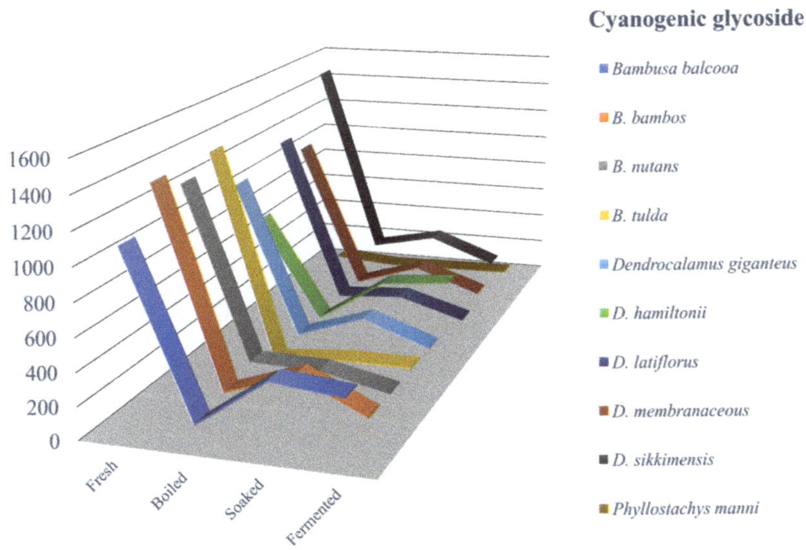

FIGURE 6.14 Effect of various processing methods on cyanogenic glycoside content (mg/kg HCN f.w.) in shoots of different bamboo species.

followed by the thickness of the shoot and treatment time. The optimum condition was 2.4% NaCl concentration, 1.25 cm thickness, 216 ml of NaCl solution and 23 mins treatment. Corresponding cyanide content was 11.2 mg/kg which is quite low and safe. The reduction of cyanide content was 98.3% at the optimum level.

6.5.2 Effect of Processing on Other Anti-Nutrients

Effect of processing on other anti-nutrients such as glucosinolates, oxalates, phytates, saponin and tannin have not been studied extensively. It is seen that most of the processing treatments such as soaking (12 hrs), boiling (20 min) and fermentation (3 months) cause a reduction in these anti-nutrients (Sharma 2018). A maximum reduction in glucosinolate content was seen in fermented shoots (67–74%) (Table 6.2).

Several other studies have also reported a similar reduction in glucosinolate content upon processing treatments such as blanching, steaming, boiling and fermentation. In the case of oxalates, the reduction was maximum in fermented shoots wherein oxalate content reduced by 48.46% in the case of *B. tulda* shoots (Table 6.2). Between boiling and soaking, boiling was more effective in reducing oxalate content whereas fermentation was found to be most effective in terms of reduction in oxalate content. Phytate content reduction is highest in the fermented samples as seen in *B. tulda* shoots (97.23%). There was no significant difference between boiling and soaking treatments in terms of the reduction of phytate content. Sarangthem and Singh (2013) also reported a reduction in phytate content in fermented shoots of *D. hamiltonii* and *B. balcooa* where it gets reduced from 35.95 to 30.67 mg/100 g in case of fresh shoots, respectively.

TABLE 6.2
Effect of Various Processing Methods on Anti-Nutrient Content (mg/100 g f.w.) in Shoots of Four Bamboo Species

Species/ Processing Treatments	Glucosinolates	Oxalates	Saponins	Phytates	Tannins
			Bambusa tulda		
Fresh	29.99 ± 0.62	283.71 ± 0.49	229.58 ± 0.88	86.25 ± 0.61	49.03 ± 0.60
Boiled	17.44 ± 0.97	233.72 ± 0.52	174.43 ± 0.92	48.11 ± 0.28	33.84 ± 0.50
Soaked	13.01 ± 0.61	299.43 ± 0.25	185.91 ± 0.58	49.33 ± 0.30	32.99 ± 0.56
Fermented	8.89 ± 0.47	146.22 ± 0.21	43.91 ± 0.52	2.39 ± 0.69	6.82 ± 0.74
			D. giganteus		
Fresh	27.02 ± 0.67	286.58 ± 0.93	232.96 ± 0.55	90.33 ± 0.51	51.14 ± 0.38
Boiled	14.72 ± 1.25	236.10 ± 0.34	177.21 ± 0.13	52.37 ± 0.38	36.26 ± 0.66
Soaked	10.85 ± 1.33	269.26 ± 0.56	190.03 ± 0.70	53.76 ± 0.58	35.32 ± 0.49
Fermented	7.75 ± 0.70	158.48 ± 0.83	48.11 ± 0.70	4.63 ± 0.44	8.14 ± 0.10
			D. latiflorus		
Fresh	26.45 ± 0.91	263.93 ± 1.08	241.96 ± 0.50	94.60 ± 0.80	40.09 ± 0.32
Boiled	14.59 ± 0.69	213.03 ± 0.34	204.97 ± 0.45	57.65 ± 0.76	27.22 ± 0.36
Soaked	9.44 ± 1.03	244.66 ± 0.84	208.57 ± 0.77	60.73 ± 0.65	26.30 ± 0.56
Fermented	6.97 ± 0.13	166.08 ± 0.73	50.85 ± 0.49	11.51 ± 0.87	2.50 ± 0.41
			D. membranaceus		
Fresh	27.52 ± 0.50	278.28 ± 0.75	246.22 ± 0.27	96.78 ± 0.69	42.68 ± 0.94
Boiled	15.92 ± 0.49	228.55 ± 0.86	210.01 ± 0.65	59.87 ± 0.64	29.56 ± 0.65
Soaked	9.89 ± 0.12	258.68 ± 0.21	212.96 ± 0.50	63.13 ± 0.87	27.93 ± 0.18
Fermented	7.13 ± 0.29	187.28 ± 0.35	53.34 ± 0.51	12.19 ± 0.43	5.83 ± 0.21

Values reported are measurement replication means ± standard deviation (n = 3 replicates).

Regarding saponin content, the maximum reduction was seen in fermented samples wherein saponin content reduced about 80% in *D. giganteus*. A similar reduction after fermentation was reported by Sarangthem and Singh (2013). These authors also determined the tannin content of fresh shoots of *D. hamiltonii* (45.49 mg/100 g) and *B. balcooa* (31.49 mg/100 g). They also reported that fermentation caused an increase in the tannin content as compared to fresh shoots. In our studies of four species, *B. tulda*, *D. giganteus*, *D. latiflorus* and *D. membranaceus*, it was found that all the processing treatments caused a reduction in the tannin content (Table 6.2). Maximum reduction in tannin content was seen in fermented shoots where the tannin content reduced by 93.76% in *D. latiflorus* (Figure 6.15).

6.6 EFFECT OF PROCESSING ON NUTRIENT CONTENT

Processing not only changes the physical attributes of the shoots such as texture, colour and flavour but also the nutrient content depending upon the processing

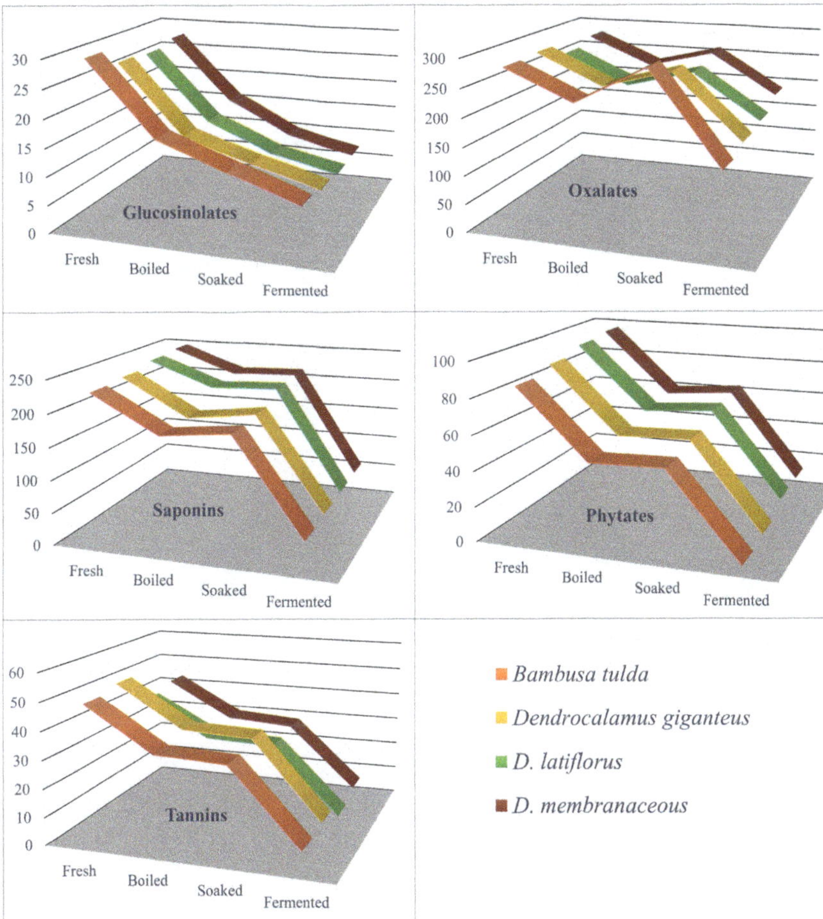

FIGURE 6.15 Effect of processing on anti-nutrient content (mg/100 g) in shoots of four bamboo species.

method used (Tables 6.1–6.6). It is preferable to use the method in which maximum nutrient is retained. A proper combination of treatment duration, temperature and concentration in the case of brine, is very important to retain the nutrients and quality of the bamboo shoots. Processing treatments viz. soaking, boiling, drying and fermentation bring about significant changes in the macronutrient content of the shoots (Bajwa et al. 2016, Rawat et al. 2016, Saini et al. 2017). Fresh shoots were boiled for different durations viz. 10 mins, 20 mins and 30 mins and soaked for 6 hrs, 12 hrs and 24 hrs for analysis. For oven-drying, fresh shoots were dried at 60°C for 24 hrs. For freeze-drying, fresh shoots are cut into cubes and frozen at –50°C for 24 hrs in deep freezer followed by vacuum freeze-drying at –50°C for 24 hrs in a lyophilizer. Freeze-drying maintained the shoot volume and was creamish, lighter weight, porous and the powder was soft with pleasant aroma as compared to the sun and oven-dried shoots (Figure 6.16.). The colour of oven-dried shoots varied from light to dark brown (Figure 6.17.). The nutrient content increased three to more than

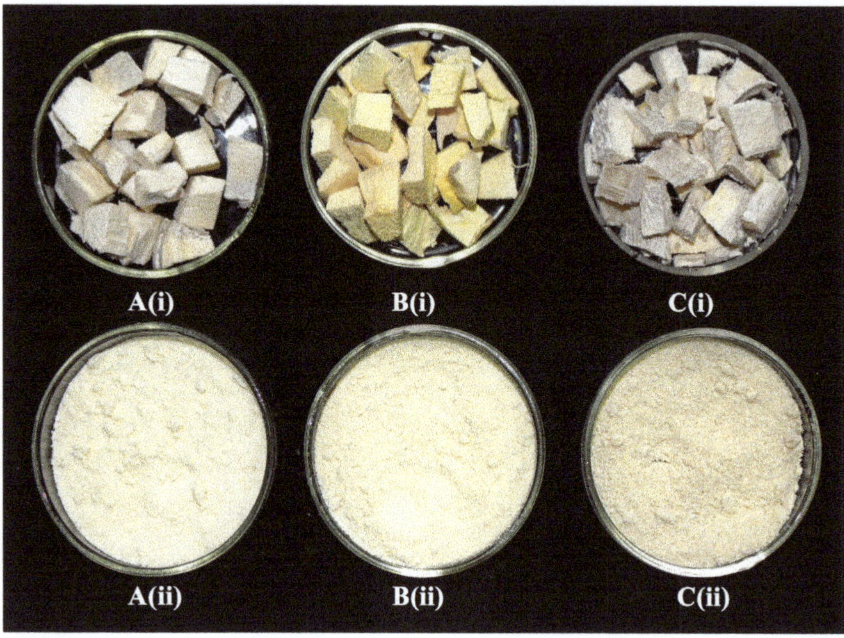

FIGURE 6.16 Freeze-dried shoot and powder of *D. hamiltonii*, A(i–ii) fresh; B(i–ii) boiled and C(i-ii) soaked.

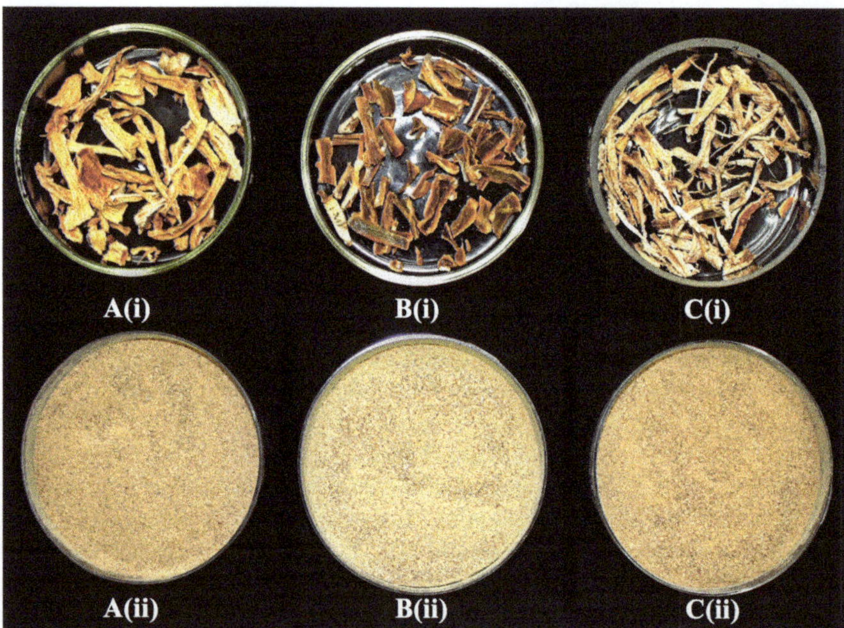

FIGURE 6.17 Oven-dried shoot and powder of *D. hamiltonii*, A(i–ii) fresh; B(i–ii) boiled and C(i–ii) soaked

ten times in freeze-dried shoots compared to the fresh shoots (Table 6.4). Boiling the shoots for 20 mins retained most of the macronutrients except amino acids, vitamin C and vitamin E, which showed an increase during fermentation (Rawat et al. 2016). A decrease in most of the macronutrients was observed when the shoots were soaked in water for 12 hrs. When shoots were subjected to different drying processes, freeze-drying was the most effective in retaining most of the nutrients as nutrient content increased four to five times compared to fresh shoots.

6.6.1 Protein

With harvesting age of shoots, the protein content reduces gradually as reported by Chongtham et al. (2007) and Pandey and Ojha (2013) in 10-day-old and 16-day-old shoots when compared with freshly harvested juvenile shoots. Blanching of shoots of *B. balcooa* for 5–30 mins reduced the protein content by 9.52 to 41% and the reduction was higher with longer blanching time and temperature (Badwaik et al. 2015). Zhang et al. (2011) studied the effect of cooking treatments on the protein content and reported higher reduction (7.38%) after ten mins boiling of shoots of *P. praecox* as compared to stir-frying and steaming (1.23%). Chongtham et al. (2008) revealed that canned shoots have the lowest (1.93%) protein content followed by fermented (2.57%) and raw shoots (3.11%) in *D. giganteus* species. Badwaik et al. (2014) analyzed fresh and fermented shoots of *B. balcooa* and found a decline in protein content after fermentation (2.56%) in comparison to fresh shoots (3.78%).

Protein content in the fresh shoots of ten investigated species ranged from a minimum of 3.03 g/100 g of fresh weight (f.w.) in *D. sikkimensis* to maximum 5.87 g/100 g in *B. bambos*. Protein reduced with all processing practices in all the species (Table 6.3, Figure 6.18). Soaking was better in retaining protein (1.65–2.97 g/100 g) in all the species with maximum retention in *D. membranaceous* (2.97g/100g) and minimum in *D. sikkimensis* (1.65g/100g). There was more retention of protein after boiling (0.65–2.17 g/100 g) than fermentation (0.32–2.71 g/100 g) in all the species except *D. giganteus, D. hamiltonii* and *D. membranaceous* which retained more protein with fermentation than boiling. With different drying processes (sun, oven and freeze), there was an increase in the protein content which ranged from 12.77 to 27.32 g/100 g dry weight. The maximum amount was observed with freeze-drying followed by sun and oven-drying of shoots in most of the species.

6.6.2 Carbohydrate

The carbohydrate content is also affected by harvesting age and processing methods in different bamboos as reported by several researchers (Chongtham et al. 2008, Pandey and Ojha 2013). The decline in carbohydrate content on boiling the shoots of four bamboo species (*B. tulda, B. bambos, D. asper, D. strictus*) for different durations (10–25 mins) in water and NaCl (1%–10%) concentration was reported by Pandey and Ojha (2014). Similarly, blanching of *B. balcooa* shoots at different temperatures and duration (5–30 mins) showed a drop in carbohydrate content (Badwaik et al. 2015). Park and Jhon (2013), detected three sugars with high fructose content

TABLE 6.3

Macronutrients (g/100 g f.w.) and Vitamins (mg/100 g f.w.) Content in Boiled—20 Mins, Soaked—12 Hrs, Fermented—3 Month Shoots

Species	Processing Treatments	Carbohydrate	Amino acid	Starch	Protein	Fat	Vit C	Vit E	Ash	Moisture
Bambusa balcooa	Fresh	3.22 ± 0.13	2.13 ± 0.03	1.21 ± 0.02	3.70 ± 0.09	0.47 ± 0.01	2.63 ± 0.02	0.42 ± 0.02	0.86 ± 0.02	90.68 ± 0.09
	Boiled	2.33 ± 0.05	1.28 ± 0.04	1.71 ± 0.08	0.82 ± 0.00	0.32 ± 0.02	1.36 ± 0.02	0.32 ± 0.00	0.80 ± 0.02	91.72 ± 0.05
	Soaked	1.50 ± 0.08	1.50 ± 0.06	1.18 ± 0.01	2.34 ± 0.12	0.28 ± 0.01	1.72 ± 0.01	0.34 ± 0.02	0.37 ± 0.01	93.60 ± 0.02
	Fermented	0.32 ± 0.01	2.46 ± 0.02	2.24 ± 0.14	0.314 ± 0.02	0.42 ± 0.02	1.79 ± 0.03	0.35 ± 0.01	1.34 ± 0.02	85.78 ± 0.14
B. bambos	Fresh	2.24 ± 0.08	2.02 ± 0.05	1.24 ± 0.08	5.87 ± 0.39	0.53 ± 0.04	1.62 ± 0.01	0.61 ± 0.01	0.88 ± 0.03	90.09 ± 0.10
	Boiled	1.6 4 ± 0.04	1.39 ± 0.01	1.37 ± 0.02	1.53 ± 0.02	0.40 ± 0.03	0.97 ± 0.01	0.47 ± 0.01	0.73 ± 0.01	92.10 ± 0.15
	Soaked	1.57 ± 0.06	1.75 ± 0.05	0.70 ± 0.04	2.12 ± 0.06	0.36 ± 0.03	1.08 ± 0.02	0.52 ± 0.01	0.69 ± 0.03	92.80 ± 0.10
	Fermented	1.25 ± 0.04	1.54 ± 0.06	0.95 ± 0.02	1.30 ± 0.02	0.79 ± 0.01	1.60 ± 0.02	0.44 ± 0.02	0.88 ± 0.01	85.87 ± 0.12
B. tulda	Fresh	3.26 ± 0.02	1.92 ± 0.02	1.20 ± 0.02	3.16 ± 0.01	0.51 ± 0.04	2.45 ± 0.04	0.58 ± 0.01	0.93 ± 0.01	83.00 ± 0.08
	Boiled	2.43 ± 0.02	1.50 ± 0.02	2.18 ± 0.01	1.16 ± 0.02	0.40 ± 0.02	1.32 ± 0.02	0.37 ± 0.01	0.89 ± 0.01	85.89 ± 0.07
	Soaked	2.26 ± 0.07	1.55 ± 0.02	0.75 ± 0.01	1.65 ± 0.02	0.33 ± 0.02	1.39 ± 0.02	0.40 ± 0.02	0.59 ± 0.02	87.71 ± 0.07
	Fermented	0.49 ± 0.01	1.94 ± 0.01	0.45 ± 0.01	0.57 ± 0.02	0.18 ± 0.01	0.72 ± 0.02	0.37 ± 0.01	1.76 ± 0.01	82.06 ± 0.06
B. nutans	Fresh	2.76 ± 0.10	3.45 ± 0.05	1.36 ± 0.08	3.47 ± 0.23	0.70 ± 0.08	1.90 ± 0.02	0.49 ± 0.01	0.82 ± 0.01	91.21 ± 0.09
	Boiled	1.90 ± 0.02	1.65 ± 0.01	1.53 ± 0.02	1.09 ± 0.02	0.57 ± 0.02	0.71 ± 0.01	0.30 ± 0.01	0.69 ± 0.02	92.72 ± 0.10
	Soaked	1.73 ± 0.04	1.99 ± 0.03	0.92 ± 0.03	1.69 ± 0.05	0.40 ± 0.03	0.98 ± 0.01	0.44 ± 0.01	0.64 ± 0.01	93.74 ± 0.11
	Fermented	1.32 ± 0.01	1.88 ± 0.03	1.09 ± 0.04	0.89 ± 0.06	0.87 ± 0.02	1.49 ± 0.02	0.31 ± 0.01	0.87 ± 0.03	89.87 ± 0.03
Dendrocalamus giganteus	Fresh	5.65 ± 0.06	2.26 ± 0.04	2.38 ± 0.04	3.64 ± 0.05	0.49 ± 0.02	2.21 ± 0.02	0.56 ± 0.03	1.03 ± 0.00	89.02 ± 0.03
	Boiled	4.11 ± 0.03	1.53 ± 0.01	2.67 ± 0.01	1.27 ± 0.01	0.39 ± 0.00	1.26 ± 0.02	0.40 ± 0.01	0.76 ± 0.01	89.64 ± 0.02
	Soaked	4.46 ± 0.05	1.78 ± 0.01	1.41 ± 0.02	1.72 ± 0.02	0.32 ± 0.01	0.81 ± 0.01	0.48 ± 0.01	0.72 ± 0.01	92.68 ± 0.04
	Fermented	1.52 ± 0.02	2.31 ± 0.03	1.45 ± 0.06	1.57 ± 0.02	0.49 ± 0.03	1.26 ± 0.04	0.24 ± 0.03	1.19 ± 0.02	87.83 ± 0.13

(*Continued*)

TABLE 6.3 (CONTINUED)
Macronutrients (g/100 g f.w.) and Vitamins (mg/100 g f.w.) Content in Boiled—20 Mins, Soaked—12 Hrs, Fermented—3 Month Shoots

Species	Processing Treatments	Carbohydrate	Amino acid	Starch	Protein	Fat	Vit C	Vit E	Ash	Moisture
D. hamiltonii	Fresh	3.33 ± 0.04	2.33 ± 0.02	1.74 ± 0.02	3.37 ± 0.03	0.42 ± 0.02	2.48 ± 0.07	0.68 ± 0.03	0.76 ± 0.02	91.33 ± 0.18
	Boiled	2.78 ± 0.12	1.47 ± 0.04	1.83 ± 0.03	1.65 ± 0.02	0.38 ± 0.02	1.11 ± 0.04	0.32 ± 0.02	0.73 ± 0.04	91.74 ± 0.02
	Soaked	2.60 ± 0.03	1.97 ± 0.03	1.03 ± 0.01	2.85 ± 0.06	0.34 ± 0.01	1.26 ± 0.02	0.37 ± 0.02	0.68 ± 0.03	92.58 ± 0.11
	Fermented	1.58 ± 0.02	2.37 ± 0.09	0.99 ± 0.01	2.71 ± 0.05	0.41 ± 0.03	1.38 ± 0.01	0.44 ± 0.01	1.72 ± 0.05	86.91 ± 0.16
D. latiflorus	Fresh	3.44 ± 0.01	2.22 ± 0.02	0.93 ± 0.01	3.47 ± 0.02	0.45 ± 0.02	2.39 ± 0.02	0.54 ± 0.01	0.80 ± 0.01	88.81 ± 0.05
	Boiled	2.83 ± 0.02	1.63 ± 0.01	1.87 ± 0.03	1.34 ± 0.01	0.37 ± 0.01	1.24 ± 0.01	0.35 ± 0.01	0.79 ± 0.01	91.92 ± 0.07
	Soaked	2.67 ± 0.05	1.74 ± 0.01	0.91 ± 0.02	2.11 ± 0.01	0.30 ± 0.01	1.27 ± 0.01	0.35 ± 0.01	0.51 ± 0.02	96.45 ± 0.09
	Fermented	0.62 ± 0.02	3.53 ± 0.02	0.71 ± 0.02	0.48 ± 0.01	0.27 ± 0.01	0.86 ± 0.02	0.25 ± 0.01	1.63 ± 0.02	86.19 ± 0.12
D. membranaceus	Fresh	3.48 ± 0.03	3.20 ± 0.02	1.49 ± 0.04	3.65 ± 0.09	0.44 ± 0.05	1.83 ± 0.04	0.65 ± 0.03	1.00 ± 0.04	89.02 ± 0.33
	Boiled	2.59 ± 0.03	2.21 ± 0.05	1.74 ± 0.02	0.65 ± 0.02	0.41 ± 0.02	0.78 ± 0.02	0.36 ± 0.01	0.98 ± 0.03	89.61 ± 0.04
	Soaked	3.11 ± 0.06	3.06 ± 0.01	1.09 ± 0.01	2.97 ± 0.04	0.36 ± 0.01	1.01 ± 0.06	0.44 ± 0.02	0.70 ± 0.04	92.59 ± 0.12
	Fermented	1.09 ± 0.02	2.29 ± 0.03	1.02 ± 0.01	2.46 ± 0.03	0.44 ± 0.01	1.48 ± 0.08	0.48 ± 0.02	1.26 ± 0.02	87.08 ± 0.18
D. sikkimensis	Fresh	2.99 ± 0.03	1.87 ± 0.02	1.13 ± 0.02	3.03 ± 0.13	0.51 ± 0.01	2.43 ± 0.03	0.59 ± 0.04	0.76 ± 0.03	91.47 ± 0.04
	Boiled	2.14 ± 0.02	1.22 ± 0.05	1.49 ± 0.02	0.94 ± 0.09	0.40 ± 0.01	1.42 ± 0.01	0.42 ± 0.01	0.56 ± 0.01	91.81 ± 0.02
	Soaked	1.95 ± 0.04	1.32 ± 0.03	0.78 ± 0.01	1.65 ± 0.02	0.35 ± 0.00	0.85 ± 0.02	0.53 ± 0.03	0.55 ± 0.03	93.79 ± 0.02
	Fermented	1.39 ± 0.06	1.30 ± 0.03	1.15 ± 0.06	0.72 ± 0.01	0.80 ± 0.02	2.46 ± 0.03	0.41 ± 0.01	0.74 ± 0.01	86.52 ± 0.22
Phyllostachys mannii	Fresh	2.73 ± 0.02	2.36 ± 0.06	1.09 ± 0.02	3.24 ± 0.03	0.44 ± 0.01	3.23 ± 0.05	0.53 ± 0.03	0.86 ± 0.01	90.34 ± 0.12
	Boiled	1.14 ± 0.05	1.09 ± 0.03	0.87 ± 0.06	2.17 ± 0.03	0.29 ± 0.02	1.01 ± 0.01	0.48 ± 0.02	0.85 ± 0.01	91.52 ± 0.14
	Soaked	0.89 ± 0.03	1.22 ± 0.02	0.60 ± 0.04	2.53 ± 0.02	0.23 ± 0.03	1.34 ± 0.04	0.48 ± 0.03	0.40 ± 0.02	95.89 ± 0.11
	Fermented	1.09 ± 0.02	1.83 ± 0.04	1.35 ± 0.07	1.28 ± 0.02	0.25 ± 0.02	1.09 ± 0.03	0.44 ± 0.01	1.21 ± 0.02	80.91 ± 0.11

Values reported are measurement replication means ± standard deviation (n = 3 replicates).

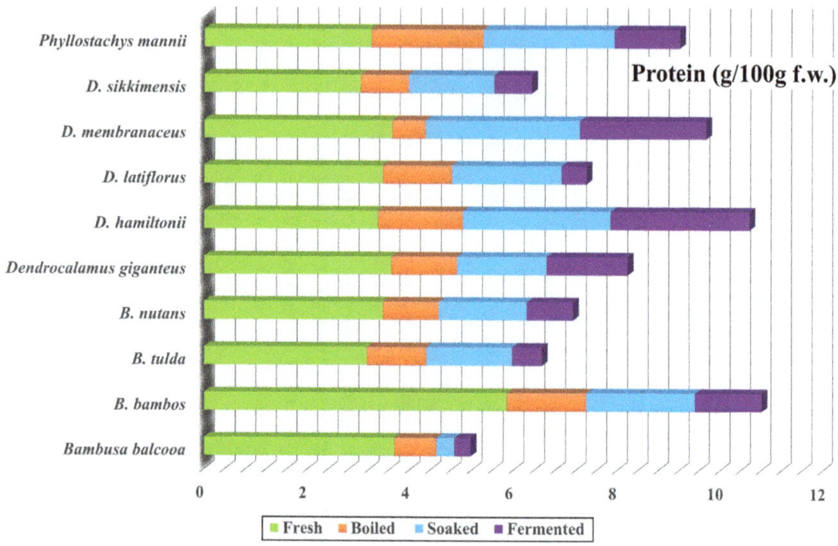

FIGURE 6.18 Effects of processing in protein (g/100 g f.w.) content in shoots of different bamboo species.

followed by glucose and galactose and also showed a reduction in these sugars with boiling except galactose in the shoots of *P. pubescens*. Bamboo shoots have been reported to maintain their firmness even after heat processing due to the presence of glucose and xylose rich low methoxyl pectin, which prevents the disintegration of polysaccharides (Fuchigami, 1990). Sun et al. (2015) examined carbohydrate composition by HPLC-ion chromatography in the dried shoots of *P. pubescens* and confirmed the presence of fructose (9.11 g/kg) as the main component followed by glucose (2.04 g/kg) and galactose (0.24 g/kg). With fermentation, carbohydrate content was reduced significantly in *B. balcooa* (Badwaik et al. 2014) and *D. giganteus* (Chongtham et al. 2008) shoots. Awol (2015) reported 73.5% of the carbohydrate content in sun-dried bamboo shoots.

In bamboo species investigated by our team, carbohydrate content in boiled, soaked, fermented, sun, oven and freeze-dried shoots were compared (Table 6.3–6.4). Boiling retained higher carbohydrates in all the species except *D. giganteus* and *D. membranaceus* where soaking was found better (Figure 6.19). Fermentation influenced conspicuously the carbohydrate content and caused higher losses than soaking and boiling in all the species. The amount was lowered maximum up to 0.32 g/100 g in *B. balcooa*. In dried shoots, carbohydrate content ranged from 7.15 to 33.47 g/100 g d.w. (Table 6.4). The amount was found maximum with freeze-drying in all the species. However, there was some variation among oven and sun-dried shoots in the studied species.

6.6.3 Total Free Amino Acids

Free amino acid profiles in the bamboo shoots have not been studied extensively and only limited bamboo species have been investigated (Zhang et al. 2011, Park and

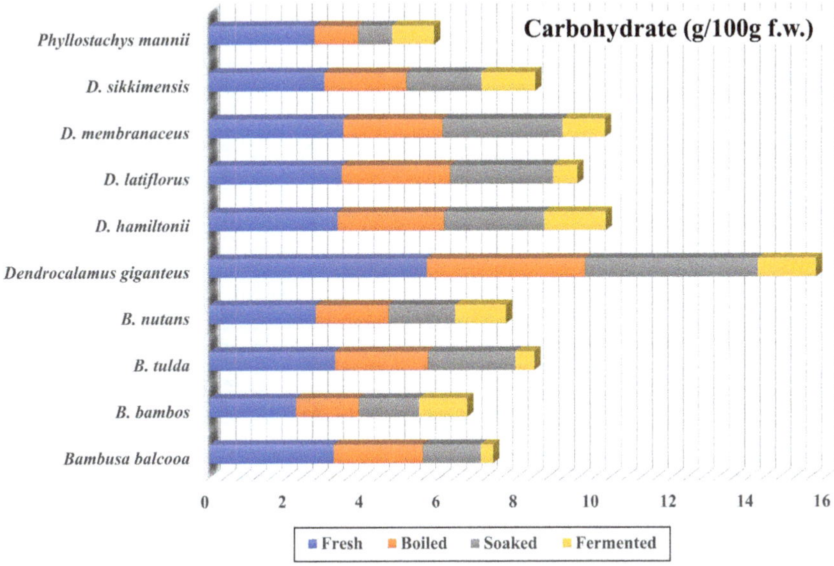

FIGURE 6.19 Effects of processing in carbohydrate (g/100 g f.w.) content in shoots of different bamboo species.

Jhon 2013, Zheng et al. 2013, Sun et al. 2015). Zhang et al. (2011) investigated the effect of three cooking treatments on *P. praecox* shoots and reported 12 free amino acids, including six non-essential (Asp, Glu, Gly, Ala, Tyr and His) and six essential (Val, Met, Ile, Leu, Phe and Lys) with predominantly highest value of tyrosine (163 mg/100g f.w). They depicted reduction in the amount of most of the free amino acids after boiling and stir-frying, despite an improvement in Glu, Gly, Tyr and Ile content after steaming. Changes in free amino acid content in the fresh shoots and after the pickling process in *D. latiflorus* was studied by Zheng et al. (2013). The studies showed aspartic and glutamic acids to be the most abundant amino acids among the 17 detected amino acids in the fresh shoots and also reported a decrease in total free amino acid content by 58% in low salt (8%) and 52% in high salt (20%) pickling process. Park and Jhon (2013) evaluated free amino acid composition in fresh and boiled shoots of two species, that is *P. pubescens* and *P. nigra*. They identified 21 amino acids, of which asparagine, tyrosine and glutamine were the most copious. Asparagine plays a vital role in ammonia detoxification, fatigue relieving, maintaining immunity, nervous system and brain functioning (Wu 2013). Tyrosine is involved in melanin synthesis, improving brain function, treating depression, sleep and brain disorders (Harmer et al. 2001). According to the reports of Park and Jhon (2013), content of different amino acids varied differently with boiling treatments. Amino acids like Cys, Asp, Asn, Ser, His, Thr, Val and Trp showed an increase while other amino acids decreased in *P. pubescens.* Our investigation of ten bamboo species revealed that the amino acid content reduced with boiling and soaking in all the species but increased with fermentation in some of the species (Figure 6.20). Soaking maintained a higher amino acid proportion in seven species (*B. balcooa, B. bambos, B. nutans, D. hamiltonii, D. latiflorus, D. membranaceus, D. sikkimensis*) compared with boiling.

TABLE 6.4

Nutrient Components in Dried Shoots (g/100 g d.w.) of Some Bamboo Species

Species	Dried forms	Carbohydrate	Protein	Fat	Ash	NDF	ADF	Lignin
Bambusa balcooa	Sun	18.22 ± 0.24	23.18 ± 1.48	6.30 ± 0.09	9.56 ± 0.18	62.11 ± 3.20	10.93 ± 0.22	2.97 ± 0.14
	Oven	14.27 ± 0.08	20.87 ± 1.70	7.47 ± 0.08	9.53 ± 0.10	67.08 ± 2.53	10.13 ± 0.56	2.09 ± 0.15
	Freeze	27.09 ± 0.46	23.88 ± 0.88	4.42 ± 0.04	9.83 ± 0.12	66.88 ± 3.11	7.84 ± 0.63	1.76 ± 0.14
B. bambos	Sun	7.92 ± 0.73	25.38 ± 0.54	4.56 ± 0.04	9.37 ± 0.12	53.65 ± 1.52	14.95 ± 0.91	2.75 ± 0.10
	Oven	12.77 ± 0.56	27.08 ± 0.73	4.65 ± 0.10	9.31 ± 0.14	53.05 ± 3.04	12.25 ± 0.49	2.61 ± 0.11
	Freeze	13.48 ± 0.44	24.18 ± 0.35	4.60 ± 0.13	9.19 ± 0.15	60.45 ± 1.81	9.10 ± 0.42	2.43 ± 0.09
B. nutans	Sun	13.64 ± 0.24	22.63 ± 0.47	6.72 ± 0.22	9.40 ± 0.14	59.90 ± 1.65	18.60 ± 0.28	4.17 ± 0.12
	Oven	16.26 ± 0.25	26.77 ± 0.20	6.70 ± 0.17	9.58 ± 0.12	53.25 ± 3.74	16.55 ± 0.27	4.07 ± 0.10
	Freeze	17.14 ± 0.54	21.98 ± 0.29	6.79 ± 0.28	9.60 ± 0.11	65.45 ± 3.46	12.95 ± 0.49	3.84 ± 0.10
B. tulda	Sun	8.79 ± 0.41	12.77 ± 0.73	4.32 ± 0.19	8.29 ± 0.31	60.03 ± 1.99	10.02 ± 0.08	2.07 ± 0.17
	Oven	7.15 ± 0.32	18.91 ± 1.01	4.55 ± 0.08	8.65 ± 0.18	56.38 ± 1.56	7.43 ± 0.29	3.63 ± 0.09
	Freeze	9.55 ± 0.77	19.20 ± 0.92	4.43 ± 0.11	8.20 ± 0.52	61.92 ± 0.81	5.37 ± 0.21	4.60 ± 0.08
Dendrocalamus giganteus	Sun	16.92 ± 1.40	21.53 ± 0.28	5.67 ± 0.10	9.51 ± 0.11	68.40 ± 3.64	11.88 ± 0.40	8.49 ± 0.14
	Oven	17.58 ± 0.41	14.42 ± 0.34	8.99 ± 0.06	9.44 ± 0.12	72.32 ± 4.12	11.69 ± 0.48	5.65 ± 0.14
	Freeze	33.47 ± 0.23	27.32 ± 0.55	4.59 ± 0.04	9.52 ± 0.17	69.48 ± 3.43	11.10 ± 0.38	3.08 ± 0.13
D. hamiltonii	Sun	20.08 ± 0.32	15.90 ± 0.59	5.61 ± 0.07	9.31 ± 0.12	64.70 ± 4.01	11.80 ± 0.31	7.77 ± 0.12
	Oven	23.36 ± 0.10	13.55 ± 0.34	6.74 ± 0.05	9.24 ± 0.16	70.05 ± 4.08	10.70 ± 0.20	3.16 ± 0.14
	Freeze	31.57 ± 0.32	21.91 ± 0.24	4.28 ± 0.03	9.82 ± 0.14	66.80 ± 3.70	10.51 ± 0.18	2.07 ± 0.15
D. latiflorus	Sun	9.74 ± 0.52	13.90 ± 0.68	4.16 ± 0.13	7.58 ± 0.71	76.68 ± 2.92	9.40 ± 0.14	3.57 ± 0.12
	Oven	8.51 ± 0.30	19.97 ± 0.83	4.23 ± 0.23	8.11 ± 0.24	73.82 ± 1.71	7.13 ± 0.05	4.67 ± 0.05
	Freeze	10.73 ± 0.35	20.55 ± 0.71	4.29 ± 0.08	8.07 ± 0.82	77.74 ± 3.06	7.17 ± 0.25	4.03 ± 0.09

(Continued)

TABLE 6.4 (CONTINUED)

Nutrient Components in Dried Shoots (g/100 g d.w.) of Some Bamboo Species

Species	Dried forms	Carbohydrate	Protein	Fat	Ash	NDF	ADF	Lignin
D. membranaceus	Sun	17.21 ± 0.28	23.26 ± 0.69	5.73 ± 0.08	9.55 ± 0.11	63.43 ± 3.22	10.58 ± 0.44	8.01 ± 0.13
	Oven	17.94 ± 0.32	21.29 ± 1.41	6.88 ± 0.03	9.54 ± 0.13	64.83 ± 3.40	9.87 ± 0.62	5.00 ± 0.13
	Freeze	27.36 ± 0.86	25.15 ± 1.00	4.32 ± 0.03	9.70 ± 0.10	64.22 ± 4.10	7.69 ± 0.47	2.60 ± 0.11
D. sikkimensis	Sun	14.26 ± 0.46	24.43 ± 0.32	4.42 ± 0.12	9.48 ± 0.09	48.61 ± 0.07	15.05 ± 0.21	4.00 ± 0.10
	Oven	16.81 ± 0.52	25.15 ± 0.51	4.50 ± 0.19	9.60 ± 0.05	43.20 ± 0.21	12.10 ± 0.14	3.89 ± 0.13
	Freeze	17.51 ± 1.02	17.84 ± 0.24	4.66 ± 0.30	9.61 ± 0.03	57.70 ± 1.14	8.70 ± 0.57	3.50 ± 0.12
Phyllostachys mannii	Sun	14.05 ± 0.06	17.32 ± 1.13	4.39 ± 0.05	8.26 ± 0.21	65.80 ± 2.64	8.50 ± 0.31	1.34 ± 0.17
	Oven	9.90 ± 0.06	18.02 ± 1.49	4.65 ± 0.03	8.40 ± 0.12	53.70 ± 3.17	7.43 ± 1.06	1.40 ± 0.17
	Freeze	14.27 ± 0.08	21.06 ± 1.83	4.53 ± 0.02	8.35 ± 0.20	67.70 ± 2.45	6.52 ± 0.98	1.04 ± 0.14

Values reported are measurement replication means ± standard deviation (n = 3 replicates).

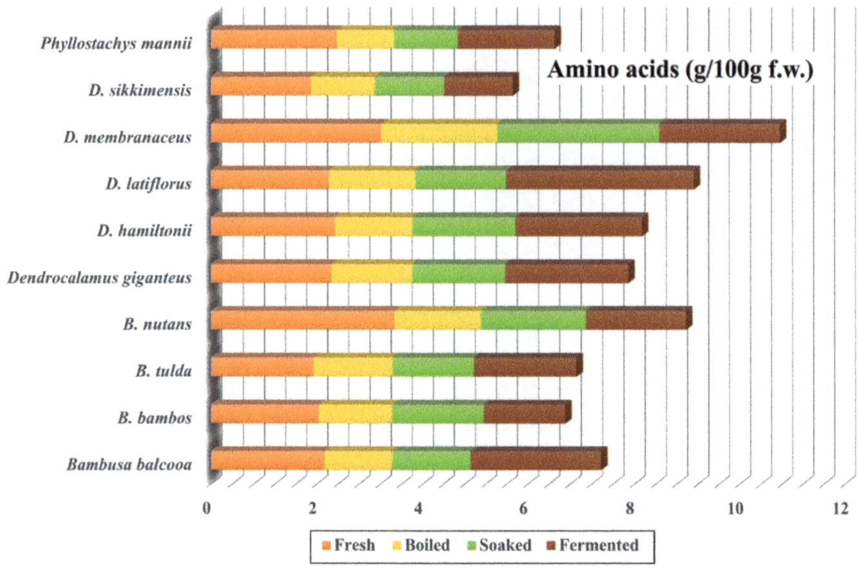

FIGURE 6.20 Effects of processing in amino acids (g/100 g f.w.) content in shoots of different bamboo species.

Fermentation increased the amino acid content in *B. balcooa*, *D. hamiltonii* and *D. latiflorus*, whereas it led to a decline in the rest of the bamboo species (Figure 6.20).

6.6.4 Starch

Starch content was estimated in processed shoots of ten species (Table 6.3, Figure 6.21). Fermentation showed a variable effect in starch content of shoots of different bamboo species. Three species (*B. balcooa*, *D. sikkimensis* and *P. mannii*) showed enhancement of starch with fermentation while others (*B. bambos*, *B. nutans*, *B. tulda*, *D. giganteus*, *D. hamiltonii* and *D. latiflorus*, *D. membranaceus*) showed a decline in the content. Boiling also elevated the starch content while soaking reduced the content in almost all the species.

6.6.5 Fat

Fat ranged from 0.42 to 0.70 g/100 g f.w. in the fresh shoots; being lowest in *D. hamiltonii* and highest in *B. nutans* (Table 6.3, Figure 6.22). Fermentation increased the fat content in *B. bambos*, *B. nutans*, *D. hamiltonii* and *D. sikkimensis* while it was reduced in the remaining species. Boiling and soaking tend to decrease the fat content in almost all the species with more retention during boiling as compared to soaking. In dried shoots, fat ranged from 4.16 to 8.99 g/100 g d.w. being minimum in *D. latiflorus* and maximum in *D. giganteus*. Among drying processes, fat content was found highest in oven-dried and least in freeze-dried shoots in the majority of studied species (Table 6.4).

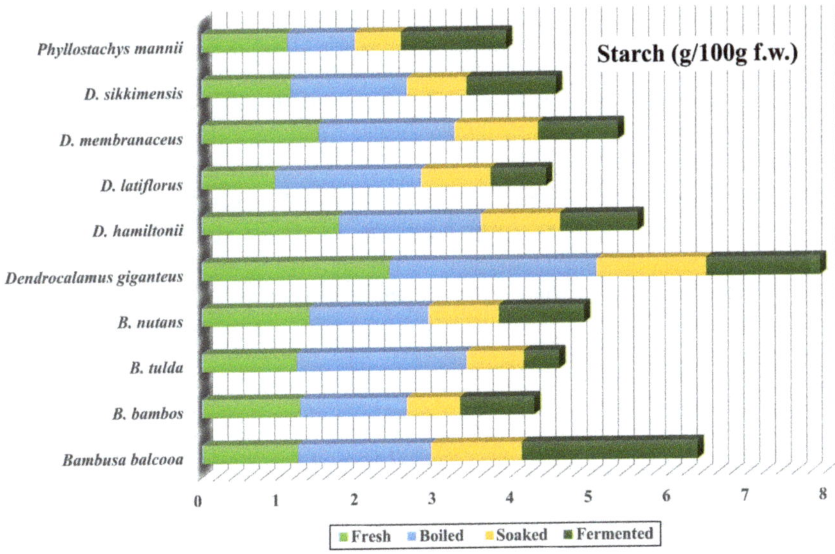

FIGURE 6.21 Effects of processing in starch (g/100 g f.w.) content in shoots of different bamboo species.

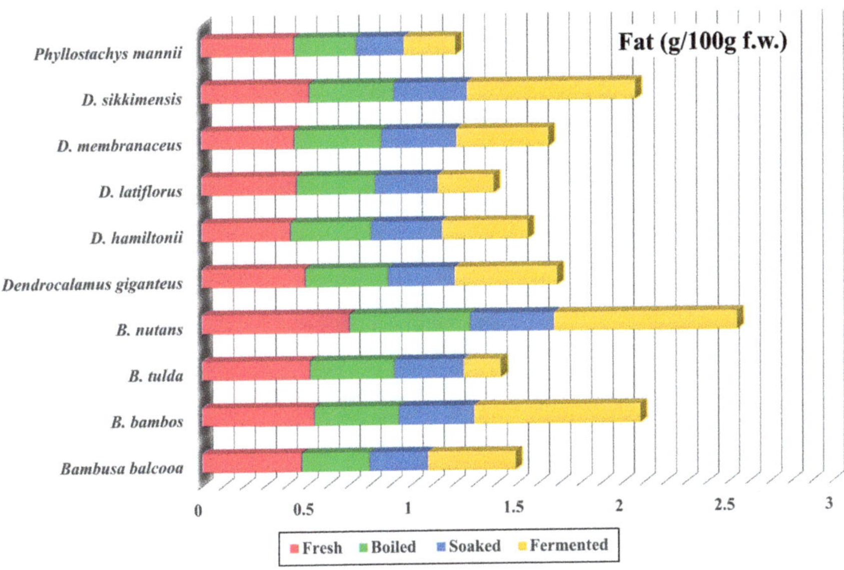

FIGURE 6.22 Effects of processing in fat (g/100 g f.w.) content in shoots of different bamboo species

6.6.6 Ash

Ash content in the fresh shoots ranged from a minimum of 0.76 g/100 g f.w. in *D. hamiltonii and D. sikkimensis* to a maximum of 1.03 g/100 g f.w. in *D. giganteus* (Table 6.3, Figure 6.23). Soaking causes greater loss in ash content than boiling in most of the studied species. However, the amount was elevated after fermentation in majority of the species. In dried shoots, ash content ranged from 8.07 to 9.83 g/100 g d.w.; the values were found highest in *B. balcooa* and least in *D. latiflorus*. The amount of ash was found maximum in freeze-dried shoots followed by sun and oven-drying but no major variation in the content was observed with different drying processes (Table 6.4).

6.6.7 Moisture

In the fresh shoots, moisture content ranged from a minimum of 83.00 g/100 g in *B. tulda* to a maximum of 91.47 g/100 g in *D. sikkimensis* shoots (Figure 6.24). Fermentation reduced the moisture content to 80.91–89.87% in all of the species. However, the water content of shoots increased with soaking as well as boiling where the increase was higher with soaking than boiling in all the investigated species.

6.6.8 Vitamins

In the unprocessed shoots, vitamin C ranged from minimum (1.62 mg/100 g f.w.) in *B. bambos* to maximum (3.23 mg/100 g f.w.) in *P. mannii*. Boiling and soaking tend to decrease vitamin C content in all the species. The amount was retained more

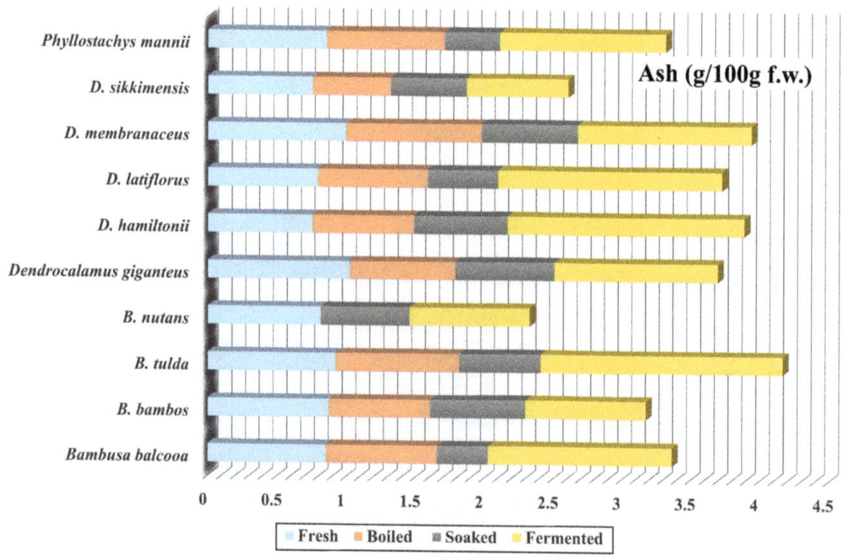

FIGURE 6.23 Effects of processing in ash (g/100 g f.w.) content in shoots of different bamboo species

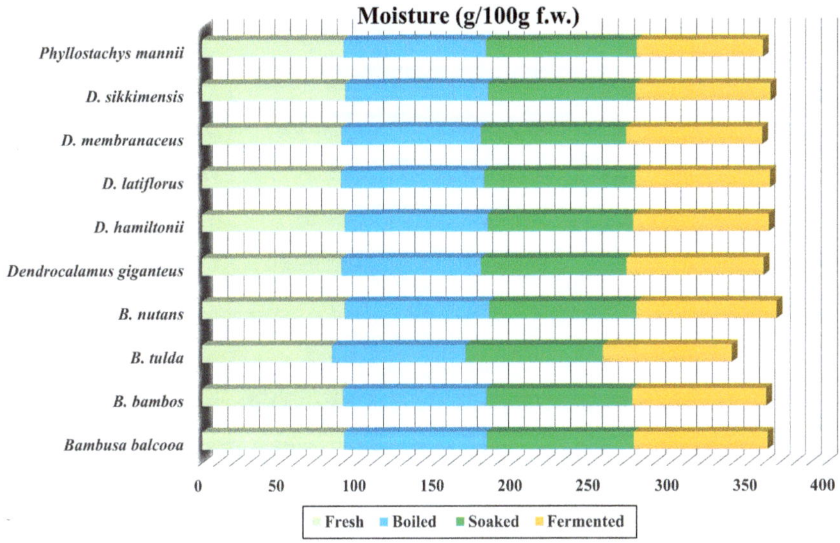

FIGURE 6.24 Effects of processing in moisture (g/100 g f.w.) content in shoots of different bamboo species.

with soaking than boiling in all the species. However, fermentation increased the content in *D. sikkimensis* and showed a reduction in the rest of the species (Figure 6.25). Vitamin E in the unprocessed shoots revealed a range of minimum (0.42 mg/100 g f.w.) in *B. balcooa* to maximum (0.68 mg/100 g f.w.) in *D. hamiltonii*. The amount decreased with all processing treatments (Figure 6.26). Soaking was better

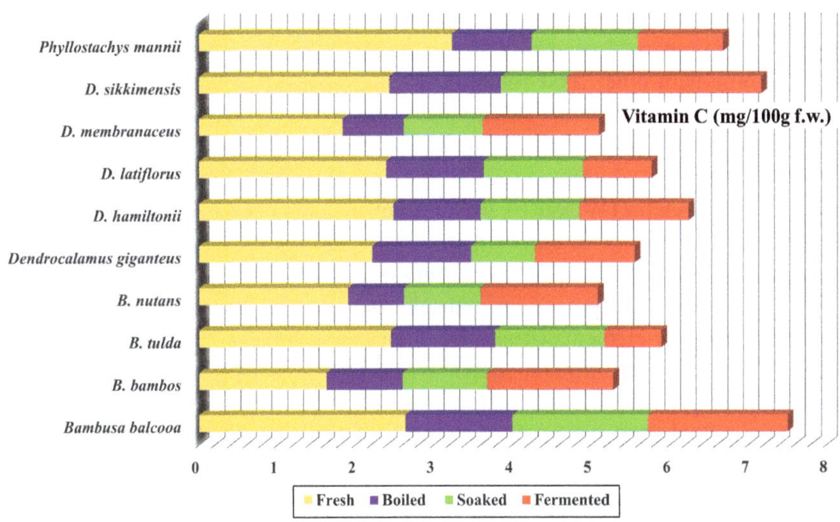

FIGURE 6.25 Effects of processing in vitamin C (mg/100 g f.w.) content in shoots of different bamboo species.

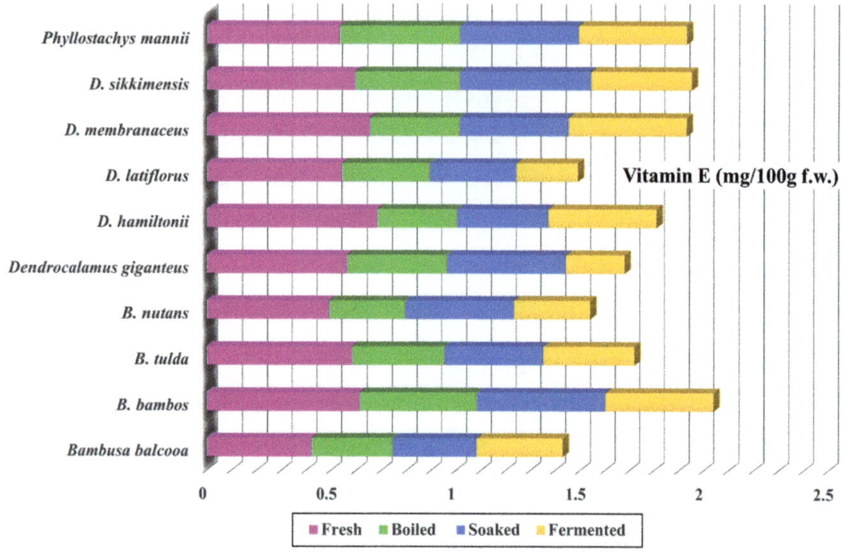

FIGURE 6.26 Effects of processing in vitamin E (mg/100 g f.w.) content of different spcies of bamboo shoots.

in retaining vitamin E content in most species. However, the rate of reduction was quite similar with no remarkable difference with soaking and boiling in the majority of studied species (Table 6.3).

6.7 EFFECT OF PROCESSING ON MINERALS

When food is processed, cooked or stored, minerals may become unavailable as they may combine with other food components. Minerals are generally not sensitive to heat during processing but are susceptible to leaching or cooking. Of all processing methods, fermentation is the best method in retaining the mineral content in the shoots (Saini et al. 2017, Bajwa et al. 2019). Using Wavelength Dispersion X-ray fluorescence spectrometry (WDXRF), mineral elements were analyzed in soaked, boiled and fermented shoots of *B. balcooa*, *B. bambos*, *B. nutans*, *B. tulda*, *D. giganteus*, *D. hamiltonii*, *D. latiflorus*, *D. membranaceus*, *D. sikkimensis* and *P. mannii*, in which macro-elements (potassium, phosphorous, magnesium, calcium, silicon and sodium) and micro-elements (iron, zinc, copper, manganese, nickel) were detected (Table 6.5). The overall mineral content was high in fresh shoots and low in the fermented shoots probably due to leaching in the form of exudates during the fermentation process. Soaked shoots retained minerals compared to the boiled shoots. Effect of different drying methods such as sun-dried, oven-dried and freeze-dried on the macro- and micro-elements were also estimated in five bamboo species (Table 6.6). Among the macro-elements detected, potassium showed the highest values ranging from 2770 to 6660 mg/100 g dry weight. Compared to the three drying methods, mineral content was highest in the freeze-dried shoots.

TABLE 6.5

Changes in Total Mineral Content (mg/100 g d.w.) during Different Processing Methods (Soaked—12 Hrs, Boiled—20 Mins, Fermented—3 Month) in the Edible Shoots Of Some Bamboo Species

		Macro-Element							Micro-Element				
Species	**Treatments**	**K**	**P**	**Mg**	**S**	**Ca**	**Si**	**Na**	**Ni**	**Cu**	**Fe**	**Zn**	**Mn**
Bambusa balcooa	Fresh	4230	560	210	230	180	150	20	0.9	2.6	8.2	6.8	2.5
	Soaked	3700	530	180	250	240	110	30	0.9	2.8	7.2	6.6	1.9
	Boiled	2700	440	120	210	230	100	20	0.8	2.0	6.8	6.0	1.4
	Fermented	3520	360	120	200	160	120	30	0.8	2.6	8.2	5.6	0.9
B. bambos	Fresh	5980	750	230	260	190	130	20	0.7	2.5	8.0	10	3.6
	Soaked	3810	590	190	290	210	90	30	0.4	2.7	7.0	10	2.8
	Boiled	2770	370	140	240	230	80	20	0.6	1.7	5.9	7.7	2.0
	Fermented	3370	350	120	200	180	90	30	0.6	2.4	8.0	9.4	1.9
B. nutans	Fresh	5350	620	230	260	140	160	30	0.8	2.5	7.3	7.8	7.0
	Soaked	4120	520	190	290	200	110	60	0.6	2.5	9.4	6.0	6.2
	Boiled	3530	430	140	240	130	110	0	0.5	2.2	10.6	4.5	-
	Fermented	4500	410	160	230	120	130	60	0.6	2.6	12	5.4	3.5
Dendrocalamus giganteus	Fresh	4590	540	190	270	210	120	40	0.8	5.1	6.9	6.1	1.3
	Soaked	3320	530	180	270	190	120	20	0.8	2.9	7.4	7.2	1.2
	Boiled	2790	490	160	250	170	110	20	0.7	2.7	7.2	6.8	1.1
	Fermented	2310	260	100	190	180	110	50	0.9	3.3	6.9	8.6	0.8
D. hamiltonii	Fresh	5230	560	200	220	150	190	40	0.7	2.6	7.4	6.8	1.2
	Soaked	4810	560	190	290	230	170	40	0.6	2.8	7.1	7.3	1.0
	Boiled	4790	540	170	220	210	150	30	0.7	2.0	5.6	6.2	1.0
	Fermented	3980	380	130	210	130	140	50	0.8	2.5	7.4	6.8	0.8

(Continued)

TABLE 6.5 (CONTINUED)

Changes in Total Mineral Content (mg/100 g d.w.) during Different Processing Methods (Soaked—12 Hrs, Boiled—20 Mins, Fermented—3 Month) in the Edible Shoots Of Some Bamboo Species

		Macro-Element							Micro-Element				
Species	Treatments	K	P	Mg	S	Ca	Si	Na	Ni	Cu	Fe	Zn	Mn
D. latiflorus	Fresh	4390	480	160	230	120	170	-	1.2	1.9	4.7	7.9	3.6
	Soaked	3930	530	160	250	180	110	60	0.9	1.9	6.2	7.8	6.4
	Boiled	3400	420	150	220	120	110	30	0.7	1.7	9.1	7.3	5.3
	Fermented	3280	350	110	210	110	150	50	0.9	1.8	7.7	7.9	1.5
D. membranaceus	Fresh	6120	620	200	240	160	150	90	0.9	2.2	6.8	8.5	1.5
	Soaked	4730	540	180	240	280	140	80	0.8	2.6	6.6	6.2	1.2
	Boiled	4430	580	180	230	210	120	60	0.9	2.2	6.5	7.0	1.1
	Fermented	5550	560	190	230	160	140	90	0.9	2.2	6.7	7.9	0.9
D. sikkimensis	Fresh	5200	540	230	260	160	150	50	1.1	2.5	8.0	7.5	3.4
	Soaked	4010	440	190	260	250	100	80	0.8	2.5	8.6	5.8	2.6
	Boiled	3320	320	140	250	150	100	0	0.6	2.3	9.8	4.2	-
	Fermented	4330	370	150	240	130	120	60	0.8	2.5	14	5.1	2.1
Phyllostachys mannii	Fresh	6660	930	230	330	130	70	60	0.8	2.6	9.1	10	9.0
	Soaked	5750	890	210	390	190	70	20	0.5	3.1	8.5	9.8	8.4
	Boiled	5710	870	210	330	180	60	10	0.8	2.5	8.4	10	7.6
	Fermented	5380	860	190	310	120	60	70	0.9	2.5	9.1	4.5	8.2

TABLE 6.6

Effect of Different Drying Methods on the Macro- and Micro-Elements (mg/100 g d.w.) on the Edible Shoots of Five Bamboo Species

Drying Methods	Species	Macro-Elements								Micro-Elements				
		K	P	Mg	Ca	S	Na	Cl	Si	Fe	Zn	Cu	Ni	Mn
Sun-Dried	*B. balcooa*	4860	550	150	200	210	90	1260	200	10	6.6	2.5	0.8	-
	D. giganteus	4610	510	170	190	280	40	630	220	6.9	6.2	4.9	0.8	-
	D. hamiltonii	6080	550	170	180	290	50	1060	390	9.1	8.6	2.6	0.9	1.2
	D. membranaceus	6240	660	210	180	290	30	1210	230	7.4	9.3	2.3	0.9	1.5
	P. mannii	6440	1100	290	180	380	50	760	70	8.7	10	2.5	0.9	9
Oven-Dried	*B. balcooa*	3870	450	130	180	180	10	1060	160	7.5	5.7	2.7	0.8	-
	D. giganteus	4320	410	140	130	240	30	610	190	5.4	6.0	5.2	0.6	-
	D. hamiltonii	5110	460	140	130	210	20	890	210	7.1	6.4	2.8	0.6	1.0
	D. membranaceus	5620	580	210	160	240	20	750	200	5.8	8.8	3.5	0.7	1.3
	P. mannii	5710	930	220	130	330	60	940	60	6.8	10	2.1	0.6	5.4
Freeze-Dried	*B. balcooa*	4230	560	210	180	230	20	1220	150	8.2	6.8	2.6	0.9	2.5
	D. giganteus	4590	540	190	210	270	40	590	120	6.9	6.1	5.1	0.8	1.3
	D. hamiltonii	5230	560	200	150	220	40	870	190	7.4	6.8	2.6	0.7	1.2
	D. membranaceus	6120	620	200	160	240	90	930	150	6.8	8.5	2.2	0.9	1.5
	P. mannii	6660	930	230	130	330	60	850	70	9.1	10	2.6	0.6	9.0

Phosphorus exhibited a range from 260 to 930 mg/100 g d.w. Among the examined species, shoots of *P. mannii* and *B. bambos* were rich in P. Ca content ranged from 110 to 280 mg/100 g d.w. while Mg ranged from 110 to 290 mg/100g d.w. being maximum in *P. manii* and minimum in *D. latiflorus* Si ranged from 60 to 390 mg/100 g d.w. with the maximum amount in *D. hamiltonii*. Na was not detected in boiled shoots of *B. nutans* and *D. sikkimensis*. Among micro-elements, in the processed shoots, higher range of values were observed for Fe (4.7–14 mg/100 g d.w.) followed by Zn (4.2–10 mg/100 g d.w.) and Cu (1.7–5.2 mg/100 g d.w.). Fe was found maximum in fermented shoots of *D. sikkimensis* (14 mg/100 g d.w.), followed by boiled shoots of *D. sikkimensis* and *D. latiflorus*.

6.8 EFFECT OF PROCESSING ON BIOACTIVE COMPOUNDS

Processing not only depletes the quality and quantity of nutrients but also affects the bioactive compounds which are already present in very low concentrations in the food matrices. Bioactive compounds lie spatially protected well within the plant tissues but processing events such as peeling, cutting, chopping, shredding, milling, etc. destroy this protection and expose these bioactive compounds to oxygen and degrading enzymes resulting in quantity and quality loss. On some occasions, though, processing treatments have been reported to enhance the bioactive potential of foods, probably because these methods cause tissue softening and breakage thereby increasing the bioavailability of bioactive compounds. Thus, a proper understanding of the mechanisms pertaining to the stability of bioactive compounds during processing is vital for modifying current processing treatments to maximize their bioavailability with minimum loss. Modern processing methods such as vacuum drying, freeze-drying, high-pressure treatments, pulsed electric field treatments, microwave cooking, etc. are very promising in this regard as they are able to retain almost all the natural ingredients and characteristics of the raw foods to their maximum potential even after processing. Several scientific studies have been conducted to analyze the effect of such processing methods on the nature and bioavailability of bamboo shoot bioactive compounds.

6.8.1 PHENOL

Different processing treatments affect the phenol content of food products. It has been reported that few processing treatments such as high-pressure treatment and fermentation tend to increase the total phenol content as compared to the unprocessed samples. This increase is mainly attributed to better extractability of phenols after such processing treatments. Other processing treatments such as cooking and blanching tend to reduce the phenol content of food products probably because of the leaching effect. Changes in phenol content during processing have been studied in some bamboo species (Badwaik et al. 2015, Rawat 2017, Sharma 2018, Devi 2018, Saini 2019). Yang et al. (2010) studied the effect of Nitric Oxide (NO) treatment and cold storage at 10°C on the total phenol content, cellulose content and lignin content in the shoots of *Phyllostachys violascens*. They found that total phenol content decreased gradually during storage whereas treatment with

NO markedly delayed the increase in lignin and cellulose content of the shoots. Zhang et al. (2011) studied the effect of three cooking methods viz. boiling steaming and stir-frying on the nutritional content and anti-oxidant properties of the *Phyllostachys praecox* shoots. Boiling and stir-frying reduced the total phenol content whereas steaming increased it slightly as compared to the fresh shoots. The total anti-oxidant activity decreased after boiling, remained unchanged after steaming and increased slightly after stir-frying. Increase in heat treatment affect the phenol content in more than one way; it can cause decomposition of the phenols which are then lost in the boiling aqueous solution (Ranilla et al. 2010); alternatively, heat treatment could cause the deactivation of polyphenol oxidases thereby preventing polyphenol decomposition (Yamaguchi et al. 2003). Reduction in anti-oxidant activity of aqueous shoot extracts after boiling is mainly due to loss of ascorbic acid and total phenols during boiling. On the other hand, increased anti-oxidant activity after stir-frying is possibly because of the occurrence of Maillard's reaction at a temperature exceeding 100°C which results in the generation of novel anti-oxidant substances (Nicoli et al. 1997). Luo et al. (2012) studied the effect of salicylic acid treatment on the shoots of *Phyllostachys praecox* f. *prevernalis* during storage at 1°C and found that salicylic acid treatment inhibited the total phenol content by 18% during storage. Pandey and Ojha (2014) analyzed the effect of boiling medium (water, 1%, 5% and 10% NaCl) and boiling durations (10, 15, 20 and 25 mins) on total phenol content in shoots of four bamboo species, that is *Bambusa bambos*, *B. tulda*, *Dendrocalamus strictus* and *D. asper.* They reported that with respect to removal of the anti-nutrient cyanogen along with retention of total phenols, the best processing method for *B. bambos* shoots was boiling shoots in 5% NaCl for 15 mins which retained 0.28 g/100 g of total phenol; for *B. tulda* it was boiling in 1% NaCl for ten mins retaining 0.38 g/100 g of total phenols; for *D. asper* it was boiling shoots in 5% NaCl for ten mins with 0.07 g/100 g retention of total phenols; and for *D. strictus* it was boiling shoots in 1% NaCl for 15 mins with 0.16 g/100 g retention of total phenols.

Badwaik et al. (2014) studied the effect of fermentation on total phenol content and anti-oxidant activity of *Bambusa balcooa* shoots. After fermentation, the total phenol content increased from 97.5 mg/100 g in fresh samples to 239 mg/100 g in fermented samples whereas total anti-oxidant activity increased from 26.67% in fresh samples to 55.30% in fermented samples. This signifies the role of fermentation in enhancing the bioactive potential of the bamboo shoots. Studies were conducted on the effect of different processing treatments (soaking, boiling, canning and fermentation) on the total phenol content in the shoots of the 12 bamboo species (Table 6.7). In fresh shoots, the total phenol content ranged from 101 mg/100 g to 721.62 mg/100 g among the species investigated. From the results, it was found that most of the processing treatments except fermentation caused a reduction in the total phenolic content of the shoots. This reduction was most severe after boiling in almost all the species except *B. balcooa, D. giganteus and D. hamiltonii* where the highest reduction in total phenol content was seen after brine treatment (21.37 mg/100 g, 44.60 mg/100 g and 34.47 mg/100 g, respectively). Fermentation, on the other hand, caused an increase in total phenol content of all the species with the highest content seen in *D. latiflorus* shoots (1027.24 mg/100g) (Table 6.7).

TABLE 6.7
Changes in Total Phenol Content (mg/100 g f.w.) during Different Processing Methods in the Edible Shoots of Some Bamboo Species.

Species	Fresh	Soaked 24 hrs	Boiled 30 mins	10 % Brine 3 months	Fermented	References
B. bambos	721.62 ± 16.86	312.98 ± 5.51	238.43 ± 3.03	342.10 ± 8.41	746.5 ± 17.81	Saini 2019
	360	-	100	-	-	Pandey and Ojha 2014
B. balcooa	362.36 ±4.80	284.27 ± 2.05	123.34 ± 1.04	143.22 ± 3.13	459.65 ± 6.39	Rawat 2017
	191.37 ± 2.62	53.07 ± 0.09	56.83 ± 1.67	21.37 ± 0.28	298.53 ± 2.50	Chongtham et al. 2014
	101.65 ± 2.75	-	39.34 ± 2.00	-	255.00 ± 4.40	Badwaik et al. 2014, 2015
B. nutans	558.96 ± 23.24	228.56 ± 13.22	204.12 ± 9.96	325.31 ± 3.11	746.5 ± 17.81	Saini 2019
B. tulda	479.22 ± 1.26	226.20 ± 0.73	180.01 ± 1.6	94.24 ± 0.88	898.39 ± 0.45	Sharma 2018
	443.97 ± 6.09	58.17 ± 0.09	120.77 ± 0.72	67.23 ± 0.67	641.73 ± 0.90	Chongtham et al. 2014
	390	-	300	-	-	Pandey and Ojha 2014
D. asper	580	-	40	-	-	Pandey and Ojha 2014
D. giganteus	609.32 ± 1.2	293.90 ± 1.04	173.04 ± 0.57	44.60 ± 0.33	1022.38 ± 0.49	Sharma 2018
	347.27 ± 2.34	187.97 ± 1.26	182.80 ± 1.19	80.36 ± 1.10	891.33 ± 7.45	Chongtham et al. 2014
D. hamiltonii	678.56 ± 2.34	315.56 ± 2.58	421.83 ± 3.46	189.09 ± 4.16	767.65 ± 15.61	Rawat 2017
	505.93 ± 1.68	56.74 ± 0.18	88.47 ± 0.88	34.47 ± 1.12	745.56 ± 1.55	Chongtham et al. 2014
D. latiflorus	659.11 ± 0.84	590.38 ± 0.46	323.25 ± 0.58	68.62 ± 1.30	1027.24 ± 1.22	Sharma 2018
D. membranaceus	596.67 ± 0.89	104.59 ± 1.47	280.83 ± 1.15	191.08 ± 2.89	878.79 ± 0.45	Sharma 2018
D. sikkimensis	450.29 ± 15.00	385.18 ± 1.31	181.15 ± 2.10	245.08 ± 2.65	472.42 ± 13.56	Saini 2019
D. strictus	630	-	50	-	-	Pandey and Ojha 2014
Phyllostachys mannii	382.23 ± 2.08	144.43 ± 2.88	106.61 ± 2.43	128.00 ± 5.29	486.14 ± 3.43	Rawat 2017

Values reported are measurement replication means ± standard deviation (n = 3 replicates).

6.8.2 Phytosterol

Phytosterols possess a bulkier, fused ring tetracyclic structure with one or more double bonds. The presence of these double bonds in their structure makes them highly sensitive to the effect of various thermal treatments such as heating, frying, roasting, etc. These thermal treatments invariably cause a reduction in total phytosterol content of the concerned food albeit to a different extent. Under the influence of these factors, phytosterol undergoes oxidation leading to the formation of phytosterol oxidation products (POPs) such as 7-hydroxy, 7-keto, epoxy, 25-hydroxysterols and triols of sterols. In bamboo shoots, the effect of only fermentation process on phytosterol has been investigated in depth. Srivastava (1990) reported an enhancement in the total phytosterol content of *Dendrocalamus giganteus* shoots from 0.39% to 2.80% after fermentation. Sarangthem and Singh (2003a) while studying the effect of fermentation on the phytosterol content in shoots of *Bambusa balcooa* and *Dendrocalamus strictus* shoots found that fermentation caused the enrichment of phytosterol from 0.18% to 0.61% in *B. balcooa* and from 0.14% to 0.42% in *D. strictus*. Sarangthem and Singh (2003b) reported an increase in phytosterol content in the shoots of *B. balcooa* from 0.12% to 0.62% after fermentation. Phytosterol level further increased in fermented bamboo shoots of *Dendrocalamus hamiltonii* from 0.19% to 0.44% (Sarangthem and Singh 2003c). Studies were conducted on the effect of processing (soaking, boiling, brine treatment and fermentation) on the phytosterol content in ten species (Table. 6.8). In fresh shoots, the total phytosterol content of different species ranged from 0.06% to 0.26% on a dry weight basis. Results showed that in all the investigated species, after each and every processing method, the total phytosterol content either remained unchanged or there was an increase in its content as compared to the fresh shoots (Table 6.8). No reduction in total phytosterol content was observed upon processing in the present studies. Among different processing methods employed, the maximum increase in phytosterols content was seen in fermented shoots of *Dendrocalamus giganteus* (Table 6.8).

6.8.3 Dietary Fibre

Muchtadi and Adawiyah (1996) reported a 4.6% reduction in crude fibre content in *Dendrocalamus asper* shoots when subjected to drying in a cabinet dryer at 60°C for 7–8 hrs. Kumbhare and Bhargva (2007) analyzed the effect of processing on the nutritional value of central Indian bamboo shoots of *Bambusa nutans*, *B. vulgaris*, *Dendrocalamus asper* and *D. strictus* and found out that crude fibre content did not change much after boiling. Luo et al. (2008) while studying the effect of cold storage on the shoots of *Phyllostachys praecox* f. *prevernalis* found out that the lignin content of bamboo shoots increased rapidly during storage at 20°C, but at 2°C it increased slowly, whereas increase in cellulose content was higher at 20°C as compared to 2°C. Chongtham et al. (2008) analyzed the effect of fermentation and canning on the concentration of different components of dietary fibre viz. NDF, ADF, lignin, hemicellulose and cellulose in the shoots of *Dendrocalamus giganteus*. NDF content increased in both fermented (4.18 g/100 g) as well as in canned shoots (3.04 g/100 g) as compared to freshly emerged shoots (2.64 g/100 g), ADF was higher in fermented

TABLE 6.8
Effect of Different Processing Methods in Total Phytosterol Content (mg/100 g d.w.) in the Edible Shoots of Some Bamboo Species

Species	Fresh	Soaked (24 hrs)	Boiled (30 mins)	10% Brine 3 months	Fermented	References
Bambusa bambos	198.69 ± 4.92	266.44 ± 1.34	250.24 ± 2.78	204.22 ± 3.09	275.29 ± 2.93	Saini 2019
B.balcooa	127.24 ± 2.86	148.14 ± 1.35	163.14 ± 2.22	-	284.73 ± 1.68	Rawat 2017
B. nutans	181.59 ± 3.88	263.50 ± 2.34	242.63 ± 2.58	186.29 ± 4.45	267.13 ± 5.13	Saini 2019
B. tulda	109.57 ± 0.69	132.19 ± 0.81	158.44 ± 0.42	50.25 ± 0.38	352.66 ± 1.49	Sharma 2018
Dendrocalamus giganteus	158.10 ± 1.27	215.73 ± 0.48	275.52 ± 1.00	71.31 ± 0.86	543.26 ± 1.37	Sharma 2018
D. hamiltonii	131.73 ± 1.68	143.38 ± 1.48	148.31 ± 1.34	-	169.18 ± 4.34	Rawat 2017
D. latiflorus	89.90 ± 0.02	85.52 ± 1.53	99.91 ± 1.20	85.39 ± 0.99	234.06 ± 1.16	Sharma 2018
D. membranaceus	178 ± 2.35	206.19 ± 0.89	238.37 ± 0.97	47.97 ± 0.71	498.80 ± 0.86	Sharma 2018
D. sikkimensis	122.08 ± 4.27	150.67 ± 4.61	135.15 ± 2.80	125.38 ± 0.82	247.98 ± 3.41	Saini 2019
Phyllostachys mannii	264.49 ± 3.16	305.23 ± 2.54	286.33 ± 2.00	-	318.65 ± 3.05	Rawat 2017

Values reported are measurement replication means ± standard deviation (n = 3 replicates).

shoots (3.28 g/100 g) but lower in canned shoots (2.02 g/100 g) than freshly emerged shoots (2.15 g/100 g). Lignin and hemicellulose content was higher in both fermented (1.39 g/100 g and 0.90 g/100 g) and canned shoots (0.78 g/100 g and 1.02 g/100 g), respectively, as compared to freshly emerged shoots (0.56 g/100 g and 0.49 g/100 g). Cellulose content increased after fermentation (1.88 g/100 g) but decreased after canning (1.24 g/100 g) as compared to the fresh shoots (1.58 g/100 g).

The effect of boiling, soaking and fermentation on dietary fibre content was evaluated in ten species (Table 6.9). It was observed that NDF increased in all species during fermentation as compared to boiling and soaking. The NDF also increased in all species during soaking except in *D. hamiltonii* and *Phyllostachys mannii*. Hence, fermentation is the best processing method for increasing the dietary fibre content in the shoots.

6.9 ORGANOLEPTIC PROPERTIES OF FRESH AND PROCESSED SHOOTS

Organoleptic properties of food play an important role in judging the censoring acceptability or rejection of food items in the market. Sensory qualities are of particular importance for complementary foods for changing consumer attitudes towards particular food products. Sensory evaluation was used for the identification of sensory characteristics of fresh and processed shoots like colour, aroma, taste, texture and overall acceptability (Tables 6.10–6.12). Fresh (unprocessed) shoots were hard/crunchy to touch, cream coloured with acrid taste but with almost no flavour. Upon boiling, colour changed to light brown/pale yellow; boiled shoots were soft to touch, sweet in taste with no particular flavour. Brine-preserved shoots became gradually hard, colour of the shoots changes from cream to light yellow while, taste of the shoots was little salty. After fermentation, colour of the shoots is light brown, texture becomes soft with a sour taste and pungent flavour. On the basis of organoleptic evaluation, it was observed that boiling is the best option for seasonal consumption of shoots. Boiled shoots can be included in our daily meal as healthy and nutritious salad and also for preparing different types of cuisines. They can also be used for value addition in a number of food products. Brine-treated shoots can be used for the preparation of different snacks, chips and fries and so on because there is no need to add extra salt to improve the taste of the food products. Fermented shoots though with a little bit pungent flavour has improved nutrient profile and increased therapeutic properties (Bajwa et al. 2019a).

Sensory evaluation was carried out for unprocessed and processed shoots of fresh weight sample and dried powder of freeze-dried and oven-dried shoots of *Dendrocalamus hamiltonii* for selected parameters which include colour, aroma, texture, taste and overall acceptability (Santosh et al. 2019). In the fresh weight sample (Table 6.11), 20 mins boiled shoots (BS) were observed to have higher acceptability in all the parameters whereas 24 hrs soaked (SS) was observed to be the least acceptable (Figure 6.27). A comparison between freeze-dried and oven-dried shoots revealed that the sensory acceptability was observed to be higher in freeze-dried shoots (Table 6.12).

TABLE 6.9
Dietary Fibre and Its Components (g/100 g Fresh Weight) in the Processed Shoots (Boiled—20 Mins, Soaked—12 Hrs, Fermented—3 Months)

Species	Processing Methods	NDF	ADF	Lignin	Cellulose	Hemicellulose
B. balcooa	Fresh	6.07 ± 0.04	0.51 ± 0.02	0.30 ± 0.02	0.21 ± 0.01	5.56 ± 0.06
	Boiled	3.99 ± 0.25	0.51 ± 0.03	0.17 ± 0.01	0.31 ± 0.02	3.50 ± 0.12
	Soaked	4.17 ± 0.30	0.58 ± 0.08	0.20 ± 0.05	0.38 ± 0.01	3.59 ± 0.04
	Fermented	14.03 ± 0.54	3.51 ± 0.14	0.32 ± 0.04	3.19 ± 0.20	10.52 ± 0.64
B. bambos	Fresh	3.95 ± 0.12	0.48 ± 0.01	0.30 ± 0.02	0.18 ± 0.01	3.47 ± 0.6
	Boiled	3.25 ± 0.08	0.49 ± 0.02	0.28 ± 0.04	0.21 ± 0.02	2.76 ± 0.02
	Soaked	3.22 ± 0.04	0.45 ± 0.05	0.26 ± 0.01	0.19 ± 0.00	2.77 ± 0.03
	Fermented	6.57 ± 0.49	2.80 ± 0.08	0.95 ± 0.03	1.85 ± 0.08	3.77 ± 0.11
B. tulda	Fresh	5.59 ± 0.28	0.73 ± 0.02	0.61 ± 0.01	0.12 ± 0.01	4.86 ± 0.26
	Boiled	4.28 ± 0.14	0.82 ± 0.02	0.15 ± 0.01	0.67 ± 0.01	3.46 ± 0.12
	Soaked	4.00 ± 0.33	0.81 ± 0.01	0.16 ± 0.02	0.65 ± 0.01	3.19 ± 0.32
	Fermented	10.22 ± 0.23	4.62 ± 0.02	1.50 ± 0.01	3.12 ± 0.01	5.60 ± 0.22
B. nutans	Fresh	5.34 ± 0.14	1.17 ± 0.06	0.78 ± 0.10	0.39 ± 0.01	4.17 ± 0.03
	Boiled	4.14 ± 0.10	1.18 ± 0.08	0.40 ± 0.02	0.78 ± 0.03	2.96 ± 0.02
	Soaked	4.36 ± 0.05	1.11 ± 0.03	0.50 ± 0.06	0.61 ± 0.02	3.25 ± 0.06
	Fermented	7.10 ± 0.48	2.93 ± 0.11	1.58 ± 0.02	1.35 ± 0.03	4.17 ± 0.14
D. giganteus	Fresh	5.60 ± 0.02	0.83 ± 0.01	0.49 ± 0.04	0.34 ± 0.02	4.77 ± 0.14
	Boiled	4.48 ± 0.01	1.02 ± 0.02	0.27 ± 0.03	0.75 ± 0.03	3.46 ± 0.14
	Soaked	4.52 ± 0.04	0.82 ± 0.01	0.34 ± 0.04	0.48 ± 0.03	3.70 ± 0.12
	Fermented	12.87 ± 0.84	3.58 ± 0.34	2.32 ± 0.22	1.26 ± 0.08	9.29 ± 0.20

(Continued)

TABLE 6.9 (CONTINUED)

Dietary Fibre and Its Components (g/100 g Fresh Weight) in the Processed Shoots (Boiled—20 Mins, Soaked—12 Hrs, Fermented—3 Months)

Species	Processing Methods	NDF	ADF	Lignin	Cellulose	Hemicellulose
D. hamiltonii	Fresh	4.78 ± 0.21	0.94 ± 0.02	0.38 ± 0.05	0.56 ± 0.02	3.84 ± 0.09
	Boiled	4.69 ± 0.04	1.01 ± 0.04	0.26 ± 0.04	0.65 ± 0.02	3.68 ± 0.10
	Soaked	4.61 ± 0.06	0.96 ± 0.02	0.31 ± 0.05	0.64 ± 0.04	3.85 ± 0.08
	Fermented	10.23 ± 0.12	5.25 ± 0.14	1.44 ± 0.06	3.81 ± 0.14	4.98 ± 0.21
D. latiflorus	Fresh	6.95 ± 0.18	0.62 ± 0.01	0.47 ± 0.01	0.15 ± 0.01	6.33 ± 0.17
	Boiled	5.52 ± 0.28	0.86 ± 0.01	0.35 ± 0.01	0.51 ± 0.03	4.66 ± 0.25
	Soaked	5.34 ± 0.14	0.87 ± 0.01	0.39 ± 0.01	0.48 ± 0.01	4.47 ± 0.02
	Fermented	11.66 ± 0.29	5.04 ± 0.02	1.02 ± 0.01	4.02 ± 0.02	6.62 ± 0.27
D. membranaceus	Fresh	5.33 ± 0.12	1.93 ± 0.07	0.37 ± 0.03	1.56 ± 0.06	3.40 ± 0.04
	Boiled	3.59 ± 0.04	1.97 ± 0.08	0.21 ± 0.02	1.77 ± 0.05	1.60 ± 0.03
	Soaked	3.77 ± 0.08	1.46 ± 0.06	0.19 ± 0.06	1.27 ± 0.02	2.31 ± 0.04
	Fermented	12.40 ± 1.08	3.23 ± 0.28	1.29 ± 0.10	1.94 ± 0.08	9.17 ± 0.14
D. sikkimensis	Fresh	4.66 ± 0.04	0.93 ± 0.00	0.51 ± 0.04	0.42 ± 0.02	3.73 ± 0.04
	Boiled	3.36 ± 0.03	1.15 ± 0.02	0.42 ± 0.01	0.73 ± 0.06	2.21 ± 0.11
	Soaked	3.53 ± 0.01	0.92 ± 0.01	0.38 ± 0.04	0.54 ± 0.02	2.61 ± 0.02
	Fermented	8.23 ± 0.31	2.95 ± 0.10	1.46 ± 0.02	1.49 ± 0.05	5.28 ± 0.17
Phyllostachys mannii	Fresh	5.72 ± 0.03	1.41 ± 0.05	0.17 ± 0.00	1.24 ± 0.01	4.31 ± 0.03
	Boiled	3.42 ± 0.03	1.41 ± 0.02	0.10 ± 0.00	1.31 ± 0.01	3.00 ± 0.02
	Soaked	4.07 ± 0.03	1.6 ± 0.05	0.17 ± 0.02	1.52 ± 0.03	2.38 ± 0.02
	Fermented	9.87 ± 0.04	3.42 ± 0.01	0.60 ± 0.01	2.82 ± 0.01	6.45 ± 0.02

TABLE 6.10
Effect of Different Processing Methods on Organoleptic Properties

Types	Methods	Parameters		
		Colour	Texture	Taste
Unprocessed	Fresh	Cream	Hard	Acrid
Precooked	Soaking	White to greyish	Medium soft	Sour
Processing	Boiling	Light yellow	Soft	Sweet
	Fermentation	Brown	Soft	Sour
Dehydration operation	Sun	Light brown	Coarse and granular	Earthy
	Oven	Medium brown	Coarse and granular	Earthy
	Freeze	White to Cream	Soft	Sweet
Refrigerated storage	In Water	Yellow	Soft	Sweet
	In Brine	Light Yellow	Coarse	Salty

TABLE 6.11
Sensory Analysis for Different Forms of *D. hamiltonii* Shoot Using 9-Point Hedonic Scale (1—Extremely Dislike to 9—Extremely Like)

	Bamboo Shoot		
Parameter	Unprocessed (US)	20 Mins Boiled (BS)	24 Hr Soaked (SS)
Colour	6.30 ± 1.33	7.90 ± 0.99	5.20 ± 1.48
Aroma	6.10 ± 0.99	6.60 ± 1.71	4.40 ± 1.51
Texture	6.70 ± 1.25	7.50 ± 0.85	6.10 ± 1.10
Taste	6.70 ± 1.25	7.50 ± 0.85	6.60 ± 0.84
Overall	5.90 ± 1.37	7.20 ± 1.23	5.30 ± 1.49

Values reported are measurement replication means ± standard deviation (n = 20 replicates).

TABLE 6.12

Sensory Analysis for Different Forms of Freeze-Dried and Oven-Dried *D. hamiltonii* Shoot Using 9-Point Hedonic Scale (1—Extremely Dislike To 9—Extremely Like)

	Freeze-Dried Shoot			Oven-Dried Shoot		
Parameter	**Unprocessed**	**20 Mins Boiled**	**24 Hr Soaked**	**Unprocessed**	**20 Mins Boiled**	**24 Hr Soaked**
Colour	6.40 ± 0.84	7.50 ± 1.35	6.20 ± 0.79	5.60 ± 1.27	5.30 ± 1.06	5.30 ± 1.52
Aroma	5.90 ± 1.10	6.10 ± 1.52	4.60 ± 1.27	5.00 ± 1.16	5.30 ± 0.68	4.30 ± 1.49
Texture	6.90 ± 1.45	7.00 ± 1.33	4.60 ± 1.27	6.10 ± 0.99	5.90 ± 0.88	6.00 ± 0.82
Taste	6.90 ± 1.45	7.10 ± 1.10	5.00 ± 0.67	6.10 ± 0.99	5.90 ± 0.88	6.00 ± 0.82
Overall	5.30 ± 1.06	6.40 ± 1.27	5.60 ± 0.52	4.50 ± 0.53	5.10 ± 0.57	4.50 ± 0.53

Values reported are measurement replication means ± standard deviation (n = 20 replicates).

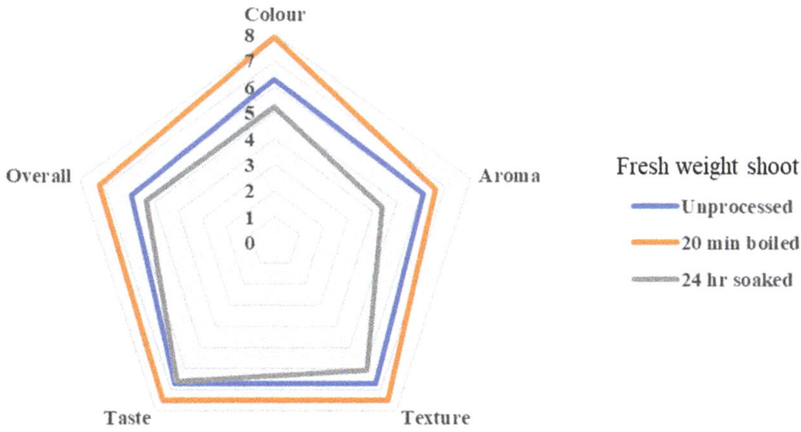

FIGURE 6.27 Radar chart of the average sensory scores of different samples of fresh weight shoot using a 9-point Hedonic scale (1–extremely dislike to 9–extremely like, n = 20 replicates).

7 Packaging and Shelf-Life Evaluation of Shoots

Since ancient times, the prime objective of food packaging has always been to uphold food quality, improve safety by averting contagions and diminish postharvest losses to provide wholesome food products to consumers while additionally gratifying their demand of innocuous handling and transport of fresh-like as well as processed agricultural products. Fresh food such as fruits and vegetables can't be kept for long because, even after harvesting, biological processes like respiration and ethylene production continue which ultimately leads to decomposition and degradation and hence shorten their shelf-life. This perishability of food which goes against increasing food demand with an increasing global population must be resolved to meet the rising interest and consciousness about exotic, ready to eat, hygienic and healthy food.

Traditional packaging systems with natural packaging material like leaves, barks, animal skin and shells perform the primary functions of containment, protection, convenience and communication, but consumer preferences toward quality and safe food with enhanced shelf-life have resulted in the development of various new trends in the packaging systems. With the evolvement of packaging with wood, paper, metal, ceramic and glass through the centuries, it progressed to canning by the invention of metal cans and the establishment of pasteurization concepts in the 19th century. One of the important factors in rapid innovations in the packaging sector is the problem of food-borne microbial outbreaks, which require the introduction of anti-microbial effects in the packaging system without compromising the quality of the food. The main triumph in this field ensued in the 20th century when aluminium foil, heat-stable cellophane films, heat-shrinkable polyvinyl chloride (PVC), nylon films, modified aluminium alloy and coated steel cans were introduced for food packaging, but the major breakthrough was expansion of plastic-based packages like jars, bottles, tubs and sheets manufactured with polyolefins, polyvinyl, polyethylene, vinylidene, vinyl chloride, in the late 20th century which provides immeasurable practices for stowing foodstuff. However, the potential influence of plastic on product safety and quality remains in question when diffusion of chemical substances from such material in food exceeds their specified limits.

7.1 BAMBOO SHOOT PACKAGING

In traditional gastronomy, bamboo shoots have arisen as contemporary nourishment and its demand is mounting comprehensively through the years due to its enormous health promotional benefits and functional properties. But the limiting factor of its distribution and marketability is (i) seasonal availability during monsoons only (ii) very short shelf-life due to high moisture content ($\geq 90\%$) which makes them highly

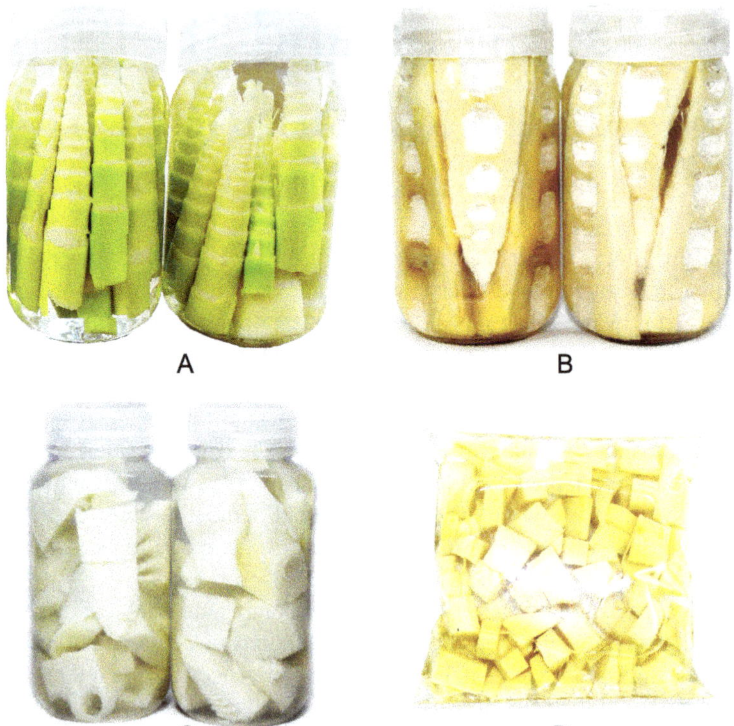

A B C D

FIGURE 7.1 Packaging of bamboo shoot in (A, B) glass bottle, (C) high density polyethylene bottle (HDPE) and (D) low density polyethylene (LDPE).

susceptible to microbial spoilage. Fresh shoots rapidly undergo discolouration and browning after harvesting probably due to the activity of enzymes polyphenol oxidase (PPO), peroxidase (POD) and phenylalanine ammonia lyases (PALs) if not processed or packaged appropriately (Chen et al. 1989). Lignification in bamboo shoots enhance briskly after harvesting like in other plant tissues under stress conditions which is due to disproportionate radical oxygen species (ROS) and ROS- scavenging system (Liu and Jiang 2006, Song et al. 2011, Zeng et al. 2015). Moreover, minimal processing of bamboo shoots like peeling of the outer sheath, cutting and slicing lead to more rapid deterioration and senescence due to elevation in respiration by $\geq$ 40% (Xu et al. 2005). The risk of microbial attack that is enhanced due to high surface water activity further shortens their stability if proper control measures are not applied (Song et al. 2013).

To inactivate inoperable enzymatic and microbial activities and to maintain quality of fresh-cut and minimally processed shoots with more pliability and extended shelf-life, different packaging materials and appropriate packaging methods should be developed and applied. In north-east India, bamboo shoots are packed in banana leaves and put in bamboo baskets or in polythene bags or plastic bottles (Figure 7.1). Now, various packaging materials are used for bamboo shoot packaging (Table 7.1, Figure 7.2).

TABLE 7.1
List of Various Packaging Materials and Modes Used for Bamboo Shoot Packaging

Bamboo Shoot Species	Material for Packaging	Mode of Packaging/Storage	Effects Studied/References
Bambusa oldhamii	Low-density polyethylene (perforated/ non-perforated), Polyvinyl chloride film	Storage at different temperatures	Respiration rate, weight loss, colour, fungal infection, microbial load and shelf-life (Kleinhenz et al. 2000)
Phyllostachys praecox	Low-density polyethylene bags	Modified atmospheric packaging	Gas components, browning index, Polyphenol content, lignification, MDA content, POD, PAL and PPO activity (Shen et al. 2006)
Dendrocalamus asper	Polyethylene, Polyvinyl chloride film	Vacuum packaging, Low temperature	Respiration rate, weight loss, lignin content, POD and PPO activity (Pongprasert et al. 2007)
Thyrsostachys siamensis	Polyethylene film	Storage at room temperature	Contamination, general features, odour, taste, texture, pH, lead level and microbial analysis (Chiangthong and Chayawat 2009)
Phyllostachys violascens	Polyethylene bags	Nitric oxide application, Storage at minus 80°C	Ethylene production, browning index, firmness, total phenol, lignin and cellulose contents, PAL, POD and PPO activity (Yang et al. 2010)
Bambusa balcooa	Edible coating	Storage at room temperature	Weight loss, colour, surface microbial count (Badwaik et al. 2014)
Phyllostachys praecox f. *prevernalis*	Edible coating wrapped with polythene film	Stored at 4°C	Respiration rate, weight loss, lignification, colour, PAL, POD, PPO, CAD activity and microbial analysis (Yang et al. 2015)

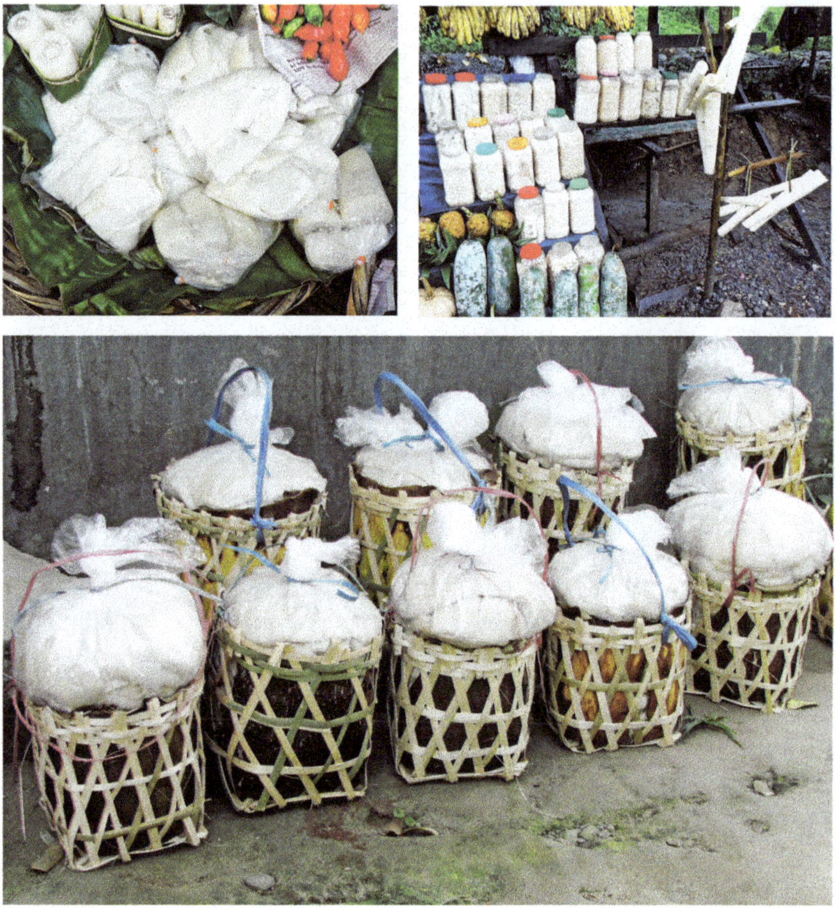

FIGURE 7.2 Packed bamboo shoot sold in a local market in north-east India.

7.1.1 Polyethylene Packaging

Formed by polymerization of ethylene, polyethylene is one of the most extensively used and inexpensive food packaging material because of its significant mechanical properties like tensile and tear strength, elasticity, weightlessness, stability, barrier to gases, moisture and chemicals, recyclability and reusability. High density polyethylene (HDPE) and low density polyethylene (LDPE) are the two categories of polyethylene. Because of its stiffness, HDPE is used for making liquid containers, margarine tubs, bags for retail, grocery and scrap and so on, whereas squeezable food bottles, bendy lids, bread and frozen food bags are made up of LDPE due to its flexible and transparent nature.

Kleinhenz et al. (2000) used LDPE film (10.5 μm thick), macro-perforated LDPE bags (45 μm thick, 8.9% area perforated), micro-perforated LDPE bags (35 μm thick, 0.01% area perforated) and LDPE bags (45 μm thick) for packaging of shoots of

Bambusa oldhamii at different storage temperatures. Experiments were conducted to study their effect on weight loss, respiration, discolouration, microbial infection and shelf-life of bamboo shoots. They observed that shoots stored in LDPE bags lost the least weight, 0.09% and 4.17% after 10 and 28 days of storage, respectively, which is significantly less compared to unpacked controlled shoots stored at 1°C temperature wherein a loss of 7.67% (10 days) and 26.96% (28 days) was observed. Respiration and transpiration rate of shoots is greatly affected by temperature irrespective of packaging. The influence of packaging on fungal infection and discolouration is insignificant and mainly depends on temperature. Considering all the parameters at 1°C, semi-permeable micro-perforated LDPE bags and LDPE film extended the shelf-life of shoots up to and more than 28 days, whereas the low permeable LDPE bag and high permeable macro-perforated LDPE bags limited the shelf-life to 21 and 17 days due to deposition of condensate and much weight loss. The shoots are still better preserved compared to control unpacked shoots, i.e.7 days only at 1°C.

Chiangthong and Chayawat (2009) reported that in *Tha-Sao* community of Thailand the shoots of *Thyrsostachys siamensis* Gamble were steamed (100°C) for 15–30 mins and wrapped in the bilayer of plastic bags to preserve and maintain the quality of bamboo shoots for 120 days. Upon analyzing the physical, chemical and biological characters scientifically, they observed that the general features like taste, odour and texture were at standard levels. The pH level (5.58–5.98) and microbes (< 10 cfu) were observed to be lower than the standard levels on keeping the shoots up to 120 days. Wang and He (1989) reported that the shelf-life of bamboo shoots prolonged for 62 days by packaging in polyethylene with the incorporation of fungicide when kept at 0°C.

Yang et al. (2010) studied the effect of nitric oxide (NO) on browning and lignification of peeled shoots of *Phyllostachys violascens*. Sodium nitroprusside (SNP 0.05 mM) was used as NO donor for treating peeled shoots, packed in perforated polyethylene bags (0.01 mm thick) and stored at 10.5°C at 90% relative humidity for 10 days. In NO treated shoots, the activity of PPO, PAL and POD reduced significantly ($p < 0.05$) along with biosynthesis of ethylene which further delayed the senescence, browning, lignin and cellulose content as compared to controlled shoots. But the actual mechanism of NO in affecting those activities is yet to be worked out.

In our studies, shoots of *Bambusa bambos, B. nutans* and *Dendrocalamus sikkimensis* were packed in three different materials viz. glass bottles, HDPE bottles and LDPE bags (55 μm thick) in the form of raw and boiled (20 mins) cubes in water and brine (Table 7.2). Shelf-life of all three species and nutrient content status of *Bambusa nutans* was studied in stored shoots. Shelf-life was evaluated externally through visible changes and internally by analyzing microbial growth in internal tissue. Visible changes in packaged shoots were analyzed by considering three parameters i.e. turbidity in the solution, discolouration of shoots and fungal infection on the surface of shoot cubes. If symptoms of any of these appeared, then packages were marked as unwell (X) and if not, they were marked as well (✓).

Microbial growth in the internal tissue of shoots was tested by using the method of Kleinhenz et al. (2000) with some modifications. After three months, there was no change in the colour of shoots; preserving solutions were translucent with no turbidity and no sign of visible fungal growth (Table 7.2). But after three months, visible changes,

TABLE. 7.2
Wellness of Shoots after Six Months of Storage in Different Packages

Packaging Material and Shoot Sample		Preserving Solution	Species					
			Bambusa bambos		*Bambusa nutans*		*Dendrocalamus sikkimensis*	
			Visible	Microbe free	Visible	Microbe free	Visible	Microbe free
Glass bottle	Raw	Water	X	X	X	X	✓	✓
		Brine	✓	✓	✓	✓	✓	✓
	Boiled	Water	✓	X	✓	X	✓	✓
		Brine	✓	✓	✓	✓	✓	✓
HDPE bottle	Raw	Water	X	X	X	X	X	✓
		Brine	✓	✓	✓	X	✓	✓
	Boiled	Water	X	X	X	X	X	✓
		brine	✓	✓	✓	✓	✓	✓
LDPE bag	Raw	Water	X	X	X	X	X	X
		Brine	✓	X	✓	X	✓	X
	Boiled	Water	X	X	X	X	X	X
		Brine	✓	X	✓	X	✓	✓

HDPE—High density polyethylene, LDPE—Low density polyethylene.

as well as microbial growth, started appearing in some samples packaged in LDPE bags. Samples that were preserved in water spoiled earlier than those preserved in brine. Whereas, in glass bottles, all the shoots were well-preserved without any visible or internal alteration. Overall it was inferred that brine, as well as packaging material, played an important role in the shelf-life extension of easily perishable bamboo shoots.

Regarding the nutrients (Table 7.3), all the nutrients gradually decreased with increasing time of storage due to leaching out in preserving solution, but proteins reduced at a faster rate than other nutrients. Brine preserved shoots retained more nutrient content as compared to water preserved except for vitamin C which was higher in water storage than brine. After three months of storage, carbohydrate and amino acid content retained maximum at 55% and 78% respectively in brine preserved raw shoots in glass and HDPE bottles. A low amount of proteins was retained after storage with maximum content (23%) in brine stored boiled shoots. The boiled shoot samples showed the highest retention of dietary fibres compared to all other nutrients with almost equal content of up to 89%. In the case of vitamins, brine preserved raw shoots retained a reasonable amount of vitamin E (31%), whereas water preserved raw shoots showed a high amount of vitamin C content (68%). It was observed that packaging material had a great influence on shelf-life of bamboo shoots but less on nutrient availability; whereas brine positively affected both the shelf-life as well as retention of nutrients in bamboo shoots in most of the cases compared to water preservation.

7.1.2 Polyvinyl Chloride Film

Polyvinyl chloride (PVC) is a moderately strong, stiff, heavy, amorphous, transparent electrically stable compound that is resistant to chemicals, grease and oils and also has a capacity to extend its flexibility to different levels. It is used more for non-food packaging but less for food packaging. Kleinhenz et al. (2000) used heat-sealed PVC film as a packaging material for shoots of *Bambusa oldhamii* along with LDPE. Weight loss in PVC packages reduced significantly to 1.59% and 5.96% on the 10th and 28th days, respectively, as compared to unpacked shoots. But high deposition of condensates visually deteriorated the quality of packages, which limited the shelf-life of shoots to just 14 days.

Pongprasert et al. (2007) packaged shoots of *Dendrocalamus asper* in foam trays (15 × 20 cm) wrapped with 13 μm PVC film having a transmission rate of 2.93×10^5 cc/m² per day for CO_2 and 8.61×10^4 cc/m² per day for O_2. They studied the effect of this packaging on postponing the deterioration of sliced shoots by evaluating CO_2 production, weight loss, browning, lignin deposition, polyphenol oxidase (PPO) and peroxidase (POD) activity during storage at low temperature. Weight loss significantly reduced from 16% in control shoots to 0.9% in PVC wrapping after eight to ten days of storage in response to dropping in the evaporation process. CO_2 was maintained at a steady rate of 1.8% during storage but O_2 reduced to 18.4%. Reduced oxygen further lowered POD activity, which was required for polymerization of a lignin precursor thereby reducing lignification of shoots in PVC packages. Storage of shoots in PVC wraps was recommended to abolish anaerobism and diminish browning and desiccation of bamboo shoots.

TABLE 7.3

Nutrient Content in Juvenile Shoots of *Bambusa nutans* after Three Months of Packaging in Different Packaging and Preservation Materials

Packaging Methods		Parameters					
		Carbohydrates (g/100g)	Proteins (g/100g)	Amino Acid (g/100g)	Dietary Fibre (g/100g)	Vitamin C (mg/100g)	Vitamin E (mg/100g)
		Unprocessed Shoot					
Water	**GB**	1.21 ± 0.03	0.40 ± 0.02	1.55 ± 0.08	4.02 ± 0.07	1.03 ± 0.03	0.10 ± 0.00
	HDPE	1.18 ± 0.02	0.42 ± 0.01	1.57 ± 0.00	3.99 ± 0.01	1.02 ± 0.02	0.10 ± 0.00
	LDPE	0.96 ± 0.03	0.37 ± 0.01	1.23 ± 0.11	4.03 ± 0.02	1.03 ± 0.02	0.11 ± 0.01
Brine	**GB**	1.52 ± 0.04	0.74 ± 0.01	1.73 ± 0.12	4.29 ± 0.05	0.75 ± 0.02	0.15 ± 0.01
	HDPE	1.53 ± 0.07	0.75 ± 0.02	1.67 ± 0.00	4.24 ± 0.06	0.75 ± 0.01	0.14 ± 0.00
	LDPE	1.02 ± 0.02	0.71 ± 0.02	1.44 ± 0.05	4.26 ± 0.05	0.73 ± 0.00	0.14 ± 0.01
		Boiled Shoots					
Water	**GB**	0.80 ± 0.02	0.41 ± 0.01	0.69 ± 0.00	4.77 ± 0.03	0.80 ± 0.01	0.12 ± 0.01
	HDPE	0.81 ± 0.01	0.42 ± 0.02	0.64 ± 0.00	4.80 ± 0.09	0.81 ± 0.02	0.11 ± 0.01
	LDPE	0.77 ± 0.02	0.39 ± 0.00	0.56 ± 0.03	4.78 ± 0.02	0.80 ± 0.01	0.11 ± 0.00
Brine	**GB**	0.97 ± 0.03	0.83 ± 0.02	0.75 ± 0.01	4.75 ± 0.08	0.72 ± 0.01	0.12 ± 0.01
	HDPE	0.95 ± 0.02	0.82 ± 0.02	0.71 ± 0.01	4.79 ± 0.04	0.71 ± 0.02	0.12 ± 0.01
	LDPE	0.92 ± 0.04	0.80 ± 0.02	0.63 ± 0.01	4.79 ± 0.01	0.73 ± 0.02	0.11 ± 0.00

Values reported are measurement replication means ± standard deviation (n = 3 replicates).
GB = Glass bottle, HDPE = High density polyethylene bottle, LDPE = Low density polyethylene bag (55μm thick)

But the plasticizers used in PVC have a possibility to leach out in food especially phthalates, use of which is banned in some countries for food packaging material due to safety concerns. There are some difficulties in the recyclability of PVC and also its destruction through ignition contributes chlorine to the atmosphere which is a problematic issue and hence its use in packaging is a matter of concern.

7.1.3 Vacuum Packaging

Vacuum packaging is a mode of packaging achieved by packing the product in a low oxygen permeable film with a secured sealing while excluding air from it. The initial environment of the package which might have slight aeration, experience change through preservation and storage due to active microbial and metabolic processes within the foodstuff.

Pongprasert et al. (2007) have implicated the technique of vacuum packaging for storing shoots of *Dendrocalamus asper* in polyethylene (PE). They reported minimal weight loss (0.8%) and an effective reduction in respiration in vacuum PE bags compared to unpacked control shoots after 10 days of storage. Low oxygen concentration in packages leads to a sharp diminution in PPO and POD activity initially which later increased gradually during storage period that might have a great influence on reducing lignification and browning of shoot slices to a remarkable level. Vacuum packaging of shoot is common in some countries (Figure 7.3.)

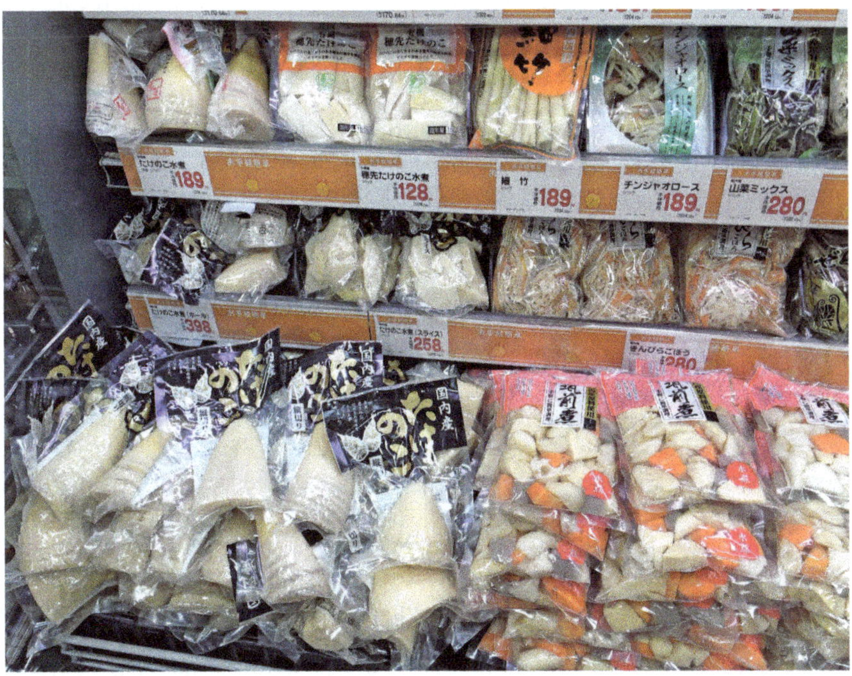

FIGURE 7.3 Vacuum-packed bamboo shoot sold at a department store in Osaka, Japan.

7.1.4 Modified Atmospheric Packaging

For extending the shelf-life of fresh fruits and vegetables, modified atmospheric packaging (MAP) has gained much popularity in recent years. MAP operationally lower down respiration, PPO, POD and phenol biosynthetic enzyme activities of food in the packages. MAP can be achieved by active or passive mode or by combining both. Through active mode, the atmosphere of the package can be modified directly by pulling a slight vacuum and replacing the former atmosphere with a preferred assortment of gases. On the other hand, passive modification depends upon physiognomies of product and packaging material. It can be accomplished by establishing a relevant relationship between packaging film and enclosed foodstuff, which in fact is affected by respiration of product, the permeability of film, the equilibrium of gases and external factors like temperature, pressure and humidity. For a MAP of fresh produce, packaging films having properties like light weights, transparency, thermal stability, non-toxicity, high tear strength, permeability to different gases and commercial suitability should be preferred.

Shen et al. (2006) studied the effect of MAP on browning and lignification of shoots of *Phyllostachys praecox*. They packaged peeled shoots in LDPE bags (0.04 mm); the control samples were stored openly while others were stored with the modified atmosphere of 2% O_2, 5% CO_2 and 93% N_2 and all treatments were kept at temperature 10 ± 0.5°C and 92% relative. MAP limited the respiration of shoots at 0.4–0.8% for O_2 and 5.1–5.8% for CO_2 during storage (10 days). Malondialdehyde (MDA) content which is related to lipid peroxidation, decreased during the first six days of storage but later increased gradually. There was a significant decline in POD ($p < 0.05$) and PAL ($p < 0.01$) activity in MAP as compared to control, whereas PPO activity was enhanced. Low oxygen and reduced MDA, POD and PAL activities were co-related to browning of shoots which was inhibited by MAP in contrary to severe browning of controlled shoots. MAP could inhibit the cellulose and lignification of shoots where lignin content was 36% less than the control, which might also be contributed by low PAL and POD activity which are the key enzymes in phenylpropanoid pathway that synthesize monomers of lignin, namely coumaryl alcohol, coniferyl alcohol and sinapyl alcohol.

7.1.5 Edible Film and Coatings

Due to disposal and environmental issues of conventional synthetic packaging, interests in the use of bio-based material for packaging has increased. The edible coating acts as a barrier to microbes on the food surface and also reduces moisture and solute migration, gas exchange, oxidation, physiological disarrays thereby ultimately extending shelf-life. The material used for edible film and coatings are commonly proteins, lipid and polysaccharides that are generally regarded as safe and approved by the FDA. These materials can be applied to food by directly immersing, spraying, brushing or wrapping the surface and have certain properties such as flexibility, tension, brightness, opacity, resistance to microbes, moisture, gas flow and sensory adequacy. Additionally, they can also enhance the value of food by the integration of colourant, flavours, nutrients, spices, anti-oxidants, anti-browning and anti-microbial additives to them.

Badwaik et al. (2014) used edible films to coat bamboo shoots and studied its effect on shoot quality. They used six combinations of starch, sodium alginate and carboxymethyl cellulose (CMC) to make edible coating where glycerol was used as plasticizer and $CaCl_2$ for strengthening. On the basis of thickness, water vapour permeability, moisture absorption (9.37%), water solubility (40%), tensile/breakage strength (977.30 g), colour, uniform surface characteristics and thermal stability (up to 200°C) of prepared films, the best combination of alginate and starch (1:2) with 15% (w/w) of CMC with incorporation of anti-oxidant and anti-microbial extract was selected for coating of *Bambusa balcooa* shoots. Shoots were immersed in the coating solution then dried and stored at 30 ± 2°C temperature and 64 ± 3% relative humidity for 5 days. This combination was effective to reduce the weight loss by 7% that might be accredited to low water vapour permeability. It maintained the colour lightness of shoots to a higher level and the colour change value also increased though at a slow rate compared to the uncoated ones which may be due to combined effect of alginate, starch and added anti-oxidants (4 ml/100ml). The microbial count also dropped significantly ($p \leq 0.05$) from 4.64 to 2.34 log cfu/cm^2 that may be due to the anti-microbial agent (27 mg/ml) added to the coating solution.

Yang et al. (2015) used chitosan which is approved by the US Food and Drug Administration (US FDA) as a food additive and chlorine dioxide (ClO_2) which is legally permitted as a food sanitizer in the United States and China for coating fresh-cut shoots of *Phyllostachys praecox* f. *prevernalis.* They used three treatments for shoots: (i) ClO_2 (28 ml/l), (ii) chitosan coating (1.5%) and (iii) a combination of (i) and (ii) along with a control and preserved them in plastic trays covered with unsealed plastic bags, kept at 4°C and 60–70% relative humidity for six days. The treatment mentioned in (iii) proved best to maintain the quality of minimally processed shoots because it significantly ($p < 0.05$) lowered the rate of respiration, weight loss and firmness of shoots. It also diminished the PAL, POD, CAD and PPO activity significantly ($p < 0.05$) till the last day of storage which might be attributed to lowered lignification and browning of the shoot in comparison to control. Growth of anaerobic bacteria (3.26 log cfu/g), yeast and mould (2.40 log cfu/g) were also retarded as ClO_2 decreased the initial population of microbes and chitosan limited the further growth. Overall, ClO_2 may be responsible for restriction of enzymatic reactions while chitosan acted as a barrier to oxygen, respiration and further oxidation of phenolic enzymes.

Some of the packaging materials mainly plastic-based are non-degradable, non-reusable and non-recyclable which augment environmental waste and there is also an issue of mobilization of low molecular weight constituents like stabilizers, plasticizers, monomers and oligomers from the packaging material to the food product. The use of biopolymers for packaging can overcome these drawbacks, like polyesters, which could either directly be extracted from proteins, lipids and polysaccharides or can be synthesized by polymerization e.g. aliphatic-aromatic copolymers, aliphatic polyesters, polylactic aliphatic copolymers. Bio-based polymers that are renewable like poly lactic acid, oil-based monomers such as polycaprolactone, micro-organisms generated material like polyhydroxyalkanoates can be used to prepare packaging material and thereafter their application on bamboo shoots can be studied. Application of nanocomposites has also been introduced for food packaging but there is limited scientific data on their toxicological effect on humans or migration of nanoparticles to food, which must further be explored.

8 Bamboo Shoots as Functional Foods and Nutraceuticals

Most foods are considered functional in terms of providing nutrients and/or energy to sustain basic life. However, in the last decade, consumer demands in the field of food have changed considerably. Rapid economic growth, urbanization and globalization are the main drivers for these changes. Different lifestyles and purchasing patterns have resulted in a change in diet which has modified production, distribution and marketing trends. With the economic development and the improvement of people's living standards, demand for natural foods, especially healthy and organic food, has greatly increased. At the same time, an increased number of working women caused a shift towards processed food, which requires less time for preparation. Moreover, increasing public awareness of the link between diet and health has boosted the consumption of these foods to unparalleled levels, particularly in countries where the population is aging and health care costs are rising. Scientific evidence and a growing awareness of the correlation between diet and health, coupled with sedentary lifestyles, an aging population, and ever-increasing health care costs have driven the interest in healthier food products (Malla et al. 2014). These products include functional or fortified foods and nutraceuticals that confer positive health benefits to consumers. Nutraceuticals and functional foods have not only captured the world food market but also the psyche of average consumers through the supply of rich nutrients to the body even by the simple popping of different supplement formats, for example, dietary supplements, capsules or pills. Both are intensively researched for their role in maintaining health and prevention of diseases. Functional foods are defined as products that resemble traditional foods but possess demonstrated physiological benefits. However, nutraceuticals are commodities derived from foods but are mostly used in the medicinal form of pills, capsules or liquids and again render demonstrated physiological benefits. In some countries, however, the term functional foods and nutraceuticals are used interchangeably. Regardless, the main focus of such products is to improve health and reduce disease risk through prevention. There is an increased interest both in functional foods and nutraceuticals, as they provide physiological and metabolic benefits by boosting the immune system and counteracting diseases and degenerative disorders. One of the most important trends in the food industry is the demand for all-natural food ingredients that are free of chemical additives and they are usually obtained from edible plants and bamboo is one such plant that can be utilized for this purpose.

8.1 FOOD FORTIFICATION AND FUNCTIONAL FOODS

Functional foods are defined as whole foods along with fortified, enriched, or enhanced foods that have a potentially beneficial effect on health when consumed as part of a varied diet on a regular basis at effective levels (Crowe 2013). Consumers today demand foods that are sustainably produced and processed, deemed safe and have nutritional value and food producers have invested resources in the development of functional foods that may provide added benefits to consumer well-being (Granato et al 2020). Such types of food include foods supplemented with bioactive and mineral substances (e.g. probiotics, anti-oxidants, iodized salt) and derived food ingredients introduced to conventional foods (e.g. prebiotics). According to FAO report, it is estimated that 2 billion people worldwide suffer from micronutrient malnutrition and micronutrient deficiencies account for approximately 7.3% of global diseases. The most effective way of combating malnutrition is food fortification which is one of the many public health interventions towards mitigating micronutrient malnutrition as well as poor growth and development of children (Alina et al. 2019, Okeyo 2019). Fortification or enrichment refers to the addition of one or several essential nutritional elements to a food product towards the prevention or correction of proven deficiencies in one or more nutrients. In many cases, fortification targets restoring nutrients and/or enhancing nutrients lost during processing, enhancing nutrient levels of food vehicles that have limited content than what is required, and adding nutrients not usually present in food to some commonly consumed food vehicles for the purposes of boosting intake of that particular nutrient (Ottaway 2008). There is a large interest in fortifying food with vitamins, minerals, organic acids, dietary fibres, phenolic compounds, essential amino acids and anti-oxidants. Although a huge world population suffers from various nutritional deficiencies, people with low income are the most affected, particularly in developing countries. The most efficient and accessible way of providing nutrients is additional fortification using these substances in popular consumer food products especially flour and bakery products.

Food fortification and supplementation with nutrients are not new and have been carried out for centuries even before the scientific rationale became available. Nutrient supplementation of food was mentioned for the first time in the year 400 BCE by the Persian physician Melanpus who suggested adding iron filings to wine to increase soldier's potency (Meija 1994). However, it was between the first and second world wars (1924–1944) that supplementation was established as a measure to prevent nutritional deficiencies in populations or to restore nutrients lost during the processing of foods. Thus, during this period, the adding of iodine to salts, vitamins A and D to margarine, vitamin D to milk and vitamins B1, B2, niacin and iron to flours and bread was established (Murphy 1996). In Central Europe during the Middle Ages, mothers were known to push iron nails into apples, leave them for a while and then feed the apples to their ailing daughters. In 1824, the indigenous population of Columbia and South America treated goiter with a special type of salt which was later found to have a high content of iodine. In Mexico, while making traditional tortillas, the corn was first soaked in lime water and a pinch of ground limestone was added to the tortilla to enrich it with calcium. In 1831, French physician Bossingault urged adding iodine to salt to prevent goiter. The first official addition of iodide to domestic salt started in Switzerland in 1900 which later spread to other countries also. Currently, food fortification encompasses a broader concept and is done for several reasons: as a tool to correct or prevent widespread nutrients inadequacies and hence, correct associated micronutrient deficiencies to balance the total nutrient profile of diets, to restore nutrients lost during processing, to add nutrients that may not be naturally present in food, to make products more appealing to consumers and to provide certain technological functions in food processing such as adding a preservative or colouring agent to processed food. Food fortification is now one of the most effective methods of preventing nutritional deficiencies and has contributed to the virtual elimination of many diseases of goiter, rickets, beriberi and pellagra. The most commonly used fortified food products include ready-to-eat breakfast cereals, cereal bars, fat spreads, bread, milk and milk products and juices.

8.2 FORTIFYING FOOD PRODUCTS WITH BAMBOO SHOOTS

The quest for finding suitable natural ingredients to make popular healthy food items is gaining momentum. In recent years, attention is being paid to foods that have valuable amounts of minerals, vitamins, micronutrients and other bioactive compounds such as fibre and anti-oxidants. The most important elements used for food fortification are iron, iodine, vitamins, calcium, selenium, fibres, proteins and fatty acids (Alina et al. 2019). The concern for healthy diets and cost-effective health care among people has prompted the food industry to search for plants rich in nutrients and have nutraceutical properties and desirable functional characteristics. Bamboo shoots have been frequently assessed for various bioactivities due to their nutritional and therapeutic importance and overall application in the food industry. The juvenile bamboo shoots being rich in nutrients, health promoting bioactive compounds (phenols, phytosterols, dietary fibre), vitamins (vitamin A, vitamin B1, vitamin B3, vitamin B6, vitamin C, vitamin E), amino acids and minerals, hence, play a significant role in maintaining good health and is being projected as health food (Hiromichi 2007, Kumbhare and Bhargava 2007, Park and Jhon 2009, Chongtham et al. 2011). Nowadays, consumer's interest has inclined towards food products that can impart health benefits, increase longevity and reduce the risks of, or delay the onset of, diseases and disorders. Thus, formulation of novel food products by incorporating nutrients, bioactive compounds, dietary fibre and anti-oxidants from bamboo shoots, as ingredients for physiological benefits or disease prevention and control has drawn the attention of researchers, nutritionists, consumers and industrialists.

Bamboo shoot dietary fibre possesses a wide range of structural diversity and favorable functional properties that makes it an ideal ingredient for various functional and health foods and is gaining popularity in the food and nutraceutical industry. The utilization of bamboo fibre in fortifying bakery products, meat, sausage, beverages, spices, pasta and ketchup have been reported (Chongtham et al. 2011). Inclusion of bamboo dietary fibre in the diet has a beneficial effect on healthy digestion and lowering of lipid profile. Fortification of dietary fibre in food also lowers the fat content in deep-fried products, which will also solve the problems of obesity and various cardiovascular diseases due to the over-ingestion of high fat-containing food items. Ge et al. (2017) analyzed the effect of extrusion on various physiochemical and functional properties of bamboo shoot dietary fibre. It was observed that extrusion cooking enhanced the functional properties of bamboo shoot dietary fibre viz. swelling capacity, water holding capacity, cholesterol absorption capacity and fat absorption capacity. Several scientific studies have been conducted to analyze the effect of bamboo shoot dietary fibre on the physical and functional properties of food fortified with bamboo shoot dietary fibre. Felisberto et al. (2017a, 2017b) analyzed the nutritional and physiochemical properties of flour prepared from *Dendrocalamus asper* young culms and reported significantly higher quantities of fibre (67–79 g/100 g) and starch (6–16 g/100 g), thus highlighting the potential of young bamboo culm flour utilization in fibre enriched bakery and other food products. Zheng et al. (2017) analyzed the effect of the addition of bamboo shoot dietary fibre (BSDF) extracted from *Dendrocalamus latiflorus* on rheological behavior, microstructure and textural properties of milk pudding. They observed that the addition of 2 g BSDF was effective in improving all these features of milk pudding which is helpful in enhancing its food-industrial value. Zhang et al. (2017) investigated the effect of bamboo shoot dietary fibre (1.0%, 1.5% and 2%) on the mechanical properties, moisture distribution and microstructure of frozen dough. Results indicated that the addition of BSDF can improve the viscoelasticity, extensibility and plasticity of frozen dough and enhance its processing qualities thereby making it more suitable for the production of various processed food products such as bread and dumplings. Hemicellulose components of *Sasa senanensis*, a mixture of xylose and xylo-oligosaccharides (XOS) isolated by steaming and subsequent water extraction are reported to be a potential raw material in the development of functional food and pharmaceutical industries. Miura et al. (2013) reported the presence of xylitol in *Phyllostachys pubescens* which is converted from hemicelluloses through microbial activity. Since the compound has several health benefits such as anti-caries, anti-inflammatory and sweetening properties, it is of great interest in the food industries.

Interest in utilizing bamboo shoot which is rich in nutrients, bioactive compounds and minerals for the production of natural functional food is gaining popularity in the food industries (Chongtham et al. 2011, Santosh et al. 2019). Processing of shoots for long term preservation and removal of anti-nutrients for the production of value-added food products have been reported (Choudhury et al. 2012, Santosh et al. 2019). Bamboo shoots are now being used for food fortification to incorporate the nutrients and bioactive compounds to make (Table 8.1) several value-added products such as pickles, candies, nuggets, crackers, chutney, chips, cookies, chappatis and buns (Pandey et al. 2012, Bisht et al. 2012, Mustafa et al. 2016, Sood et al. 2013, Choudhary et al. 2012). Shoots can be used as fresh, dried or fermented for making various food items as described next.

8.2.1 Biscuits/Cookies

It is well established that malnutrition in early life can compromise the development potential of children and their later health and productivity as adults. To address the nutritional needs of young school going children and provide social protection to families, global efforts have largely focused on school feeding and school-based

TABLE 8.1

Contemporary Food Items Fortified with Bamboo Shoots

Fortified Product	Bamboo Species	Form Used	References
Amaretti cookies	Not mentioned	Bamboo fibre	Farris and Piergiovanni 2008
Crackers, Nugget, Pickle	*Bambusa bambos, B. tulda, Dendrocalamus asper, D. strictus*	Brine-treated boiled shoot	Pandey et al. 2012
Chicken nuggets	*B. auriculata*	Fermented for two months	Das et al. 2013
Candy, Chutney, Chukh, Cracker, Nugget	*D. hamiltonii*	Boiled shoot	Sood et al. 2013
Pork Nuggets	*B. polymorpha*	Brine-treated boiled and fermented for six months	Thomas et al. 2014
Biscuit	*B. balcooa*	Boiled, dried and powdered	Choudhury et al. 2015
Chips	*B. vulgaris*	Shoot boiled for two hours	Maroma 2015
Pork Pickles	Not mentioned	Minced shoot exposed to sun and fermented for 21 days, dried and powdered	Chavhan et al. 2015
Candies	Not mentioned	Boiled shoot	Nimisha et al. 2015
Cookies	Not mentioned	Boiled shoot, dried and powdered	Mustafa et al. 2016
Pork Nuggets	*B. polymorpha*	Brine-treated boiled shoot extract	Thomas et al. 2016
Battered and breaded fish balls	*Not mentioned*	Bamboo shoot fibre	Zeng et al. 2016
Fried potato chips	*Bambusa balcooa*	Bamboo shoot powder and bamboo shoot extract	Shanmgam et al. 2016
Frozen dough	Not mentioned	Bamboo shoot fibre	Zhang et al. 2017
Milk pudding	*D. latiflorus*	Shoot fibre extracted with cellulase and papain enzyme method	Zheng et al. 2017
Biscuit	*D. hamiltonii*	Freeze-dried powder of fresh, boiled and soaked shoots	Santosh et al. 2018
Biscuit	*D. hamiltonii*	Fresh, boiled and soaked shoot paste	Santosh et al. 2019
Cookies	*D. asper*	Bamboo culm treated with meta-bisulphite, dried and powdered	Felisberto et al. 2019

fortification approaches (Adams et al. 2017). Biscuits represent a good candidate for the addition of functional ingredients because they are popular, daily consumed bakery items and have long shelf-life. Many functional biscuits have been formulated with anti-oxidant and/or prebiotic properties (Pasqualone et al. 2015, Obafaye and Omoba 2018). Daily consumption of fortified biscuits by primary school children had a significant positive impact on mean levels of iron, folic acid, vitamin B12, retinol and vitamin D. Bamboo shoots with its high nutrient content and health promoting bioactive compounds have been used for fortifying biscuits (Bisht et al. 2015, Choudhury et al. 2015, Mustafa et al. 2016, Santosh et al. 2018, 2019). Influence of bamboo shoot powder fortification on physico-chemical, textural and organoleptic characteristics of biscuits have been studied (Choudhury et al. 2015). Shoots of *B. balcooa* were sliced, boiled, dried, powdered, analyzed for nutritional status and used for making biscuits. Different concentrations of bamboo shoot powder (BSP) along with other necessary ingredients were mixed to make biscuits followed by an analysis of protein, fibre, fat, ash, phenolics, anti-oxidant activity, hardness, colour and sensory acceptability. Biscuits enriched with BSP showed higher phenolics, fibres and protein contents than the control. It was concluded that up to 10% BSP could be incorporated in the formulation of biscuits without affecting the overall quality.

Effect of ingredients and process conditions on important characteristics of bamboo fibre fortified Amaretti cookies, a popular Italian food product was studied by Farris et al. (2008). Fructose, bamboo fibre and egg white were used as ingredients and their effects along with baking time and baking temperature on quality responses such as hardness, water activity, moisture content and colour of cookies were measured by using a fractional factorial design in a screening test. It was observed that the addition of bamboo fibre contributed to beneficial textural properties and improved mouthfeel. Choudhury et al. (2015) investigated the influence of fortifying biscuits with the shoots of *Bambusa balcooa* for physicochemical, texture and organoleptic characteristics. The shoot was processed by blanching 30 mins, which was then dried and the powder was used for the formulation of 5%, 10% and 15% shoot-fortified biscuit. The study observed an increased level of water absorption capacity whereas gluten content decreased with the increased fortification level in the dough sample. Fortified biscuits also showed an increase in moisture, fibre, protein, fat and ash content with an increase in fortification level. There was a decrease in the phenolic and anti-oxidant properties of bamboo shoot powder during processing, however, the increase was observed in the fortified products with increasing level of formulation. Sensory observation for appearance, colour, texture, flavor, mouthfeel and overall acceptability was also analyzed and a decrease in acceptability was found with increasing the percentage of fortification. Incorporation of 10% shoot powder was recommended due to overall consumer acceptability.

Mustafa et al. (2016) studied the effect of bamboo powder supplementation on the physicochemical and organoleptic characteristics of fortified cookies. They studied physical characteristics like diameter, thickness and spread factor and observed a significant reduction in the spread factor with an increase in bamboo shoot powder. Physical characteristics depicted exceptional dough making characteristics when mixed with wheat flour. Sensory evaluation revealed that the cookies prepared with 6% and lower concentration of bamboo shoot powder was acceptable.

Santosh et al. (2018, 2019) developed bamboo shoot–fortified functional biscuits by using freeze-dried bamboo shoot powder and paste from *Dendrocalamus hamiltonii* (Figure 8.1). Nutrients, bioactive compounds and minerals were increased in bamboo shoot–fortified biscuits as compared to control biscuits. Nutritional content was observed to be maximum in fresh freeze-dried fortified biscuits with 0.30 g/100 g amino acids, 1.27 g/100 g protein, 20.45 g/100 g carbohydrate, 0.22 g/100 g phenol, 0.18 g/100 g phytosterol, 62.44 g/100 g neutral detergent fibre (NDF) and 5.16 g/100 g acid detergent fibre (ADF). Anti-nutrient content in all the fortified biscuits was much below the permissible level. Both the bamboo shoot paste and freeze-dried powder fortified biscuits scored high on sensory analysis and overall acceptability indicating that bamboo shoot supplementation in biscuits is a convenient vehicle for imparting nutrients and health promoting bioactive compounds into people's diet.

8.2.2 Nuggets

Value-added edible products such as nuggets, pickle and papad have been made from fresh bamboo shoots of four species *Bambusa bambos*, *B. tulda*, *Dendrocalamus strictus* and *D. asper* (Pandey et al. 2012). The nuggets were made by mixing boiled shoots, soaked chickpea, green gram, soybean and black gram with spices and salt as per taste. The mixture was then ground to a coarse paste and small equal sized balls were made and dried in oven for three days at 45–50°C. Organoleptic, sensory and chemical evaluation revealed that the products were good in taste, texture and quality for six months from the date of processing at ambient conditions and polypropylene and glass containers. Sood et al. (2013) modified this method and made nuggets by mixing bamboo shoots with soaked green gram and black gram along with spices

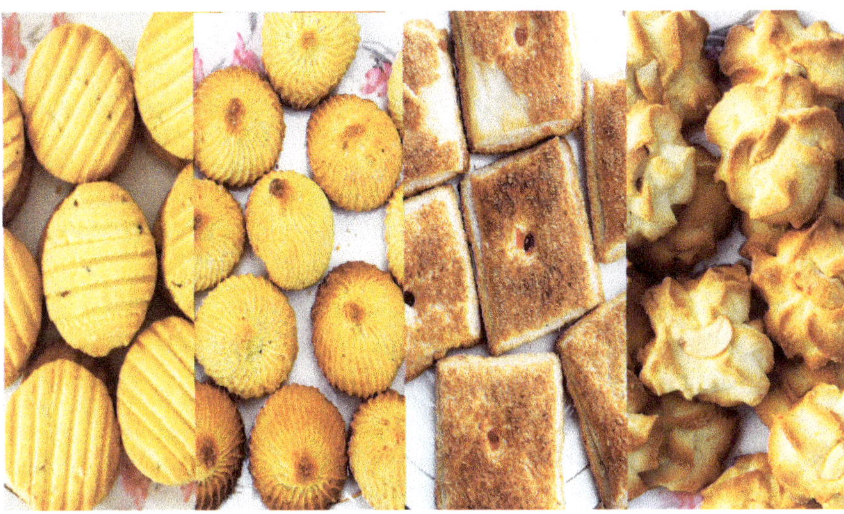

FIGURE 8.1 Bamboo shoot–fortified biscuits developed in the laboratory of Department of Botany, Panjab University and Department of Environmental Studies, North-Eastern Hill University, India.

in a different proportion and ground it to make a coarse paste. This paste was made into small equal sized balls and transferred directly to preheated and greased oven trays and dried in an oven for 24 hrs at 45–50°C.

Das et al. (2013) prepared nuggets from the relatively tough and fibrous meat of desi "spent" hen using fermented bamboo shoot (FBS) as a phyto-preservative in order to enhance the physicochemical, microbiological and keeping quality of the nuggets. The meat was minced and blended along with other non-meat ingredients and 10% fermented bamboo shoot. The emulsion was filled in metallic moulds and steam cooked and cut into pieces. Ready-to-eat nuggets thus prepared were packed in sterilized LDPE zip bags and stored at 4 ± 1°C for up to 15 days for quality evaluation. Emulsion stability (%), cooking yield (%) and proximate composition were studied on the day of preparation, while estimation of pH, TBA values, microbial load and sensory evaluation were carried out at an interval of five days and up to 15 days of storage. The emulsion stability (%), cooking yield (%), moisture (%), crude protein (%) and total ash (%) of FBS treated nuggets differed significantly from the control products. It was concluded that FBS fortified nuggets were superior to the control product and addition of 10% FBS gave the most promising physicochemical, microbial and sensory qualities in the nuggets and could be suitably stored for 15 days under refrigeration.

Pork nuggets were made by incorporating fermented bamboo shoot mince (FBSM) and their physicochemical, microbiological and sensory characteristics evaluated during 35 days' storage at refrigeration temperature (Thomas et al. 2014, 2016). The addition of fermented bamboo shoot significantly affected the pH, moisture, protein, fat fibre and texture profiles of nuggets. Addition of FBSM significantly retarded quality deterioration during refrigeration temperature storage, especially lipid oxidation and microbiological characteristics. Also, incorporation of 8% FBSM increased the storage life of pork nuggets by two weeks without impairing different physicochemical and sensory attributes and improved their microbiological characteristics. Chavhan et al. (2015) used fermented bamboo shoot as a preservative for the preparation of pork pickles and analyzed the physicochemical, microbial and shelf-life qualities of the products. Bamboo shoot–fortified pork pickle was studied in different formulations using fermented bamboo shoot extract, fermented bamboo shoot paste, dried powder of fermented bamboo shoots at the level of 50 to 100% with or without vinegar. The shelf-life of all the products was recorded maximum up to 90 days without any physicochemical and microbial effects except for the formulation of pork pickle with dried fermented powder for 30 days.

8.2.3 Candies

Tender bamboo shoots were used for preparing candies by Sood et al. (2013) and Nimisha et al. (2015). Fresh bamboo shoots were washed with tap water and the outer sheath was removed using a sharp stainless-steel knife. The inner edible portion was cut into uniform size cubes (1.5 cm). The cut cubes were washed thoroughly with tap water and subjected to boiling in steam-jacketed kettles for 30 mins followed by changing the water two to three times to ensure complete removal of HCN. Cubes were dipped in sugar syrup of required solute (sugar) strength and citric acid.

Thereafter, cubes candy was prepared by gradually increasing the solute concentration in the aqueous medium by heating 40°brix to 70°brix with 0.25% citric acid till equilibrium persists. Candy cubes to hypertonic sugar syrup ratio 1:2 were considered best because it gave complete dispersion of tender bamboo shoot (TBS) cubes into the sugar syrup and was easy to stir. Some desired flavors were also added to the syrup after equilibrium. Thereafter, preservative (KMS, 40 ppm) was added to have better preserving effect for candies cubes for the prolonged storage period. The equilibrated candy was dried at 55°C until 24–26% moisture content was retained and then packed in a pre-sterilized glass bottle.

8.2.4 Chips

Young shoots of *Bambusa vulgaris* were used for making chips with the aim to make a healthy snack by Maroma (2015). Shoots were harvested, washed and then sanitized in chlorinated water for 1 hr. The bamboo shoots were cut into half, and each sheath separated from one another and washed thoroughly. Then it was boiled in two litres of water for 1 hr. After boiling, the shoots were cut into 50 mm × 250 mm strips, coated with cornstarch and deep fried in 150°C palm oil until golden brown. The product was subjected to microbiological analysis and sensory evaluation to determine the safety and acceptability of the product and was found to be safe and liked by consumers. Such chips can also be prepared using gram flour (Figure 8.2).

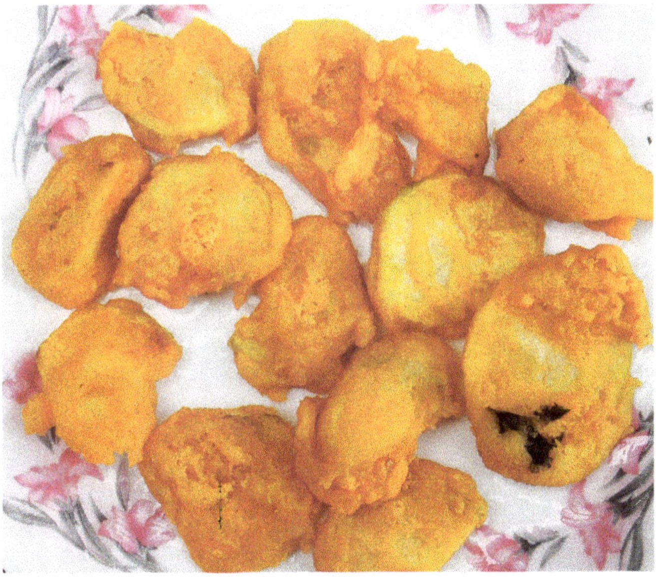

FIGURE 8.2 Bamboo shoot chips coated with gram flour.

8.2.5 Crackers

Papad is a thin, circular, crispy wafer-like a popular snack in India. It is generally roasted or fried and served with a traditional Indian meal. Bamboo papad was made mixing one part (200 g) of boiled shoots, one part (200 g) of boiled potatoes, ½ teaspoon red chili powder, ½ teaspoon black pepper powder, ½ teaspoon cumin seeds and salt to taste (Pandey et al. 2012). The mixture was then ground and the dough was prepared. Equal sized balls were made from dough and rolled on a rolling board with the help of rolling pins in circular movements to make round papads. Papads were then dried in an oven for 2 days at 45–50°C. Dried papads were then stored in an airtight container. A modified version was also made by Sood et al. (2013). The papads had higher nutritive value than the control.

8.2.6 Pickles

Pickling is one of the most popular preservation methods that not only extends a food's shelf-life but also enhances its taste and flavor. Foods that are pickled include meats, fruits, eggs and vegetables. Bamboo shoot pickles (Figure 8.3) are quite popular in some parts of India. Pandey et al. (2012) made pickles from tender shoots of *B. bambos*, *B. tulda*, *D. strictus* and *D. asper*. Shoots were cut into small pieces, boiled and dried in air for about 1 hr and mixed with appropriate spices. The shoots were then transferred to a sterile glass container and hot mustard oil was poured over it before putting on the lid and kept unopened for a week.

High perishability of meat and meat products is a serious problem in tropical countries due to the prevailing climatic conditions and pickling is a suitable method for preserving these products. Chavhan et al. (2015) studied the effect of incorporation of the fermented bamboo shoot on physiochemical and microbial quality of pork pickle. Fermented bamboo shoot (FBS) extracts, paste and powder were incorporated in the pork pickle at the level of 50% to 100% with or without vinegar and stored at room temperature for 90 days.

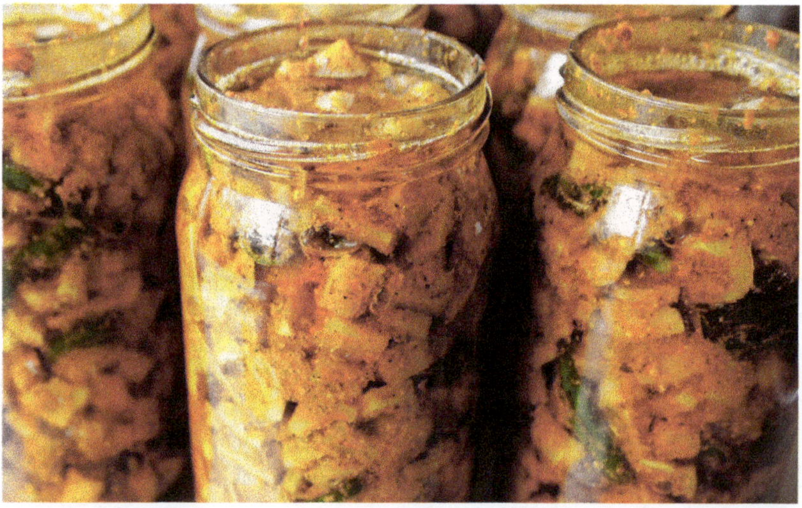

FIGURE 8.3 Bamboo shoot pickle prepared in North Eastern Hill University, Shillong, India.

No significant differences were observed with respect to proximate composition, that is percentage of moisture, protein, fat and ash contents among the products except with 100% FBS powder which had significantly lower moisture content. Except for the product with 100% FBS powder which could be stored for 30 days only, other products could be stored up to 90 days without and physiochemical and microbial problems thereby indicating that natural and organic FBS extract and paste can be used successfully replacing the conventional chemical preservative like vinegar for preparation of pork pickle and preserved for more than 90 days at room temperature.

8.3 NUTRACEUTICALS

Nutraceutical is a broad term that describes a substance extracted from food sources with additional health benefits along with basic nutritional value already present in them. The term nutraceutical was coined in 1989 by Stephen DeFelice, founder and chairman of Foundation for Innovation in Medicine, Cranford, New Jersey, by combining nutrition and pharmaceutical for any substance that is a food or part of a food and provides medical or health benefits, including the prevention and treatment of disease. The health ministry of Canada later modified the meaning of nutraceutical as 'a product isolated or purified from the food, generally sold in a medicinal form not associated with food and demonstrated to have a physiological benefit'. So, in essence, nutraceuticals differ from functional foods mainly in the manner of their consumption. Although both are consumed for their perceived health benefits courtesy to their bioactive compounds, nutraceuticals are utilized mainly in the form of pills, tablets, capsules, powders and tinctures, whereas the functional foods are always consumed as normal food formulations. Apart from capsule and pill forms, nutraceuticals are also marketed in the form of herbal and dietary supplements. With ever-increasing public health consciousness, demand for nutraceutical and related health products has grown tremendously over the past few decades. This rise in the popularity of nutraceuticals has been backed by the modern scientific research which has provided conclusive evidence toward the beneficial role of nutraceuticals against several chronic diseases such as cancer, heart diseases, hypertension, high cholesterol, osteoporosis, diabetes, arthritis, indigestion, macular degeneration, cataracts, treating headaches and migraines resulting from stress. The nutraceuticals hold the key for the food industries to create reliable health products in the future, providing a suitable and more natural alternative to consumers dissatisfied with drug cost and conventional health care systems for the prevention and treatment of chronic diseases.

The modern nutraceutical market began to develop in Japan during the 1980s. In contrast to the natural herbs and spices used as a folk medicine for centuries throughout Asia, the nutraceutical industry has grown alongside the expansion and exploration of modern technology. The global nutraceutical market is growing rapidly and is expected to grow from USD 198.1 billion in 2016 to USD 285.0 billion by 2022 as per recent reports. India has also started to strengthen its position in the functional food and nutraceutical sector, with its nutraceutical industry set to cross USD 6 billion from the current USD 2.8 billion by 2020 (ASSOCHAM, 2017).

This rise in the popularity of nutraceuticals has been backed by the modern scientific research which has provided conclusive evidence towards the beneficial role of nutraceuticals against several chronic diseases such as cancer, heart diseases, hypertension, high cholesterol, osteoporosis, diabetes, arthritis, indigestion, muscular degeneration, cataracts, headaches and migraines resulting from stress. Bioactive compounds comprise an excellent pool of molecules for the production of nutraceuticals, functional foods and food additives (Joana Gil-Chávez et al. 2013). Natural bioactive compounds are being searched for the treatment and prevention of human diseases because of their health benefits (Table 8.2). These compounds efficiently interact with proteins, DNA and other biological molecules to produce desired results, which can then be used for designing natural therapeutic agents. Hence, pharmaceutical and food domains have a common interest to obtain new natural bioactive components that can be used as drugs, functional food ingredients, or nutraceuticals (Joana Gil-Chávez et al. 2013).

8.4 BAMBOO SHOOTS AS NUTRACEUTICALS

Bamboo shoots, which make a delicious vegetable, apart from being highly nutritious are also a rich source of various bioactive compounds like phytosterols, dietary fibres and phenolic compounds as discussed in Chapter 4. The presence of these bioactive compounds makes bamboo shoots an excellent source for developing natural nutraceutical products. These bioactive compounds have been shown to be

TABLE 8.2
Bioactive Compounds Used in Nutraceuticals and Their Health Benefits

Bioactive Compounds	Health Benefits
Alkaloids (e.g. Quinine, Coumarin etc.)	Anti-malarial, hypoglycaemic, anti-depressant, heart tonic
Carotenoid terpenoids/ Isoprenoids (e.g. α-carotene, Lycopene, Lutein etc.)	Anti-oxidants, anti-carcinogenic, anti-cataract
Non-carotenoid terpenoids (e.g. Saponins, Terpenol etc.)	Anti-carcinogenic Reduces cholesterol levels in blood
Flavonoid polyphenolics (e.g. Anthocyanins, Catechins, Quercetin etc.)	Anti-oxidants, anti-sitaminic, reduces blood cholesterol
Phenolic acids (e.g. Ellagic acids)	Anti-oxidant, anti-cancer, anti-microbial, lower blood glucose
Phytosterols (β-sitosterol, stigmasterol, campestanol etc.)	Decrease LDL cholesterol level, anti-cancer activity, modulate the immune function and inflammation
Vitamins	Anti-oxidant, anti-tumor, hypocholesterolemic potential Prevention of cardiovascular disease and angiogenic disorders
Proteins and peptide	Anti-hypertensive, anti-microbial, anti-inflammatory and immune-stimulating activities, anti-oxidant, anti-cancerous properties
Dietary fibres	Prevention of cardiovascular diseases, hypertension, diabetes, obesity, cancer and gastrointestinal disorders and improvement of bowl movement

effective against several chronic disorders like cancer, diabetes, obesity and cataracts. Phytosterols from bamboo shoots have been found to be very effective in lowering the LDL and serum cholesterol levels. Bamboo shoot fibre has several health benefits and is useful in the management of hypertension and obesity and is associated with decreased low-density lipoprotein cholesterol, increased stool bulk, increased laxative properties and so on. Li et al. (2016) reported that bamboo shoot dietary fibre prevented obesity in mice by modulating the gut microbiota and also improved the host metabolism. Recent studies have indicated the nutraceutical potentials of bamboo (Table 8.3) and many nutraceutical products have been developed (Table 8.4).

Fresh bamboo shoots are also rich in potassium, which helps prevent cardiovascular diseases and blockage of blood vessels. A healthy diet including bamboo shoots is also key to blood sugar management and preventing or treating diabetes. We conducted studies on shoot extracts of the edible bamboo *Dendrocalamus*

TABLE 8.3
Nutraceutical Potential of Bamboo Proven by Scientific Experiments in Laboratories

Potential Benefit	Species	References
Anti-cancerous	*Sasa sinensis, Pseudosasa japonica, Caulis bambusae, S. quelpaertensis, Phyllostachys pubescens*	Tsunoda et al. 1998, Panee 2009, Seki et al. 2010, Hong et al. 2010, Kim et al. 2013, Hiromichi 2007
Anti-diabetic	*Phyllostachys pubescens, Sasa borealis, Pseudosasa japonica, Bambusa vulgaris*	Ding et al. 2008, Oh and Lim 2009, Senthilkumar et al. 2011, Koide et al. 2011, Nam et al. 2013
Anti-obesity	*Sasa borealis, S. quelpaertensis*	Yang et al. 2010, Li et al. 2016
Anti-inflammatory	*Bambusa arundinacea, S. quelpaertensis*	Hu et al. 2000, Lu et al. 2005, Muniappan and Sundararaj 2003, Hwang et al. 2007, Carey et al. 2009
Anti-fatigue	*Bambusa tuldoides, Phyllostachys nigra, Pseudosasa japonica,*	Zhang and Tang 1997, You et al. 2006, Zhang et al. 2006
Anti-hyperlipidemic	*Phyllostachys pubescens*	Ding et al. 2010
Anti-hypertensive	*Phyllostachys pubescens*	Liu et al. 2013
Anti-microbial	*Bambusa arundinacea, Phyllostachys pubescens, P. nigra, P. heterocycla*	Fujimura et al. 2005, Park and Jhon 2010, Tanaka et al. 2011, Singh et al. 2010, Zhanwang et al. 2005, Jin et al. 2011
Cardiovascular diseases	*Phyllostachys pubescens, P. nigra*	Fu et al. 2006, Liu et al. 2012, 2013
Cholesterol-lowering	*P. pubescens, P. nigra, P. edulis, B. oldhamii, D. latiflorus*	Park and Jhon 2009, Lachance and He 1998

TABLE 8.4
Nutraceutical Products from Bamboo

Product Name	Content	Health Benefits/Health Claims
Bamboo Silica/Silice de Bambou®	Bamboo Silica	Anti-aging, build healthy bones, nails, teeth and skin wrinkle free and beautiful
World Organic Bamboo Extract Capsule®	Bamboo Silica, Vegetable, Gelatin, Rice Flour, Magnesium Stearate	Prevent premature aging, preserves skin youthfulness, builds healthy bones and teeth and promotes growth of strong hair
Solaray Bamboo Extract®	Bamboo Silica, Cellulose and Magnesium Stearate	Dietary supplement, stimulates collagen synthesis in bone and connective tissue, remineralization effect
My Kind Organics® Organic Plant Collagen Builder	Bamboo Silica, Pomegranate, Green and Rooibos Tea, Citrus Bioflavonoids and Turmeric	Helps restore and maintain youthful levels of collagen, keratin and elastin, three proteins responsible for promoting body's healthy, natural glow
Congshengzhu Bamboo Juice®	Fresh Bamboo Shoot Juice (Zhuli), contains essential amino acids and flavonoids	Dietary supplement, nourishes blood and improves eyesight
Congshengzhu Green Bamboo Dietary FibrePowder®	Green Bamboo Dietary Fibre Powder	Dietary supplement, improve the digestive system
Lesen® Bamboo Shoot Extract Powder	Food Grade Bamboo Shoot Extract	Dietary supplement, improve digestive system
Nutra Green® Bamboo Shoot Extract Powder	Bamboo Shoot Dietary Fibre	Dietary supplement, treatment for cough and fever, dissipate phlegm
Just Fibre®	Vegetable Fibre Derived From Bamboo	Herbal tonic, reduces fat and calories
Sanacel bamboo®	Bamboo dietary fibre	Dietary supplement, improve digestive system
GuoZhen Bamboo Leaf Essence®	Bamboo Leaf Extract	Regulates blood fat, purifies blood, strengthen heart and protect brain
Fenioux Bambou Tabashir	Bamboo Silica	Maintains balance of connective tissue, strengthens bones and improves endurance, increases immunity and fights fatigue
Lamberts® Natural Source Silica	Bamboo Silica	Contributes to the structure and resilience of connective tissue, synthesis of bone collagen and cartilage, recommended for healthy skin
Hawlik® Cappilary active capsules	Bamboo Shoot Extract and Polypore Umbellate Fungal Extract	Improves hair health by restructuring hair surface layer

(Continued)

TABLE 8.4 (CONTINUED)

Nutraceutical Products from Bamboo

Product Name	Content	Health Benefits/Health Claims
Vigorous® Bamboo Shoot Extract	Bamboo Shoot Powder/ Fibre	Stimulate appetite, relieve constipation, improve immune system
Yancheng Goodex Bamboo shoot powder	Bamboo Shoot Powder/ Fibre	Improve skin health, protect the blood vessel of brain and heart, adjust blood lipid, low the blood viscidity, enhance immunity, anti-fatigue action
Aladdin® Bamboo shoot extract	Bamboo Shoot Extract	Promote intestinal peristalsis, help digestion, prevent constipation and has the effect of prevention of colorectal cancer, useful for weight loss
Herblink® Bamboo Shoot Extract Powder	Bamboo Shoot Powder	Reduce fever and dissipate phlegm, relieve pressure and prevent or arrest vomiting, improve blood cholesterol level, improve digestive health
Health Ingredients® Natural Silica	Bamboo Leaf, Shoot Extract	Organic silica plays an important role in keeping the skin and hair healthy
Organic Bamboo Tea®	Bamboo Leaves	Bamboo leaf tea is rich in silica, fibre and anti-oxidants, useful to improve bone health, strengthen hair and nails, improve dental health and make skin more elastic and healthier
Bonusan Forte®	Tabashir Exudates	Reduces fatigue, supports energy, metabolism, good for nervous system
Bamboolex	Bamboo Leaves	Anti-oxidant, anti-bacterial, anti-acrylamide

hamiltonii. When ethanol extract of shoots was analyzed using GC-MS spectroscopy (Figure 8.4), it showed the highest presence of fatty acid amide namely 13-Docosenamide (Z) (25.02%), which has anti-microbial activity. It also acts as an anti-static agent and is used in the manufacturing of food packaging material, personal daily care products like perfumes, deodorant, lotions, moisturizers, talcum powder, soaps, toothpaste, etc. Other main components were 4H-Cyclopropa [5',6'] benz [1',2':7,8] azuleno [5,6] oxiren-4-one,8,8a-bis(acetyloxy)-2a-[(acetyloxy) methyl]-1,1a,1b, 1c,2a,3,3a,6a, 6b,7,8,8a-dodecahydro-6b-0 hydroxy-3a- methoxy-1,1,5,7-tetramethyl- (9.18%), Propanoic acid, 3-chloro,4-formylphenyl ester (8.63%), ç-Sitosterol (4.43%) and 1-Monolinoleoylglycerol trimethylsilyl ether (2.43%). 1-Monolinoleoylglycerol trimethylsilyl ether has anti-microbial, anti-oxidant, anti-inflammatory, anti-arthritic and anti-asthmatic activity. The health beneficial properties of 9, 12, 15-Octadecatrienoic acid, 2, 3-bis [(trimethylsilyl)oxy] propyl ester, (Z,Z,Z)-(Linolenic acid ester) include anti-inflammatory, hypocholesterolemic, anti-arthritic, nematicide and hepatoprotective. Similarly, ç-Sitosterol, an important steroid found in shoots has cholesterol-lowering and anti-inflammatory activity (Table 8.5).

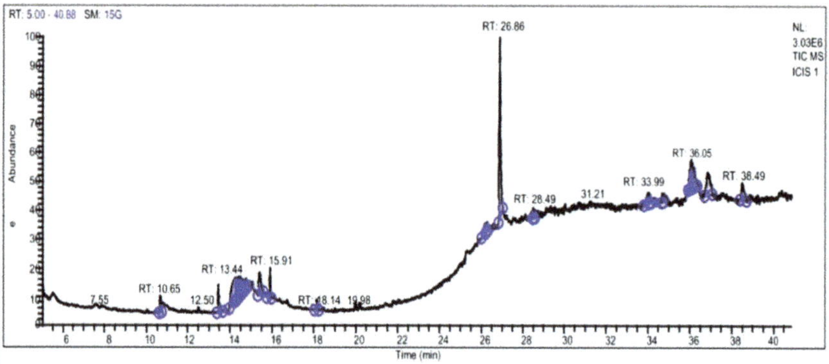

Qual Peak Table

RT	Peak Area	Area %	Peak Height
10.65	876095.92	2.52	172599.40
13.44	1258257.19	3.62	287805.18
14.19	2999709.93	8.63	250838.52
14.27	1011559.29	2.91	250452.30
14.33	971689.75	2.80	228351.38
14.41	986083.20	2.84	218053.61
14.48	816434.77	2.35	196753.69
14.57	736601.88	2.12	155332.15
14.66	482240.48	1.39	107799.21
14.74	415234.05	1.20	110657.15
15.41	1719015.49	4.95	234190.33
15.91	863565.41	2.49	322622.77
18.14	405946.14	1.17	115208.56
26.14	845785.03	2.43	118084.69
26.26	241192.24	0.69	103457.90
26.86	8691582.74	25.02	1901516.20
28.49	372798.27	1.07	110490.64
33.99	1019214.64	2.93	120396.67
34.07	368146.60	1.06	111999.62
34.68	303211.76	0.87	102784.10
35.97	832363.68	2.40	216876.22
36.05	1538626.49	4.43	304454.14
36.11	699944.95	2.01	262119.43
36.19	1369209.86	3.94	208936.19
36.84	3187703.59	9.18	241184.12
38.49	1726771.21	4.97	183825.58

FIGURE 8.4 GC-MS spectra of ethanol extract of juvenile shoots of *D. hamiltonii*.

8.4.1 Anti-Oxidant Activity of Bamboo

Phenolic compounds from bamboo shoots are known to possess potent anti-oxidant properties. Anti-oxidant rich foods have generated a lot of interest and attention as it plays an important role in disease prevention. Anti-oxidants are substances or compounds which inhibit the oxidation of other molecules in our body and prevent the formation of free radicals by scavenging them. Most of the health benefits of anti-oxidants arise from their anti-inflammatory properties within the body. The important role of anti-oxidants is to promote cardiovascular health, to inhibit the growth of cancerous tumors, to slow the aging process in the brain and nervous system and to lessen the risk and severity of neurodegenerative disease including Alzheimer

TABLE 8.5
Major Phytochemicals Identified in the Ethanolic Extract of Juvenile Shoots of *D. hamiltonii* by GC-MS

Retention Time	Peak Area (%)	Molecular Formula	Name of the Compound	Health Benefits
10.65	2.52	$C_{11}H_{24}O$	1-Undecanol	Anti-fungal
13.44	3.62	$C_{16}H_{32}O$	Hexadecen-1-ol, Trans-9-	Anti-inflammatory
14.74	1.20	$C_{14}H_{42}O_7Si_7$	Cycloheptasiloxane, tetradecamethyl-	Anti-inflammatory, anti-psychotics, anti-neoplastics
15.91	2.49	$C_{13}H_{26}$	Cyclotridecane	Anti-asthmatics
18.14	1.17	$C_{17}H_{36}O$	n-Heptadecanol-1	Anti-bacterial
26.14	2.43	$C_{27}H_{54}O_4Si_2$	1-Monolinoleoylglycerol trimethylsilyl ether	Anti-microbial, anti-oxidant, anti-inflammatory, anti-arthritic, anti-asthma, Diuretic
26.26	0.69	$C_{27}H_{52}O_4Si_2$	9,12,15-Octadecatrienoic acid, 2,3-bis[(trimethylsilyl)oxy] propyl ester, (Z,Z,Z)-	Hypocholesterolemic, Cancer preventive, Hepatoprotective, Nematicide, Insectifuge Anti-histaminic, Anti-arthritic, Anti-coronary, Anti-eczemic, Anti-acne, 5-Alpha reductase inhibitor Anti-androgenic
26.86	25.02	$C_{22}H_{43}NO$	13-Docosenamide, (Z)-	Anti-microbial
33.99	2.93	$C_{30}H_{50}O_6$	Olean-12-ene-3,15,16,21,22,28-hexol	Anti-cancer, anti-inflammatory, anti-diabetogenic, anti-microbial
36.05	4.43	$C_{29}H_{50}O$	ç-Sitosterol	Anti-cancer, anti-inflammatory, anti-diabetogenic, anti-microbial
36.19	3.94	$C_{32}H_{50}O_6$	Dodecanoic acid, 1a,2,5,5a,6,9, 10,10a-octahydro-5,5a-di hydroxy-4-(h ydroxymethyl)-1,1,7,9-tetramet hyl-11-oxo-1H-2,8a-methanocyclopenta[a] cyclopropa[e]cyclodecen-6-yl ester	Anti-obesity, cholesterol-lowering

disease and Parkinson disease. Anti-oxidants are also of immense importance in industries dealing with petrochemicals, food, cosmetics and medicine where they are used for stabilization of polymeric products. In the food and pharmaceutical industries, anti-oxidants are used to prevent deterioration, rancidity and discolouration caused by oxidation during processing and storage. There are several known natural compounds with anti-oxidant properties that can be extracted from plants, which are mainly phenols, polyphenols, vitamin C, vitamin E, beta-carotene, flavonoids, amino acids and amines that are known to have the potential to reduce disease risk. However, due to the lack of natural anti-oxidants, nowadays most food and pharmaceutical products contain synthetic anti-oxidants that cause concerns about their adverse effect on health. Hence, more emphasis is given to the use of natural anti-oxidants (Schillaci et al. 2013, Chongtham et al. 2018).

Although bamboo is known for its therapeutic properties, it is rarely considered for its anti-oxidant properties. Studies have revealed that bamboo is a rich source of anti-oxidants and regular consumption of bamboo-based products may reduce the risk of age-related chronic diseases including cardiovascular diseases, Alzheimer disease, Parkinson disease, cancer and diabetes. The main anti-oxidants in bamboo leaves and shoots are phenols, flavonoids, vitamin C and E and mineral elements such as selenium, copper, zinc, iron and manganese (Chongtham et al. 2018). Several identified anti-oxidants derived from bamboo shoot and leaves, display certain biological roles, including anti-oxidative (Hu et al. 2000), anti-cancer (Shi and Yang 1992), anti-hypertensive (Akao et al. 2004) and anti-bacterial (Fujimura et al. 2005) functions. Research on bamboo shoot anti-oxidants began with a study by Ishii and Hiroi (1990) that identified a compound namely, diferuloyl arabinoxylan hexasaccharide containing 5-5-linked diferulic acid from bamboo shoots and reported that ferulic acid is a naturally occurring anti-oxidant present in the plant-based products. At present, natural anti-oxidants are in great demand as synthetic anti-oxidants being used in food and pharmaceuticals may be deleterious to health. Hence, bamboo a fast-growing plant with huge biomass can serve as an alternative for the production of natural anti-oxidants.

Trace elements in bamboo shoots associated with anti-oxidant defense systems are selenium, zinc, copper, iron and manganese. Selenium is an essential trace element and co-factor for an enzyme, glutathione peroxidase. Chinese scientists discovered a disease, namely 'Keshen disease', that occurs due to the severe deficiency of dietary selenium (Yang et al. 1983). Copper, zinc, iron and manganese are other indispensable metals, which are required for the activities of anti-oxidant enzymes such as superoxide dismutase (SOD). Iron is the most abundant trace element in the body and almost all iron occurs bound to proteins. Dietary deficiency of proteins promotes reactive oxygen species production, lipid peroxidation and oxidative stress (Dabbagh et al. 1994). There have been only a few studies that evaluated the content of selenium in bamboo shoots (see Chapter 3).

It is well known that phenolic compounds in the plants are very important anti-oxidants and bamboo shoots are one of the best sources of phenolic compounds in the plants. Several direct and indirect health benefits have been attributed to the presence of phenolic compounds in bamboo shoots. Their action on the regulation of apoptosis, neuroprotective activity and anti-oxidant properties has been studied in detail. Several bamboo species have also been analyzed for their total phenolic content and anti-oxidant activities such as *Dendrocalamus asper*, *D. hamiltonii*, *Bambusa tulda*, *B. vulgaris*, *B. balcooa*, *B. pallida* and *Phyllostachys* species, using different anti-oxidative assays to acquire comprehensive information about the anti-oxidant capacity of bamboo shoots (Satya et al. 2009, Park and Jhon 2010, Nemenyi et al. 2015). Soesanto (2016) analyzed the total flavonoids, total polyphenols, vitamin E content and anti-oxidant activity of shoots of two bamboo species viz. *Bambusa vulgaris* and *Gigantochloa apus* and found that one- to two-week-old freeze-dried shoots of *G. apus* had the highest concentration of total flavonoids, total polyphenols and vitamin E content. It was also observed that the anti-oxidant activity of one- to two-week-old freeze-dried shoots of *G. apus* is higher as compared to the shoots of *Bambusa vulgaris*. In one of the studies, it was found that bamboo shoots contributed 46% of the daily anti-oxidant activity intake among different vegetables consumed in China (Yang et al. 2005). Anti-oxidant activity is represented as IC_{50} of DPPH/ABTS (µg/ml). The value signifies the concentration of the test sample that can scavenge 50% reduction of the DPPH/ABTS free radicals. With the increased value of IC_{50}, the decrease in anti-oxidant activity was indicated, since it required a higher test sample to achieve a 50% reduction of the DPPH/ABTS. Thus, with the decease in IC_{50} values, it indicates an increased potential of anti-oxidant activity as lower concentration or amount of test sample is able to achieve a 50% reduction of DPPH/ABTS solution. Juvenile shoots of *Dendrocalamus hamiltonii* were analyzed for their total phenols, total flavonoids and in-vitro and in-vivo anti-oxidant activities (Bajwa et al. 2018). In-vitro anti-oxidant activity of the aqueous extract of young shoots (Figure 8.5) was measured by DPPH free radical and ABTS radical cation assay. The IC_{50} values were

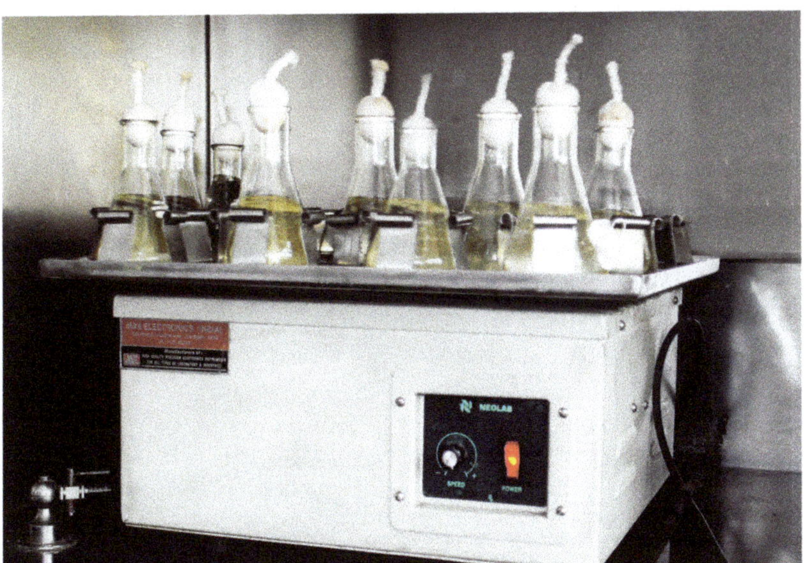

FIGURE 8.5 Bamboo shoot extract preparation for determining anti-oxidant activity.

568.18 μg/ml and 66.48 μg/ml, respectively. Butylated 4-hydroxytoluene (BHT) was used as standard. Its IC_{50} value for DPPH free radical and ABTS radical cation was 277.28 μg/ml and 12.67 μg/ml, respectively (Table 8.6).

8.4.2 *In-vivo* Studies in Balb/c Mice

Several in-vivo studies have shown that regular consumption of bamboo shoots is an effective and safe way to meet all anti-oxidant requirements. Shoots reduce the risk of arteriosclerosis, cardiovascular problems and some forms of cancer. Our team conducted studies to evaluate the effect of bamboo shoot extract on body and organ weight, blood glucose level, lipid profile, hepatic function, kidney function and anti-oxidant defense system in Balb/c mice. Mice were randomly assigned into two groups (N = 6). Group-1 served as a control group and to another group, an aqueous extract of *D. hamiltonii* shoots (BSE) was administered at the concentration of 800 mg/kg body weight for six weeks (Figure 8.6). The control group was given tap water and feed *ad libitum*. The results obtained are discussed next.

8.4.3 Effect of Bamboo Shoots on Body and Organ Weight

Involuntary weight gain worsens all elements of the cardiovascular risk profile, including dyslipidemia, hypertension, insulin-resistant glucose intolerance, left-ventricular hypertrophy, hyperuricemia and elevated fibrinogen. The degree of overweight is related to the rate of development of the cardiovascular disease. Diet plays a very important role in weight management. In the present study, individual body weight was recorded once a week during the experimental period. Mean body weight gain was calculated for each group. The body weight of both the groups increased normally but the highest increase in the body weight during the experimental period was observed in the control group. However, no significant change was observed in the weight of the liver and kidney of the BSE-treated group when compared with the control group (Table 8.7).

TABLE 8.6
Phenols, Flavonoids and Anti-Oxidant Activity of Aqueous Extract of Shoots of *D. hamiltonii*

Parameter	Bamboo Shoot	BHT (Standard)
Total phenols (mg of GAE/g of extract)	67.50 ± 0.01	–
Total flavonoid (mg of QUE/g of extract)	7.92 ± 0.05	–
ABTS, IC_{50} (μg/ml)	66.48 ± 3.11	12.67 ± 0.60
DPPH, IC_{50} (μg/ml)	568.18 ± 0.02	277.28 ± 0.02

Values reported are measurement replication means ± standard deviation (n = 3 replicates). BHT-Butylated Hydroxytoluene, GAE- Galic Acid Equivalent, QUE- Quercetin, ABTS- 2,2 – zino- bis (3-ethylbenzothiazolin- 6- sulfonic acid), DPPH- 2,2- diphenyl- 1- picrylhydrazyl.

TABLE 8.7
Effect of Bamboo Shoot Extract on Body and Organ Weight of Balb/c Mice

Weight (g)	Control	BSE (800 mg/kg b.w.) Treated Group
Initial body weight	31 ± 0.58	29 ± 0.55
First week	34 ± 0.93	27 ± 0.33
Second week	35 ± 0.37	28 ± 0.98
Third week	34 ± 0.88	28 ± 1.00
Fourth week	36 ± 0.91	30 ± 1.31
Fifth week	36 ± 0.11	31 ± 0.76
Sixth week	37 ± 0.43	31 ± 1.27
Liver weight	1.31 ± 0.25	1.32 ± 0.31
Kidney weight	0.31 ± 0.09	0.27 ± 0.04

Values reported are measurement replication means ± standard deviation (n = 3 replicates).
BSE = Bamboo shoot extract, b.w.—body weight

8.4.4 Effect of Bamboo Shoots on the Anti-Oxidant Defense System

In the present study, the activity levels of GSH, SOD, CAT, GR and GPx were detected. In the normal control mice, the level of reduced glutathione (GSH) content in the serum was 0.897 ± 0.07 (nmol/mg proteins). But the level of GSH increased significantly after administering the animals with bamboo shoot extract. The activity of enzyme glutathione reductase (GR) and catalase (CAT) was decreased while; a significant increase was seen in the activity of superoxide dismutase (SOD) in the treatment group. In contrast, no significant change was seen in the activity of glutathione peroxidase (GPx) in the treatment group when compared with the control group (Table 8.8). Bamboo anti-oxidants may thus offer promising avenues to prevent and control oxidative-stress related chronic and degenerative diseases.

8.4.5 Effect of Bamboo Shoots on Glucose and Lipid Profile

Blood glucose level is the amount of sugar present in the blood of a human or animal. The digestive system breaks the food into glucose, which is a primary source of energy for the body. Glucose then travels in the bloodstream to cells throughout the body. This causes a rise in blood sugar levels. The pancreas releases insulin to help cells in absorbing glucose for energy. When the body is in a fasting state, it relies on stored energy. The body naturally regulates blood glucose levels as a part of metabolic homeostasis. Many factors affect blood sugar levels. A healthy diet is key to blood sugar management and preventing or treating diabetes. The results of the present study confirmed the hypoglycemic properties of aqueous extract of *D. hamiltonii* shoots. In the normal control mice, non-fasting serum glucose level was 97 ± 1.56 (mg/dl) while, fasting serum glucose level was 68 ± 2.14 (mg/dl). Treatment

TABLE 8.8
Effect of Aqueous Extract of Bamboo Shoots on Anti-Oxidant Defense System in Balb/c Mice

Parameter	Group I	Group II
GSH (nmol/mg protein)	0.897 ± 0.07	1.03 ± 0.06
Glutathione reductase (nmol of NADPH consumed/min/mg protein)	19.86 ± 2.31	15.76 ± 2.63
Glutathione peroxidase (nmol of NADPH oxidized/min/mg protein)	14.87± 2.00	14.89 ± 1.25
Catalase (μmol H_2O_2 reduced/min/mg proteins)	1.53 ± 0.23	0.569 ± 0.04
Superoxide dismutase (IU/mg protein)	2.73 ± 0.68	4.21 ± 0.82

Values reported are measurement replication means ± standard deviation (n = 3 replicates).

Group I: Control, Group II: Bamboo shoot treated, GSH—Glutathione reductase, H_2O_2—hydrogen peroxide, NADPH—Nicotinamide adenine dinucleotide phosphate

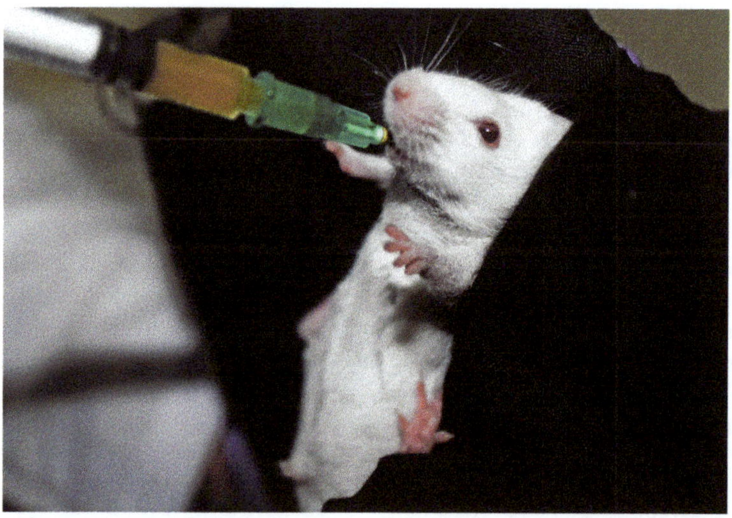

FIGURE 8.6 Administration of aqueous extract of bamboo shoot in Balb/c mice.

with aqueous extract of bamboo shoots at concentration 800 mg/kg, body weight for six consecutive weeks resulted in a slight increase in serum glucose level (72 ± 2.38 mg/dl) in fasting group while a significant decrease was observed in non-fasting animals (81 ± 1.77 mg/dl) when compared with the control group (Figure 8.6, Table 8.9). Less fall in blood sugar level in fasting mice after administration of BSE as compared to control mice which were receiving normal animal diet might be due to high fibre content present in bamboo shoots. According to Haber et al. (1977) the removal of fibre from food and also its physical disruption, can result in faster and easier ingestion, decreased satiety and disturbed glucose homeostasis which is

TABLE 8.9
Effect of Fresh Shoot Extract on Glucose Level and Lipid Profile

Parameter (mg/dl)	Control	BSE (800 mg/kg b.w.) Treated Group
Glucose	97 ± 1.56 (Non-fasting) 68 ± 2.14 (Fasting)	81 ± 1.77 (Non-fasting) 72 ± 2.38 (Fasting)
Total cholesterol	124 ± 2.71	98 ± 2.65
HDL	88 ± 0.74	94 ± 0.63
LDL	19 ± 2.24	13 ± 1.42
Triglycerides	221 ± 0.64	161 ± 1.15

Values reported are measurement replication means ± standard deviation (n = 3 replicates).
BSE = Bamboo shoot extract, HDL—High Density Lipoprotein, LDL—Low Density Lipoprotein

probably due to inappropriate insulin release. These effects favor overnutrition and if often repeated, might lead to diabetes mellitus. This is based on the findings when ten normal subjects were provided with three kinds of apple-based diet (fibre-free apple juice, apple puree and intact apples), plasma-glucose rose to similar levels. But there was a striking rebound fall in blood sugar level after apple juice and to a lesser extent after puree but was not seen after consuming intact apples because serum-insulin rose to higher levels after juice and puree than after apples. It has also been proved that juice could be consumed eleven times faster than intact apples and four times faster than fibre-disrupted puree. This indicates that the regular consumption of a high-fibre diet like bamboo shoots could help in maintaining the serum-insulin level and also the energy level of the body even in the fasting state.

The levels of total cholesterol (TC), triglycerides (TG), low-density lipoproteins (LDL) and high-density lipoproteins (HDL) in the serum of animal groups were also tested to evaluate the anti-oxidant effect of bamboo shoots (Table 8.9). It was found that the treatment groups that received the aqueous extract of bamboo shoots had decreased levels of TC, TG and LDL as compared to the control group. The level of HDL in the treatment groups was slightly higher than that of the control group. The cholesterol-lowering effects of bamboo shoots have been attributed to inhibition of cholesterol absorption and increase of cholesterol excretion (Lu et al. 2010).

8.4.6 Effect of Bamboo Shoots on Liver Function

The effect of bamboo shoots was also studied on various parameters that determine the health of the liver. Liver functions were monitored by analyzing the levels of serum bilirubin, total proteins, albumin, globulin, alkaline phosphatase, serum glutamic-oxaloacetic transaminase (SGOT), serum glutamic-pyruvic transaminase (SGPT) and lactate dehydrogenase (LDH) (Table 8.10). Bilirubin is an endogenous

TABLE. 8.10

Effect of Fresh Shoot Extract on the Liver Function in Balb/c Mice

Parameter	Control	BSE (800 mg/kg b.w.) Treated Group
Billirubin (mg/dl)	0.235 ± 0.08	0.236 ± 0.05
Proteins (mg/dl)	81 ± 2.52	79 ± 1.72
Albumin (mg/dl)	19 ± 1.31	19 ± 1.08
Globulin (mg/dl)	63 ± 0.96	52 ± 1.12
Alkaline phosphatase (U/L)	59 ± 3.32	73 ± 4.52
SGOT (U/L)	108 ± 3.22	93 ± 3.40
SGPT (U/L)	53 ± 3.68	44 ± 2.90
LDH (U/L)	991 ± 21.5	984 ± 31.2

Values reported are measurement replication means ± standard deviation (n = 3 replicates).

anion derived from hemoglobin degradation from the RBC. When the liver function tests are abnormal and the serum bilirubin levels more than 17μmol/L, it suggests underlying liver disease (Friedman et al. 2003). The measurement of proteins is another useful indicator of hepatic functions because the liver is the major source of most of the serum proteins. A total serum protein test measures the total amount of protein, albumin and globulin in the blood. Albumin is quantitatively the most important protein in plasma synthesized only by the liver. Albumin synthesis is affected not only in liver disease but also by nutritional status, hormonal balance and osmotic pressure (Rosalki and Mcintyre 1999). Globulins are produced by the liver and the immune system. High serum globulin levels may be indicative of some liver problems. The serum glutamic pyruvate transaminase (SGPT) and serum glutamate oxaloacetic transaminase (SGOT) is the most widely used liver enzymes that are sensitive to abnormalities in the liver. These liver enzymes form a major constituent of the liver cells and are the most frequently utilized and specific indicators of hepatocellular necrosis. These enzymes catalyze the transfer of the α-amino acids of aspartate and alanine, respectively, to the α-keto group of ketoglutaric acid. SGPT is primarily localized to the liver but the SGOT is present in a wide variety of tissue like the heart, skeletal muscle, kidney, brain and liver (Rosen and Keeffe 2000; Friedman et al. 2003). The SGPT and SGOT levels are increased to some extent in almost all liver diseases. Similarly, elevated levels of LDH, in the blood indicate acute or chronic cell damage. Results of the study revealed that bilirubin, protein and albumin content of the BSE-treated animals remained unchanged while, some alterations were seen in the level of globulin, alkaline phosphatase, serum glutamic-oxaloacetic transaminase (SGOT), serum glutamic-pyruvic transaminase (SGPT) and lactate dehydrogenase (LDH) as compared to the control group.

Similarly, phytomodulatory effects of fresh and processed shoots of *Dendrocalamus hamiltonii* on the anti-oxidant defense system in mouse liver were studied by Bajwa et al. (2019a). The study revealed a significant increase in glutathione content in the liver tissues of all the groups administered with extract of boiled and fermented bamboo shoots except the mice that received brine preserved shoot extract, where content decreased by 19%. Glutathione reductase (21%), glutathione peroxidase (20%) and catalase (69%) activity decreased significantly in the group administered with the extract of fresh shoots. The fermentation process was recognized as the most valuable process to improve the activity of hepatic superoxide dismutase (23%), glutathione peroxidase (27%) and catalase (29%). The results indicated that fresh, boiled and 5% brine preserved shoots significantly decreased the anti-oxidant status of the liver. Conversely, the activity of anti-oxidant enzymes increased remarkably after the administration of fermented shoot extract. It was thereby concluded that fermented shoots are best for improving the nutritional and pharmaceutical qualities and also effective utilization of bamboo shoots to their full potential as food and medicine.

8.4.7 Effect of Bamboo Shoots on Kidney Function

Kidney functions in all the experimental groups were monitored by analyzing the levels of serum creatinine, blood urea and blood urea nitrogen (BUN) which are commonly measured to determine kidney health. Creatinine is a breakdown product of creatine phosphate in muscles and is usually produced at a fairly constant rate by the body. It passes into the bloodstream and is usually passed out in the urine. Urea is also a waste product formed from the breakdown of proteins and passed out in the urine. BUN tests measure the amount of nitrogen in the blood. Urea nitrogen is a breakdown product of protein. Generally, a high blood level of creatinine, urea and BUN indicate that the kidneys may not be working properly. In a study carried out by Bajwa et al (2017), the nonsignificant increase was observed in the level of serum creatinine, blood urea and blood urea nitrogen as compared to the control group (Table 8.11). This might be due to the presence of high-protein content in

TABLE 8.11
Effect of Fresh Shoot Extract on the Kidney Function in Balb/c Mice

Parameter (mg/dl)	Control	FBSE (800 mg/kg b.w.) Treated Group
Creatinine	0.332 ± 0.02	0.348 ± 0.05
Blood urea	51± 0.34	55 ± 0.92
BUN	25 ± 0.09	27 ± 0.31

Values reported are measurement replication means ± standard deviation (n = 6 replicates).
BUN—Blood urea nitrogen

juvenile bamboo shoots. It has been reported that a high-protein diet is associated with increased glomerular filtration rate (GFR), serum creatinine, urea, urinary calcium excretion and serum concentrations of uric acid.

It is concluded that bamboo shoot being rich in nutrients, anti-oxidants and bioactive compounds has all the ideal characteristics for being used as a food additive and also exhibit potential as raw materials for the pharmaceutical, nutraceutical and food industries (Chongtham et al. 2018). In recent years, there has been considerable emphasis on the use of natural products as preservatives in foods, cosmetics and medical products as synthetic chemical compounds have caused health concerns to consumers. Bamboo is endowed with several health beneficial properties due to which its application in the pharmaceutical industry is gaining much importance. Anti-oxidants have a long history of use in nutrition, health and in the food industry (Chongtham et al. 2018). In the past, anti-oxidants were used to control oxidation and retard spoilage but today, many are used because of putative health benefits. The understanding is that anti-oxidants improve health by removing reactive species that may otherwise exert harmful metabolic effects. Many dietary compounds are capable of negating the danger of ROS—vitamin C, tocopherols, carotenoids, polyphenols, etc. It has been suggested that including these compounds in foods and medicine will enhance their capacities to support protection against ROS damage and reduce the risk of chronic diseases. The emergence of natural products with less harmful effects has become highly desirable. Natural anti-oxidants derived from plant products have been proposed as replacements for synthetic anti-oxidants to prevent spoilage. In addition, anti-oxidant activities of different agents have claimed to have potential health functions for reducing aging and possible prevention of cancer and heart diseases. Phenolic compounds are known for their anti-oxidant activity and bamboo is rich in these compounds.

Epilogue

Bamboo is a group of simple and humble plants comprising approximately 1,575 species which are perennial and evergreen and of tremendous utility, particularly in countries of east and south-east Asia. Bamboo is extremely versatile. The application of bamboo is not only limited to substitute wood in a variety of applications; it also plays an important role in soil erosion control and climate change mitigation. It is poor man's timber, on the one hand, and on the other, "green gold for countries like China, Vietnam and Thailand. A plant with tremendous potential for development of a "Green Economy", it also competes with plastic and steel in the 21st century. In fact, bamboo is deeply ingrained and interwoven in the life and culture of all classes and age groups of people in Asia: that is the origin for the saying 'To know Asia is to know bamboo'. Basically, bamboo has originated and spread from this region only after establishing land connection between Indian and Eurasian plates. Even the origin of the word *'Bambusa'* of Linneaus and 'Bamboo' in English is from the word 'Mambu' which is from India. In some parts of this region, particularly in China and Japan, bamboo is not considered to be a plant but instead is an emotional friend and spiritual teacher and guide. In the Meetei culture of Manipur, India, a bamboo grove is a must in the courtyard of a house for good luck and well-being of the family. In many other parts of north-east India, such as Tripura and Arunachal Pradesh, bamboo is revered as a deity. Rightly, bamboo is considered to be *Kalpavriksha* or a wish-fulfilling divine tree in India. Due to its many applications, including climate change mitigation, bamboo is poised to become the saviour of the earth; therefore, bamboo can be called the 'Plant for the Planet'.

In addition to its various other uses, bamboo is also being used for food and medicine since centuries in the region, particularly in China and India. In old Indian literature, around 10,000 years ago *Tabasheer* or *Banslochan*, an amorphous substance collected from the internodes of the culm, was used for rejuvenation of health and well-being. Today, with the help of modern scientific tools and techniques, bamboo has been found to be rich in silica and various other minerals. In China, several parts of bamboo including leaves, seed, roots, branches and juice are used to treat phlegm, fever, laryngitis, nose bleeding and vomiting. In Korea and China, bamboo leaf tea, particularly using the green leaves, is very common, and soothes and relaxes. In fact, these simple leaves are a rich source of a number of bioactive compounds and anti-oxidants which help in neutralizing or removing various molecules and radicals termed as reactive oxygen species (ROS) from the body.

Bamboo shoots, the young culms, have been a delicacy and important food commodity for many centuries in China, Japan and Korea, Thailand, Myanmar and north-eastern and other parts of India. Though bamboo shoots are not a part of the traditional cuisine in North America, Europe and other countries, the popularity of Chinese and Thai restaurants worldwide has given an opportunity to people in many countries to taste the edible bamboo shoots. In some countries, particularly in China, bamboo shoot processing has become a multibillion-dollar export business supplying shoots to countries including Japan, the United States, Australia and many European countries. Scientific studies have proved that this traditional food is one of the best health foods with all necessary nutrients for good health. A growing awareness of the correlation between diet and health, coupled with a sedentary lifestyle, an aging population and ever-increasing health care costs, has driven people towards health food with high nutrients packed with minerals, vitamins, anti-oxidants and fiber with health beneficial phytochemicals, also known as 'superfoods'. Superfoods increase the vitality of the human body and improve overall health by strengthening the immune system, thereby preventing a multitude of chronic diseases such as cardiovascular diseases, diabetes, obesity, osteoporosis and cancer. Bamboo shoots in particular possess all of the properties that signify a superfood—nutrients including vitamins and minerals, phytochemicals with anti-oxidant properties and fiber.

Since ancient times, bamboo shoots have been an important source of food for both animals and humans. Animals including the giant panda (*Ailuropoda melanolueca*), red panda (*Ailurus fulgens*), greater (golden) bamboo lemur (*Prolemur simus*) and mountain gorilla (*Gorilla beringei beringei*) as well as some monkeys in Ethiopia, Uganda and Rwanda survive mainly on bamboo. Although the giant panda is a carnivore and its digestive tract is short and specialized for the digestion of flesh, it has totally adapted to a vegetarian diet, eating bamboos only. The taste of bamboo shoots compels mountain gorillas to leave their protected enclosures in Congo and other African countries during the rainy season to search for young juvenile shoots.

Bamboo shoots have always been a delicacy in many Asian countries. The Japanese prefer boiled bamboo shoots, whereas in Thailand, Myanmar and India, people add a lot of spices to shoots to make a curry or pickles. In Chinese cuisine, bamboo shoots are generally used in stir fry or soups. Bamboo shoots have become a popular food throughout the world and are used in various forms.

Bamboo shoots are exceptionally rich in minerals, bioactive compounds, vitamins, amino acids and dietary fibers. Young shoots are particularly rich in potassium, silica, magnesium, iron and manganese. Potassium, which is good for the heart, ranges from 4,390 to 6,660 mg/100g dry weight. Bamboo is the richest known source of natural silica, containing around 70% of organic silica. The highest level of silica content is reported in oat bran (23.36 mg/100 g) or fruits like dried dates (16.61 mg/100 g), whereas in bamboo shoot the silica content ranges from 70 to 170 mg/100 g of fresh weight. The average intake of silica is around 20–25 mg/day and just 50 to 100 g of bamboo shoots per day are sufficient to provide the required amount of silica. Silicon provides strength, integrity and flexibility to connective tissues of skin, bones, hairs and is also considered to be an anti-aging nutrient. Minerals such as iron, phosphorus, magnesium and copper are also available in good amounts in bamboo shoots. Shoots are one of the best sources of dietary fiber, ranging from 2.25 to 6.07 g/100 g. Dietary fiber regulates bowel movement, prevents constipation, removes toxins and prevents long stay of microbes in the colon. Shoots have all of the amino acids, including eight essential ones, in the range of 1.65 to 4.61 mg/100 g fresh weight. The best part is that bamboo shoots are all organic as they can grow naturally without addition of chemical fertilizers or insecticides.

Anti-oxidants in bamboo shoots have generated a lot of interest and attention. The main anti-oxidants in bamboo shoots are phenols, vitamin C and E and mineral elements including selenium, copper, zinc, iron and manganese which have anti-oxidative, anti-cancer, anti-hypertensive and anti-bacterial properties. The phenol content ranges from 357.11 to 907.39 mg/100 g fresh weight which is higher than that in other superfoods including apple, almonds, cherry and green tea. It is well known that phenolic compounds play a significant role as anti-oxidant, neutralizing the reactive oxygen species, scavenging the free radicals or chelation of transition metals and preventing the formation of compounds which are responsible for causing chronic diseases such as cancer and cardiovascular diseases. Phytosterols which have gained a lot of acclaim in recent times due to their potential implications on human health is another important bioactive compound present in bamboo shoots. The content ranges from 91.37 to 265.49 g/100 g dry weight in the shoots of different species of bamboo. Phytosterols are similar in structure to cholesterol, and they help greatly in reducing the absorption of 'bad' cholesterols (lower density lipoprotein cholesterol) in the bloodstream, providing protection from atherosclerosis and stroke. Many health beneficial compounds have been isolated from fresh and processed bamboo shoots.

Bamboo shoots contain very few calories, about 27 Kcal in 100 g, which is also one of the important reasons why they are considered to be a superfood. The consumption of high-energy food is making people obese or overweight, which is a cause of various new age diseases like cancer, coronary artery disease and type 2 diabetes, and also leads to a significant increase in early mortality. According to a World Health Organization (WHO) report, obesity has tripled since 1975 and in 2016 around 39% adults age 18 were overweight and 18% were obese. Bamboo shoots can be a part of a natural low-calorie food commodity with low fat (0.3 g/100 g) as they are loaded with nutrients, minerals, fiber and anti-oxidants. The high dietary fiber content of bamboo shoots provide satiety, thereby limiting the overconsumption of food.

Most foods are considered to be functional in terms of providing nutrients and/or energy to sustain basic life. However, in the last decade, consumer demands have changed considerably due to rapid economic growth, urbanization and globalization, and the demand for natural, especially healthy and organic, food has greatly increased. Our research of 18 years has indicated that bamboo shoots are natural functional food rich in nutrients, health promoting bioactive compounds such as dietary fibers, phytosterols and phenols which have anti-oxidant properties and are fairly retained after processing or fortification and blend well with various other food items. Biscuits fortified with dried bamboo shoot powder and paste showed overall improvement in food quality. Several companies produce bamboo shoot–fortified food and nutraceuticals with health benefits. The health beneficial properties of bamboo shoots include weight loss, improved digestion, lowered cholesterol level and diseases prevention. Thus, bamboo shoots with all of properties of a superfood can be used as a vegetable, as a food additive and also as an ingredient in pharmaceutical, nutraceutical and food production. Bamboo shoot is indeed a 'superfood'

Glossary of Scientific Names

A

Abelmoschus esculentus
Acidosasa spp.
A. edulis
A. hirsute
A. hirtiflora
A. lingchuanensis
Acinetobacter spp.
Agrobacterium spp.
A. radiobacter
A. rhizogenes
Ailuropoda melanolueca
Ailurus fulgens
Allium porrum
Arachis hypogaea
Arundo arbor
Arundinaria spp.
A. aristata
A. callosa
A. hirsuta
Ascaris suum
Aspergillus spp.
A. fumigatus
A. niger
Amaranthus gangeticus
Aulonemia aristulata

B

Bacillus subtilis
Bambusa spp.
B. affinis
B. arundinacea
B. auriculata
B. balcooa
B. bambos
B. blumeana
B. breviflora
B. burmanica
B. cacharensis
B. edulis
B. glaucescens
B. jaintiana
B. khasiana
B. kingiana
B. longispiculata
B. manipureana
B. merrilliana
B. mizorameana
B. multiplex
B. nana
B. nutans
B. oldhamii
B. oliveriana
B. pallida
B. philippinensis
B. polymorpha
B. textilis
B. tulda
B. tuldoides
B. vulgaris
B. vulgaris var. *vittata*
Bambusiculmus makumensis
Bambusiculmus tirapensis
Bambusium arunachalense
Bambusium deomarense
Bashania fangiana
Beta vulgaris
Bifidobacterium spp.
B. adolescentis
B. animalis
B. bifidum
B. longum
Brassica spp.
B. oleracea var. *botrytis*

B. oleracea var. *capitata*
B. oleracea var. *italic*
Brassica oleracea var. *capitata*

C

Candida spp.
C. albicans
C. glabrata
C. tropicalis
Caulis bambusae
Cephalostachyum spp.
C. capitatum
C. fuchsianum
C. pergracile
Chimonobambusa spp.
C. angustifolia
C. armata
C. armata
C. callosa
C. grandifolia
C. hejiangensis
C. hookeriana
C. lactistriata
C. marmoreal
C. microfloscula
C. neopurpurea
C. pachystachys
C. quadrangularis
C. szechuanensis
C. szechuanensis var. *flexuosa*
C. utitis
C. yunnanensis
Chimonocalamus spp.
C. delicates
C. dumosus
C. dumosus var. *pygmaeus*
C. fimbriatus
C. longiligulatus
C. makuanensis
C. montanus
C. pallens
C. tortuosus
Chusquea spp.
C. bambusoides
C. capituliflora
C. culeou
C. meyeriana
Cicer arietinum
Citrobacter spp.
Clavibactor michiganensis
Curtobacterium flaccumfaciens
Cucumis sativus
Cucurbita maxima

D

Daucus carota
Dendrocalamopsis spp.
D. beecheyana
D. beecheyana var. *pubescens*
D. bicicatricata
D. daii
D. edulis
D. oldhami
D. stenoaurita
D. validus
D. vario-striata
Dendrocalamus spp.
D. asper
D. brandisii
D. calostachyus
D. farinosus
D. flagellifer
D. fugongensis
D. giganteus,
D. hamiltonii
D. hamiltonii var. *edulis*
D. hookeri
D. latiflorus
D. longispathus
D. manipureanus
D. membranaceus
D. pachystachys
D. polymorpha
D. semiscandens
D. sericeu
D. sikkimesis
D. stocksii
D. strictus
D. tibeticus
D. yunnanicus

Dinochloa spp.
Drepanostachyum sp.

E

Enterobacter spp.
E. aerogenes
Enterococcus spp.
E. durans
E. faecalis
E. spp.
Equisetum
Eragrostis cynosuroides
Erwinia carotovora
Escherichia spp.
E. coli

F

Fargesia spp.
F. angustissima
F. brevissima
F. canaliculate
F. denudate
F. dracocephala
F. edulis
F. emaculata
F. ferax
F. fractiflexa
F. fungosa
F. jiulongensis
F. lincangensis
F. mairei
F. murielae
F. nitida
F. oblique
F. orbiculate
F. pagyrifera
F. pauciflora
F. pleniculmis
F. porphyea
F. qinlingensis
F. robusta
F. ruta
F. scabrida
F. tenuilignea
F. utilis
F. yulongshaensis
F. yunnanensis
Flavobacterium
Fusarium spp.
F. oxysporum
F. oxyporum

G

Geotrichum candidum
Gigantochloa spp.
Gigantochloa albociliata
G. apus
G. atroviolacea
G. atter
G. felix
G. levis
G. ligulata
G. nigrociliata
G. pseudoarundinaria
G. rostrate
Guadua spp.
G. angustifolia
G. sarcocrpa
Gorilla beringei beringei

I

Indosasa spp.
I. angustata
I. glabrata
I. ingen
I. patens

K

Klebsiella spp.
K. pneumoniae

L

Lactobacillus spp.
Lb. acidophilus
Lb. brevis
Lb. curvatus

Lb. plantarum
Lagenaria siceraria
Lens culinaris
Leuconostoc mesenteroides

M

Melocalamus spp.
M. compactiflorus
M. indicus
Melocanna spp.
M. baccifera
M. bambusoides
Merostachys pluriflora
Musa paradisiaca

N

Neomicrocalamus mannii

O

Oxytenanthera spp.
O. abyssinica
O. albociliata
O. parvifolia

P

Pediococcus pentosaceus
Penicillium citrinum
Phaseolus vulgaris
Phrynium pubenerve
Phyllostachys spp.
P. acuta
P. amarus
P. angusta
P. arcane
P. assamica
P. atrovaginata
P. aurea
P. aureosulcata
P. aureosulcata f. aureocaulis
P. aureosulcata f. spectabilis
P. aurita
P. bambusoides
P. bambusoides var. *castillonis,*
P. bissetii
P. concave
P. dulcis
P. edulis
P. elegans
P. fimbriligula
P. flexuosa
P. fluorescens
P. glauca
P. glauca var. *variabilis*
P. heteroclada
P. heterocycla
P. heterocycla var. *pubescens*
P. humilis
P. incarnate
P. iridescens
P. kwanglsiensis
P. makinoi
P. mannii
P. meyeri
P. mitis
P. nidularia
P. nigra
P. nigra var. *henonis*
P. nigra var. *nigra*
P. nuda
P. parvifolia
P. platyglossa
P. praecox
P. praecox
P. praecox f. prevernalis
P. prominens
P. propinqua
P. pubescens
P. rigida
P. rivali
P. robustiramea
P. rubromarginata
P. rutile
P. spp.
P. sulphurea
P. sulphurea var. *sulphurea*
P. tianmuensis
P. violascens
P. viretla

P. viridiglaucescens
P. viridis
P. vivax
P. vivax f. aureocaulis
P. yunhoensis
P. nigra var. *henonis*
Pleioblastus amarus
Prolemur simus
Prunus spp.
P. amygdalus
P. avium
Pseudomonas spp.
P. aeruginosa
P. fluorescens
Pseudosasa spp.
P. japonica
P. longiligula
Pseudostachyum polymorphum
Pseudoxytenanthera bourdillonii
Pyricularia grisea
Pyrus malus

Q

Qiongzhuea spp.
Q. communis
Q. macrophylla
Q. rigidula,
Q. tumidinoda
Quillaja Saponaria

R

Raddiella vanessiae
Raphanus sativus

S

Saccharomyces cerevisiae
Salmonella spp.
S. choleraeduis
S. enteritidis
Sasa spp.
S. borealis
S. coreana
S. quelpaertensis
S. senanensis
S. sensanensis
S. sinensis
S. veitchii
Schizostachyum spp.
S. annulatum
S. capitatum
S. dullooa
S. funghomii
S. pingbianensis
Scutellaria baicalensis
Sinarundinaria spp.
S. elegans
S. hirsute
S. hookeriana
S. intermedia
Sinoarundinaria nigra
Sinobambusa elegans
Staphylococcus spp.
S. aureus
S. epidermidis
Solanum melongena
Solanum tuberosum
Spinacea oleracea

T

Teinostachyum wightii
Thamnocalamus spp.
T. aristatus
T. falconeri
Thyrsostachys spp.
T. oliveri
T. regia
T. siamensis
Trichoderma viride

V

Verticillium albo-atrum

Y

Yucca schidigera
Yushania spp.
Y. alpina

Y. brevipaniculata.
Y. cava
Y. crassicollis
Y. glauca
Y. jaunsarensis
Y. lineolate
Y. mitis
Y. oblonga
Y. qiaojiaensis

References

Adams, A.M., Ahmed, R., Latif, A.M. et al. 2017. Impact of fortified biscuits on micronutrient deficiencies among primary school children in Bangladesh. *PLoS One* 12(4):0174673.

Adhikari, U. 2013. *Bamboo Flowering Human Security and the State: A Political Ecological Study of the Impact of Cyclical Bamboo Flowering on Human Security and the Role of State in Mizoram.* A thesis submitted to the University of North Bengal, West Bengal.

Ahmed, M.M. and Singh, K.P. 2011. Traditional knowledge of kidney stones treatment by Muslim maiba (herbalists) of Manipur, India. *Notulae Scientia Biologicae* 3(2):12–15.

Akao, Y.N., Seki, Y., Nagakawa, H. et al. 2004. A highly bioactive lignophenol derivative from bamboo lignin exhibit a potent activity to suppress apoptosis induced by oxidative stress in human neuroblastoma SH-SY 5Y Cells. *Bioorganic and Medicinal Chemistry* 12(18):4791–4801.

Akinlabi, E.T., Anane-Fenin, K. and Akwada, D.R. 2017. *Bamboo: The Multipurpose Plant.* Springer, Cham, Switzerland.

Alina, V.R., Carmen, M.C., Sevastita, M. et al. 2019. Food fortification through innovative technologies. *Food Engineering.* Intech open. DOI: 10.5772/intechopen.82249

Ambika, K. and Rajagopal, B. 2017. In vitro antimicrobial and antiproliferative activity of Bambusa vulgaris. *International Journal of Pharmacy and Pharmaceutical Research* 9(1):10–22.

Anantachote, A. 1987. Flowering and seed characteristics of bamboos in Thailand. In A.N. Rao, G. Dhanarajan and C.B, Sastry (Eds) *Recent Research on Bamboos.* Chinese Academy of Forestry, Chnina and International Development Research Centre, Canada, pp. 136–145.

Anderson, J.W. 2008. Dietary fibre and associated phytochemicals in prevention and reversal of diabetes. In: V.K. Pasupuleti and J.W. anderson (Eds.) *Nutraceuticals, Glycemic Health and Type 2 Diabetes.* Blackwell Publishing, Iowa, IA, pp. 111–142.

Anping, L. 2005. The regulation role of fermenting bamboo-shoots dietary fiber in the intestinal flora and constipation of mice. *Science and Technology of Food Industry* 7:064.

Arens, J. and Beurden, J.V. 1978. *Jhagraphur: Poor Peasants and Women in a Village in Bangladesh.* Third World Publications, Birmingham, p. 180.

ASSOCHAM 2017. *Indian Nutraceuticals Industry: Current Scenario and Future Trends.* ASSOCHAM India, New Delhi.

Awol, A. 2015. Nutrient, mineral and bioactive constituent evaluation of bamboo shoots grown in Masha area, South-West of Ethiopia. *American Scientific Research Journal for Engineering, Technology, and Sciences* 7(1):15–25.

Awuchi, C.G., Victory, I.S., Ikechukwu, A.O., and Echeta, C.K. 2020. Health benefits of micronutrients (vitamins and minerals) and their associated deficiency diseases: A systematic review. *International Journal of Food Sciences* 3(1):1–32.

Azmi, A.F.M.N., Mustafa, S., Hashim, D.M. and Manap, Y.A. 2012. Prebiotic activity of polysaccharides extracted from Gigantochloa levis (Buluh Beting) shoots. *Molecules* 17(2):1635–1651.

Badwaik, L.S., Borah, P.K., Borah, K., Das, A.J., Deka, S.C. and Sharma, H.K. 2014. Influence of fermentation on nutritional compositions, antioxidant activity, total phenolic and microbial load of bamboo shoot. *Food Science and Technology Research* 20(2):255–262.

Badwaik, L.S., Borah, P.K. and Deka, S.C. 2014. Antimicrobial and enzymatic anti-browning film used as coating for bamboo shoot quality improvement. *Carbohydrate Polymers* 103:213–220.

Badwaik, L.S., Choudhury, S., Borah, P.K. and Deka, S.C. 2012. Optimization of osmotic dehydration process of bamboo shoots in mixtures of sucrose and sodium chloride solutions. *Journal of Food Processing and Preservation* 37(6):1068–1077.

Badwaik, L.S., Choudhury, M., Dash, K.K., Borah, P.K. and Deka, S.C. 2013. Osmotic dehydration of bamboo shoots enhanced by centrifugal force and pulsed vacuum using salt as osmotic agent. *Journal of Food Processing and Preservation* 38(5):2069–2077.

Badwaik, L.S., Choudhury, S., Borah, P.K., Sit, N. and Deka, S.C. 2014. Comparison of kinetics and other related properties of bamboo shoot drying pretreated with osmotic dehydration. *Journal of Food Processing and Preservation* 38(3):1171–1180.

Badwaik, L.S., Gautam, G. and Deka, S.C. 2015. Influence of blanching on antioxidant, nutritional and physical properties of bamboo shoot. *Journal of Agricultural Sciences* 10(3):140–150.

Bahadur, M. 2013. *The Art of Bamboo; Bamboo in Manipuri Cultural Life India, Bangladesh and Myanmar, Cane and Bamboo Crafts of NE India, Bangladesh, Myanmar and Thailand.* Mutua Museum Publication, Imphal.

Bailey, R.L., West, Jr, K.P. and Black, R.E. 2015. The epidemiology of global micronutrient deficiencies. *Annals of Nutrition and Metabolism* 66(2):22–33.

Bajwa, H.K. 2017. Phytomodulatory effects of fresh and processed shoots of Dendrocalamus hamiltonii on lipid profile and antioxidant defense system. A Ph.D. thesis submitted to the Panjab University, Chandigarh.

Bajwa, H.K., Chongtham, N., Koul, A. and Bisht, M.S. 2015. Effects of processing and preservation on phenols and phytosterols content in bamboo shoots. In: *Proceedings of the 10th World Bamboo Congress*, Damyang, Korea.

Bajwa, H.K., Chongtham, N., Koul, A. and Bisht, M.S. 2016. Changes in organoleptic, physicochemical and nutritional qualities of shoots of an edible bamboo Dendrocalamus hamiltonii Nees Arn. & Ex Munro during processing. *Journal of Food Processing and Preservation* 40(6):1309–1317.

Bajwa, H.K., Santosh, O., Koul, A., Bisht, M.S. and Chongtham, N. 2018. Antioxidant content and antioxidant activity of aqueous extract from processed shoots of an edible bamboo Dendrocalamus hamiltonii nees & arn. ex Munro and their effect on hepatic lipid peroxidation levels in Balb/c mice. *Journal of Pharmacognosy and Phytochemistry* 7(5):3248–3255.

Bajwa, H.K., Santosh, O., Koul, A., Bisht, M.S. and Chongtham, N. 2019a. Phytomodulatory effects of fresh and processed shoots of an edible bamboo Dendrocalamus hamiltonii Nees & Arn. Ex Munro on antioxidant defense system in mouse liver. *Journal of Food Measurement and Characterization* 13(4):3250–3256.

Bajwa, H.K., Santosh, O., Koul, A., Bisht, M.S. and Chongtham, N. 2019b. Quantitative determination of macroelement and microelement content of fresh and processed bamboo shoots by wavelength dispersive X-ray fluorescence spectrometry. *X-Ray Spectrometry* 48(6):637–643.

Bal, L.M., Karb, A., Satya, S. and Naik, S.N. 2010. Drying kinetics and effective moisture diffusivity of bamboo shoot slices undergoing microwave drying. *International Journal of Food Science and Technology* 45(11):2321–2328.

Banik, R.L. 1997. The edibility of shoots of Bangladesh bamboos and their continuous harvesting effect on productivity. *Bangladesh Journal of Forest Science* 26(1):1–10.

Banout, J. and Ehl, P. 2010. Using a Double-Pass Drier for drying of bamboo shoots. *Journal of Agriculture and Rural Development in Tropics and Subtropics* 111(2):119–127.

Baroni, M.V., Naranjo, R.D.D.P., García-Ferreyra, C., Otaiza, S. and Wunderlin, D.A. 2012. How good antioxidant is the red wine? comparison of some in vitro and in vivo methods to assess the antioxidant capacity of Argentinean red wines. *LWT-Food Science and Technology* 47(1):1–7.

Bernhoft, A. 2010. *A Brief Review on Bioactive Compounds in Plants, in: Bioactive Compounds in Plants- Benefits and Risks for Man and Animals.* The Norwegian Academy of Science and Letters, Oslo.

Bersalona, C.B. 2015. Bamboo leaves as chicken feed and fodder. In: *Proceedings of the 10th World Bamboo Congress, Theme: Food andPharmaceuticals*, September 17–22, 2015, Damyang, Korea.

Bhargava, A., Kumbhare, V., Srivastava, A. and Sahai, A. 1996. Bamboo parts and seeds for additional source of nutrition. *Journal of Food Science and Technology* 33(2):145–146.

Bhatt, B.P., Singh, K. and Singh, A. 2005. Nutritional values of some commercial edible bamboo species of the north eastern Himalayan region, India. *Journal of Bamboo and Rattan* 4(2):111–124.

Bhatt, B.P., Singha, L.B., Sachan, M.S. and Singh, K. 2004. Commercial edible bamboo species of the North-Eastern Himalayan Region, India. Part I: Young shoot sales. *Journal of Bamboo and Rattan* 3(4):337–364.

Bhatt, B.P., Singha, L.B., Sachan, M.S. and Singh, K. 2005. Commercial edible bamboo species of North Eastern Himalayan Region, India, Part II: Fermented, roasted and boiled bamboo shoots sale. *Journal of Bamboo and Rattan* 4:13–31.

Bhatt, B.P., Singha, L.B., Singh, K. and Sachan, M.S. 2003. Some commercial edible bamboo species of North East India: Production, Indigenous Uses, Cost-Benefit and Management Strategies. *Science and Culture* 17(1):4–20.

Bisht, M.S., Chongtham, N and Meetei, O.S. 2015. Bamboo shoots for food in North-East India: Conventional and contemporary. In: *Proceedings of the 10th World Bamboo Congress, Theme: Food and Pharmaceuticals.*

Bisht, M.S., Chongtham, N. and Nongdam, P. 2012. Bamboo shoot as a resource for health food and socio-economic development in North-East India. In: *Proceedings of the IXth World Bamboo Congress*, April 10–13, Antwerp, Belgium, pp. 393–402.

Bystriakova, N. and Kapos, V. 2006. Bamboo diversity: The need for a red list review. *Biodiversity* 6(4):12–16.

Bystriakova, N., Kapos, V., Lysenko, I. and Stapleton, C.M. 2003. Distribution and conservation status of forest bamboo biodiversity in the Asia-Pacific Region. *Biodiversity and Conservation* 12(9):1833–1841.

Caasi-Lit, M.T. 1999. Bamboo as food. In: *Bamboo+Coconut [Kawayan+Lubi].* Philippine Coconut Research and Development Foundation, Inc., Pasing City, Philippines, p. 82.

Caasi-Lit, M.T. and Punzalan, D.B.T. 2015. Bamboo shoots as food sources in the Philippines: Status and constraints in production and utilization. In: *Proceedings of the 10th World Bamboo Congress*, Damyang, South Korea.

Căpriţă, R., Căpriţă, A. and Julean, C. 2010. Biochemical aspects of non-starch polysaccharides. *Scientific Papers Animal Science and Biotechnologies* 43(1):368–374.

Carey, W.M., Dasi, J.M.B., Rao, N.V. and Gottumukkala, K.M. 2009. Anti-inflammatory activity of methanolic extract of Bambusa vulgaris leaves. *International Journal of Green Pharmacy* 3(3):234–238.

Catherwood, D.J., Savage, G.P., Mason, S.M., Scheffer, J.J.C. and Douglas, J.A. 2007. Oxalate content of cormels of Japanese taro (*Colocasia esculenta* (L.) Schott) and the effect of cooking. *Journal of Food Composition and Analysis* 20(3):147–151.

Chandra, A., Singh, L., Ghosh, S. and Pearce, E. 2012. Role of bamboo-shoot in the pathogenesis of endemic goiter in Manipur, North East India. *Endocrine Practice* 19(1):36–45.

Chandra, A.K., Ghosh, D., Mukhopadhyay, S. and Tripathy, S. 2004. Effect of bamboo shoot, *Bambusa arundinacea* (Retz.) Willd. on thyroid status under conditions of varying iodine intake in rats. *Indian Journal of Experimental Biology* 42(8):781–786.

Chandramouli, S. and Viswanath, S. 2015. Nutritional composition of edible bamboo shoots of some commercially important bamboo species in Peninsular India. *International Journal of Basic and Life Sciences* 3(6):275–287.

Changkija, S. 1999. Folk medicinal plants of the Nagas in India. *Asian Folklore Study* 58:205–230.

Chauhan, K.N., Shah, B. and Mehta, A.A. 2017a. Antioxidant activity of different fractions of methanolic extract of young shoots of Bambusa arundinacea. *World Journal of Pharmacy and Pharmaceutical Science* 6(8):2492–2503.

Chauhan, K.N., Shah, B., Nivsarkar, M. and Mehta, A.A. 2017b. Hepatoprotective activity of methanolic extract of young shoots of Bambusa Arundinaceae in thioacetamide induced liver injury in rats. *The Journal of Phytomarmacology* 6(2):140–148.

Chaveerach, A., Mokkamul, P., Sudmoon, R. and Tanee, T. 2006. Ethnobotany of the genus *Piper* (Piperaceae) in Thailand. *Ethnobotany Research and Applications* 4:223–231.

Chavhan, D.M., Hazarika, M., Brahma, M.L., Hazarika, R.A. and Rahman, Z. 2015. Effect of incorporation of fermented bamboo shoot on physicochemical and microbial quality of pork pickle. *Journal of Food Science and Technology* 52(2):1223–1227.

Chen, C.J., Qiu, E.F., Huang, R.Z., Fan, H.H. and Jiang, J.X. 1999. Study on the spring shoot nutrient content of Phyllostachys pubescens of different provenances. *Journal of Bamboo Research* 18:6–11.

Chen, Y., Jin, L., Li, Y., Xia, G., Chen, C. and Zhang, Y. 2018. Bamboo-shaving polysaccharide protects against high-diet induced obesity and modulates the gut microbiota of mice. *Journal of Functional Foods* 49:20–31.

Chen, Y., Quin, W., Li, X., Gong, J. and Ni, M. 1985. Study on chemical composition of ten species of bamboo. *Chemistry and Industry of Forest Products* 5:39–46.

Chen, Y.S., Wu, H.C., Liu, C.H., Chen, H.C. and Yanagida, F. 2010. Isolation and characterization of lactic acid bacteria from jiang-sun (fermented bamboo shoots), a traditional fermented food in Taiwan. *Journal of the Science of Food and Agriculture* 90(12):1977–1982.

Chen, Y.Z. and Wang, Y.R. 1989. A study on peroxidase in litchi pericarp. *Acta Botanica Sinica* 5:47–52.

Cheng, H.P. 2006. Vacuum Cooling combined with hydro cooling and vacuum drying on bamboo shoots. *Applied Thermal Engineering* 26(17–18):2168–2175.

Chew, F.S. 1988. Biological effects of glucosinolates, in biologically active natural products: Potential use in agriculture. In: H.G. Cutler (Ed.) *American Chemical Society Symposium*, pp. 155–181.

Chiangthong, K. and Chayawat, L. 2009. Bamboo shoot steam processing by Tha Sao community, Sai Yoke District, Kanchanaburi Province. In: *Abstracts of the Research and Thesis. 13th BRT Annual Conference*, October 12–14, 2009, Chiang Mai.

Choi, Y.J., Lim, H.S., Choi, J.S. et al. 2008. Blockade of chronic high glucose–induced endothelial apoptosis by Sasa borealis bamboo extract. *Experimental Biology and Medicine* 233(5):580–591.

Chongtham, N. and Bisht, M.S. 2017. 10th WBC Reports: Bamboo: A prospective ingredient for functional food and nutraceuticals. *Bamboo Journal* 30:82–99.

Chongtham, N., Bisht, M.S., Bajwa, H.K. and Santosh, O. 2018. Bamboo: A rich source of natural antioxidants and its applications in the food and pharmaceutical industry. *Trends in Food Science and Technology* 77:91–99.

Chongtham, N., Bisht, M.S. and Haorongbam, S. 2011. Nutritional properties of bamboo shoots: Potential and prospects for utilization as a health food. *Comprehensive Reviews in Food Science and Food Safety* 10(3):153–169.

Chongtham, N., Bisht, M.S. and Laishram, M. 2014. Bioactive compounds in bamboo shoots: Health benefits and prospects for developing functional foods. *International Journal of Food Science and Technology* 49(6):1425–1431.

Chongtham, N., Bisht, M.S. and Premlata, T. 2013. Germplasm evaluation in bamboos: from chromosomes to molecular markers. *Plant Cell Biotechnology and Molecular Biology* 14:115–127.

Chongtham, N., David, E. and Sharma, M.L. 2007. Changes in nutrient components during ageing of emerging juvenile bamboo shoots. *International Journal of Food Sciences and Nutrition* 58(8):612–618.

Chongtham, N., Sharma, M.L. and David, E. 2008. A comparative study of nutrient components of freshly harvested, fermented and canned bamboo shoots of Dendrocalamus giganteus Munro, *Bamboo Science and Culture, Journal of American Bamboo Society* 21(1):41–47.

Chongtham, N., Sheena, H. and David, E. 2009. Bamboo Shoots: A rich source of dietary fibres. In: F. Klein and G. Moller (Eds.) *Dietary Fibres, Fruit and Vegetable Consumption and Health*, Nova Science Publishers: Hauppauge, NY, pp. 15–30.

Choudhury, D., Sahu, J.K. and Sharma, G.D. 2012. Value addition to bamboo shoots: A review. *Journal of Food Science and Technology* 49(4):407–414.

Choudhury, M., Badwaik, L.S., Borah, P.K., Nandan, S. and Deka, C.S. 2015. Influence of bamboo shoot powder fortification on physico-chemical, textural and organoleptic characteristics of biscuits. *Journal of Food Science and Technology* 52(10):6742–6748.

Christian, A.L., Knott, K.K., Vance, C.K. et al. 2015. Nutrient and mineral composition during shoot growth in seven species of Phyllostachys and Pseudosasa bamboo consumed by giant panda. *Journal of Animal Physiology and Animal Nutrition* 99(6):1172–1183.

Clark, L.G. 1997. Bamboos: the centrepiece of the grass family. In: G.P. Chapman (Ed.) *The Bamboos*. Academic Press, London, pp. 237–248.

Clark, L.G., Londoño, X. and Ruiz-Sanchez, E. 2015. Bamboo taxonomy and habitat. In: *Bamboo*. Springer International Publishing, pp. 1–30.

Clarke, J.D., Riedl, K., Bella, D., Schwartz, S.J., Stevens, J.F. and Ho, E. 2011. Comparison of isothiocyanate metabolite levels and histone deacetylase activity in human subjects consuming broccoli sprouts or broccoli supplement. *Journal of Agricultural and Food Chemistry* 59(20):10955–10963.

Clayton, W.D. and Renvoize, S.A. 1986. *Genera Graminum*. Kew Bulletin Additional Series XIII, London, p. 389.

Crouzet, Y. 1998. *Bamboo*, 1st ed., Benedict Taschen Verlag GmbH First Edition Translations. Ltd., Cambridge.

Crowe, K.M. 2013. Designing functional foods with bioactive polyphenols: Highlighting lessons learned from original plant matrices. *Journal of Human Nutrition and Food Science* 1(3):1018.

Dabbagh, A.J., Mannion, T., Lynch, S.M. and Frei, B. 1994. The effect of iron overload on rat plasma and liver oxidant status in vivo. *The Biochemical Journal* 300(3):99–803.

Das, A.N. and Mitchell, C.P. 2005. Beliefs, superstitions and taboos associated with bamboos in Nepal and its implications. *Banko Janakari* 15(2):63–71.

Das, A., Nath, D.R., Kumari, S. and Saha, R. 2013. Effect of fermented bamboo shoot on the quality and shelf life of nuggets prepared from desi spent hen. *Vetenary World* 6(7):419–423.

Dattagupta, S., Gupta, A. and Ghose, M. 2014. Diversity of non-timber forest products in Cachar District, Assam, India. *India. Journal of Forestry Research* 25(2):463–470.

Delzenne, N.M., Olivares, M., Neyrinck, A.M. et al. 2019. Nutritional interest of dietary fiber and prebiotics in obesity: Lessons from the mynewgut consortium. *Clinical Nutrition* DOI: 10.1016/j.clnu.2019.03.002.

Devi, P.T. 2018. *Edible Bamboos of Manipur: Analysis of Nutrients, Antinutrients and Bioactive Compounds in Young Shoots.* A thesis submitted to Panjab University, Chandigarh, India.

Ding, H.X., Gao, Y.Y., Chao, H.J. and Xia, D.H. 2008. Study on hypoglycemic effect of polysaccharide from Moso bamboo leaves. *Food Science* 28(12):446–449.

Ding, H.X., Gao, Y.Y., Chao, H.J. and Xia, D.H. 2010. Effect of polysaccharide from Moso bamboo leaves on blood lipid of Mice with hyperlipemia. *Food Science* 9:60.

Diver, S. 2001. Bamboo: A multipurpose agroforestry crop. A project of the national center for appropriate technology, U.S. department of agriculture. ATTRA Publication. http://www.eaglerising.net/files/bamboo.pdf.

Dransfield, S. and Widjaja, E.A. 1995. *Plant Resources of South-East Asia* (Vol. 7). Pudoc. Backhuys Publishers: Leiden, Germany.

Duke, J.A. and Atchley, A.A. 1986. *Handbook of Proximate Analysis Tables of Higher Plants.* CRC Press: Boca Raton, FL.

Elangbam, D. 2006. *Nutritive Components of Juvenile Edible Shoots of Some Indian Bamboos.* A thesis submitted at the Department of Botany, Panjab University, Chandigarh.

Elleuch, M., Bedigian, D., Roiseux, O., Besbes, S., Blecker, C. and Attia, H. 2011. Dietary fibre and fibre-rich by-products of food processing: Characterization, technological functionality and commercial applications: A review. *Food Chemistry* 124(2):411–421.

Elliott, S. and Brimacombe, J. 1987. The medicinal plants of Gunung Leuser National Park, Indonesia. *Journal of Ethnopharmacology* 19(3):285–317.

ERG 2005. Report on process, market and business opportunity report on edible bamboo shoot. Report submitted to NMBA. Engineering Resources Group, Bangalore in association with CPF, FRESH and Delphi (Internet). http://www.bambootech.org/files/ERG%20report%20on%20 shoots.pdf. Accessed on 24 April 2009.

Eti, M., Chandana, M.P., Roopkala, B.M. and Nagarathnamma, R. 2016. Knowledge of obesity and its effects on cardiometabolic and reproductive health in women. *International Journal of Reproduction, Contraception, Obstetrics and Gynecology* 5(1):143–147.

Fahey, J.W., Wehage, S.L., Holtzclaw, W.D., Kensler, T.W., Egner, P.A., Shapiro, T.A. and Talalay, P. 2012. Protection of humans by plant glucosinolates: Efficiency of conversion of glucosinolates to isothiocyanates by the gastrointestinal microflora. *Cancer Prevention Research* 5(4):603–611.

FAO 2007. *World Bamboo Resources: A Thematic Study Prepared in the Framework of the Global Forest Resources Assessment 2005. Non-wood Forest Products # 18*, ed. Lobovikov M., Paudel S., Piazza M., Ren H. and Wu J. ed. Food and Agriculture Organisation of the United Nations, Rome.

FAO 2010. *Global Forest Resources assessment 2010: Main Report.* Food and Agriculture Organization of the United Nations, Rome.

FAO 2017. *The State of Food Security and Nutrition in the world 2017. Building Resilience for Peace and Food Security.* FAO, Rome.

Farris, S. and Piergiovanni, L. 2008. Effects of ingredients and process conditions on 'Amaretti'cookies characteristics. *International Journal of Food Science and Technology* 43(8):1395–1403.

Farris, S., Piergiovanni, L. and Limbo, S. 2008. Effect of bamboo fibre and glucose syrup as new ingredients in the manufacture of amaretti cookies. *Italian Journal of Food Science* 1:75–90.

Felisberto, M.H.F., Beraldo, A.L. and Clerici, M.T.P.S. 2017a. Young bamboo culm flour of Dendrocalamus asper: Technological properties for food applications. *LWT-Food Science and Technology* 76:230–235.

Felisberto, M.H.F., Miyake, P.S.E., Beraldo, A.L. and Clerici, M.T.P.S. 2017b. Young bamboo culm: Potential food as source of fiber and starch. *Food Research International* 101:96–102.

Felisberto, M.H.F., Miyake, P.S.E., Beraldo, A.L., Fukushima, A.R., Leoni, L.A.B. and Clerici, M.T.P.S. 2019. Effect of the addition of young bamboo culm flour as a sugar and/or fat substitute in cookie formulations. *Food Science and Technology* 39(4):867–874.

Fernandez, M.L. 2001. Soluble fibre and non-digestible carbohydrate effects on plasma lipids and cardiovascular risk. *Current Opinion in Lipidology* 12(1):35–40.

Ferreira, V.L.P., Moraes, M.A.C., De Mantovani, D.M.B. and Paschoalino, J.E. 1992. Chemical composition, processing and evaluation of bamboo shoots. *Coletanea Inst Technol Aliment* 22:177–193.

Ferreira, V.L.P., Yotsuyanagi, K. and Carvalho, C.R.L. 1995. Elimination of cyanogenic compounds from bamboo shoots Dendrocalamus giganteus Munro. *Tropical Science* 35:342–346.

Friedman, S.F., Martin, P. and Munoz, J.S. 2003. Laboratory evaluation of the patient with liver disease. In: T.D. Zakim and D. Boyer (Ed.) *Hepatology, A Textbook of Liver Disease*. Saunders Publication, Philedelphia, PA, pp. 661–709.

FSANZ (Food Standards Australia New Zealand) 2004. Cyanogenic glycosides in cassava and bamboo shoots: A human health risk assessment, technical report Series No. 28. Food Standards Australia New Zealand, p. 24.

Fu, X.C., Wang, M.W., Li, S.P. and Wang, H.L. 2006. Anti-apoptotic effect and the mechanism of orientinon ischaemic/reperfused myocardium. *Journal of Asian Natural Products Research* 8(3):265–272.

Fuchigami, M. 1990. Differences between bamboo shoots and vegetables in thermal disintegration of tissues and polysaccharides fractionated by successive extraction. *Journal of Food Science* 55(3):739–745.

Fujimura, M., Ideguchi, M., Minami, Y., Watanabi, K. and Tadera, K. 2005. Amino acid sequence and antimicrobial activity of chitin binding peptides, Pp-AMP 1 and Pp-AMP2, from Japanese bamboo shoots (Phyllostachys pubescens). *Bioscience, Biotechnology, and Biochemistry* 69(3):642–645.

Gamble, J.S. 1896. *The Bambuseae of British India*. Bengal Secretariat Press, Calcutta, p. 133.

Ge, Q., Mao, J.W., Cai, C. et al. 2017. Effects of twin-screw extrusion on physicochemical properties and functional properties of bamboo shoots dietary fiber. *The Journal of Bio Based Materials and Bioenergy* 11(4):385–390.

Geil, W.E. 1904. *A Yankee on the Yangtze: Being a Narrative of a Journey from Shanghai through the Central Kingdom to Burma*. AC Armstrong and Son: Burma.

Giada, M.D.L.R. 2013. *Food Phenolic Compounds: Main Classes, Sources and their Antioxidant Power. Oxidative Stress and Chronic Degenerative Diseases-A Role for Antioxidants*. In Tech, pp. 87–112.

Giri, S.S. and Janmejoy, L. 1992. Nutrient composition of three edible bamboo species of Manipur. *Frontier in Biology* 4:53–56.

Goh, S., Kim, D., Choi, M.H., Shin, H.J. and Kwon, S. 2019. Effects of bamboo stem extracts on adipogenic differentiation and lipid metabolism regulating genes. *Biotechnology and Bioprocess Engineering* 24(3):454–463.

Gong, J., Huang, J., Xiao, G. et al. 2016. Antioxidant capacities of fractions of bamboo shaving extract and their antioxidant components. *Molecules* 21(8):996.

Gonzãlez-Gallego, J., Sãnchez-Campos, S. and Tunon, M.J. 2007. Anti-inflammatory properties of dietary flavonoids. *Nutricion Hospitalaria* 22(3):287–293.

Gopalan, C.B., Ramasastri, V. and Balasubramanion, S.C. 1978. *Nutritive Value of Indian Foods*. National Institute of Nutrition, ICMR, Hyderabad (India), p. 204.

Goyal, A.K., Middha, S.K., Usha, T. and Sen, A. 2017. Analysis of toxic, antidiabetic and antioxidant potential of Bambusa balcooa Roxb. Leaf Extracts in alloxan-induced diabetic rats. *3 Biotech* 7(2):120.

Granato, D., Barba, F.J., Bursać Kovačević, D., Lorenzo, J.M., Cruz, A.G. and Putnik, P. 2020. Functional foods: Product development, technological trends, efficacy testing, and safety. *Annual Review of Food Science and Technology*, 11:93–118.

Greiner, R. and Konietzny, U. 1999. Improving enzymatic reduction of myo-inositol phosphates with inhibitory effects on mineral absorption in black Beans (Phaseolus vulgaris var. preto). *Journal of Food Processing and Preservation* 23(3):249–261.

Gunckel, H. 1948. La floración de la quila y del colihue en la Araucania. *Ciencia e Investicación* 4:91–95.

Guoging, L. 1985. Improved cultivation techniques of bamboos in north china. Recent research on bamboos. In: *Proceedings of the International Bamboo Workshop*, Hangzhou, People's Republic of China.

Haber, G.B., Heaton, K.W. and Murphy, D. 1977. Depletion and disruption of dietary fibre: Effects on satiety, plasma-glucose, and serum-insulin. *The Lancet* 310(8040):679–682.

Hailu, A.A. and Addis, G. 2016. The content and bioavailability of mineral nutrients of selected wild and traditional edible plants as affected by household preparation methods practiced by local community in Benishangul Gumuz Regional State, Ethiopia. *International Journal of Food Science*:1–7. Article ID 7615853. DOI: org/10.1155/2016/7615853

Han, H. and Baik, B.K. 2008. Antioxidant activity and phenolic content of Lentils (*Lens culinaris*), Chickpeas (*Cicer arietinum* L.), Peas (*Pisum sativum* L.) and Soybeans (*Glycine max*) and their quantitative changes during processing. *International Journal of Food Science and Technology* 43(11):1971–1978.

Haorongbam, S., Elangbam, D. and Chongtham, N. 2009. Cyanogenic glucosides in juvenile edible shoots of some Indian bamboos. In: *Proceedings of the 8th World Bamboo Conference*, Bangkok, Thailand.

Haque, M. and Bradbury, J.H. 2002. Total cyanide determination of plants and foods using the picrate and acid hydrolysis methods. *Food Chemistry* 77(1):107–114.

Harmer, C.J., Mctavish, S.F.B., Clark, L., Goodwin, G.M. and Cowen, P.J. 2001. Tyrosine depletion attenuates dopamine function in healthy volunteers. *Psychopharmacology* 154(1):105–111.

Hartayanie, L., Lindayani, L. And Murniati, M.P. 2016. Antimicrobial activity of lactic acid bacteria from bamboo shoot pickles fermented at 15°C. *Microbiology Indonesia* 10(2):71–77.

Hayes, J.D., Kelleher, M.O. and Eggleston, I.M. 2008. The cancer chemopreventive actions of phytochemicals derived from glucosinolates. *European Journal of Nutrition* 47(Suppl 2):73–88.

He, S., Wang, X., Zhang, Y. et al. 2016. Isolation and prebiotic activity of water-soluble polysaccharides fractions from the bamboo shoots (Phyllostachys praecox). *Carbohydrate Polymers* 151:295–304.

He, Y.H. and Lachance, P.A. 1998. Effects of dietary bamboo shoot on fecal neutralsterols and bile acid excretion in the rat. *The Journal of Federation of American Societies of Experimental Biology* 12(4):210.

Hinsui, J., Ignatius, B., Kronseder, K., Kärkkäinen, J., Pingoud, P. and Sandra, E. 2008. *Non Timber Forest Products in Northern Thailand*. University of Helsinki, Finland.

Hiromichi, H. 2007. Use of an antitumor agent. European Patent EP1413208.

Hong, E.J., Jung, E.M., Lee, G.S. et al. 2010. Protective effects of the pyrolyzates derived from bamboo against neuronal damage and hematoaggregation. *Journal of Ethnopharmacology* 128(3):594–599.

Horiuchi, Y., Kimura, R., Kato, N. et al. 2003. Evolutional study on acetylcholine expression. *Life Sciences* 72(15):1745–1756.

Hoyweghen, L.V., De Bosscher, K., Haegeman, G., Deforce, D. and Heyerick, A. 2014. In vitro inhibition of the transcription factor NF-κB and cyclooxygenase by Bamboo extracts. *Phytotherapy Research* 28(2):224–230.

Hu, C.H., Zhang, Y. and David, D.K. 2000. Evaluation of antioxidant and prooxidant activities of bamboo Phyllostachys nigra var. henonis leaf extract in vitro. *Journal of Agricultural and Food Chemistry* 48(8):3170–3176.

Hwang, J.H., Choi, S.Y., Ko, H.C. et al. 2007. Anti-inflammatory effect of the hot water extract from Sasa quelpaertensis leaves. *Food Science and Biotechnology* 16(5):728–733.

INBAR 2007. *Chinese Experts for the Training Workshop on Bamboo Cultivation and Utilization: Project Report.* Addis Ababa, Ethiopia, p. 43.

INBAR 2012. *International Network for Bamboo and Rattan, (INBAR),* Beijing, China, ISBN: 978-92-95098-44-2.

INBAR 2019. Bamboo promoted for land restoration at UNCCD. https://www.inbar.int/press-release-bamboo-promoted-for-land-restoration-at-unccd/. Accessed on 28–30 January 2019.

Ingudam, M. and Sarangthem, K. 2016. Phytosterols content in different bamboo species of Manipur, India. *International Journal of Current Microbiology and Applied Sciences* 5(8):943–948.

Ishii, T. and Hiroi, T. 1990. Linkage of phenolic acids to cell wall polysaccharides of bamboo shoot. *Carbohydrate Research* 206(2):297–310.

Ito, Y., Akao, Y., Shimazawa, M., Seki, N., Nozawa, Y. and Hara, H. 2007. Lig-8, A highly bioactive lignophenol derivative from bamboo lignin, exhibits multifaceted neuroprotective activity. *CNS Drug Reviews* 13(3):296–307.

Jackson, J.K. 1987. *Manual of Afforestation in Nepal Forestry Research Project.* Department of Forest, Kathmandu.

Jankowsky, L., de Lira, S.P., Tanaka, F.A.O. and, Pontes, I. 2018. Antimicrobial activity of the methanolic fraction of bamboo pyroligneous liquor. *Journal of Pharmacy and Pharmacology* 6(10):924–934.

Jaworska, G. 2005. Nitrates, nitrites, and oxalates in products of spinach and New Zealand spinach: Effect of technological measures and storage time on the level of nitrates, nitrites, and oxalates in frozen and canned products of spinach and New Zealand spinach. *Food Chemistry* 93(3):395–401.

Jeyaram, K., Romi, W., Singh, Th.A. and, Devi, A.R. 2010. Bacterial species associated with traditional starter cultures used for fermented bamboo shoot production in Manipur State of India. *International Journal of Food Microbiology* 143(1–2):1–8.

Jeyaram, K., Singh, T.A., Romi, W. et al. 2009. Traditional fermented foods of Manipur.*Indian Journal of Traditional Knowledge* 8(1):115–121.

Jiayan, Y. 2014. A comparative study of bamboo culture and its applications in China, Japan and South Korea 8–10 September 2014- Istanbul, Turkey. In: *Proceedings of the SOCIOINT14- International Conference on Social Sciences and Humanities.* ISBN: 978-605-64453-1-6.

Jimenez-Escrig, A., Santos-Hidalgo, A.B. and Saura-Calixto, F. 2006. Common sources and estimated intake of plant sterols in the Spanish diet. *Journal of Agricultural and Food Chemistry* 54(9):3462–3471.

Jin, Y.C., Yuan, K. and Zhang, J. 2011. Chemical composition, and antioxidant and antimicrobial activities of essential oil of Phyllostachys heterocycla Cv. Pubescens Varieties from China. *Molecules* 16(5):4318–4327.

Joana Gil-Chávez, G., Villa, J.A., Fernando Ayala-Zavala, J., Basilio Heredia, J., Sepulveda, D., Yahia, E.M. and González-Aguilar, G.A. 2013. Technologies for extraction and production of bioactive compounds to be used as nutraceuticals and food ingredients: An overview. *Comprehensive Reviews in Food Science and Food Safety* 12(1):5–23.

Joint, F.A.O. and WHO Expert Committee on Food Additives and World Health Organization 2012. *Safety Evaluation of Certain Food Additives and Contaminants: Prepared by the Seventy Fourth Meeting of the Joint FAO/WHO Expert Committee on Food Additives (JECFA).* World Health Organization.

Jones, D.A. 1998. Why are so many plants cyanogenic? *Phytochemistry* 47(2):155–162.

Jones, P.J. and AbuMweis, S.S. 2009. Phytosterols as functional food ingredients: Linkages to cardiovascular disease and cancer. *Current Opinion in Clinical Nutrition and Metabolic Care* 12(2):147–151.

Jones, P.J., MacDougall, D.E., Ntanios, F. and Vanstone, C.A. 1997. Dietary phytosterols as cholesterol-lowering agents in humans. *Canadian Journal of Physiology and Pharmacology* 75(3):217–227.

Ju, J., Song, J.L. and Park, K.Y. 2015. Antiobesity effects of bamboo salt in C57BL/6 mice. *Journal of Medicinal Food* 18(6):706–710.

Juajun, O., Vanhanen, L., Sangketkit, C. and Savage, G. 2012. Effect of cooking on the oxalate content of selected Thai vegetables. *Food and Nutrition Sciences* 3(12):1631–1635.

Judprasong, K., Charoenkiatkul, S., Sungpuag, P., Vasanachitt, K. and Nakjamanong, Y. 2006. Total and soluble oxalate contents in Thai vegetables, cereal grains and legume seeds and their changes after cooking. *Journal of Food Composition and Analysis* 19(4):340–347.

Judziewicz, E.J. and Sepsenwol, S. 2007. The world smallest bamboo: Raddiella vanessiae (Poaceae: Bambusoideae: Olyreae), A new species from French Guiana. *Journal of the Botanical Research Institute of Texas* 1(1):1–7.

Kalaiarasi, K., Prasannaraj, G., Sahi, S.V. and Venkatachalam, P. 2015. Phytofabrication of biomolecule-coated metallic silver nanoparticles using leaf extracts of in vitro-raised bamboo species and its anticancer activity against human PC3 cell lines. *Turkish Journal of Biology* 39(2):223–232.

Kalita, C., Ganguly, M. and Devi, A. 2016. Evaluation of antioxidant capacity and antimicrobial properties of ethnic Bambuseae species and identification of the active components. *International Journal Pharmaceutical and Biological Archive* 7:61–71.

Kang, S.I., Shin, H.S., Kim, H.M. et al. 2012. Anti-obesity properties of a Sasa quelpaertensis extract in high-fat diet-induced obese mice. *Bioscience, Biotechnology, and Biochemistry* 76(4):755–761.

Karakaya, S., El, S.N. and Tas, A.A. 2001. Antioxidant activity of some foods containing phenolic compounds. *International Journal of Food Sciences and Nutrition* 52(6):501–508.

Karanja, P.N., Kenji, G.M., Njoroge, S.M. et al. 2016.Variation of nutrients and functional properties within young shoots of a bamboo species (Yushania alpina) growing at Mt. Elgon region in Western Kenya. *Journal of Food and Nutrition Research* 3(10):675–680.

Katayama, N., Kishida, O., Sakai, R. et al. 2015. Response of a wild edible plant to human disturbance: Harvesting can enhance the subsequent yield of bamboo shoots. *PLoS One* 10(12):E0146228.

Kaur, K., Gupta, R., Saraf, S.A. and Saraf, S.K. 2014. Zinc: The metal of life. *Comprehensive Reviews in Food Science and Food Safety* 13(4):358–376.

Kaur, C. and Kapoor, H.C. 2002. Anti-oxidant activity and total phenolic content of some Asian vegetables. *International Journal of Food Science and Technology* 37(2):153–161.

Keng, P.C. and Wang, Z.P. 1996. Flora republicae popularis sinicae. Thomus, Beijing: Science Press of China 9(1):612–620.

Kennard, W.C. and Freyre, R.H. 1957. The edibility of shoots of some bamboos growing in Puerto Rico. *Economic Botany* 11(3):235–243.

Kensler, T.W., Chen, J.G., Egner, P.A. et al. 2005. Effects of glucosinolate-rich Broccoli sprouts on urinary levels of aflatoxin-DNA adducts and phenanthrene tetraols in a randomized clinical trial in He Zuo Township, Qidong, People's Republic of China. *Cancer Epidemiology, Biomarkers and Prevention Research* 14(11–1):2605–2613.

Khokhar, S. and Magnusdottir, S.G.M. 2002. Total phenol, catechin and caffeine contents of teas commonly consumed in the United Kingdom. *Journal of Agricultural and Food Chemistry* 50(3):565–570.

Kim, D.S., Kim, S.H. and Cha, J. 2016. Antiobesity effects of the combined plant extracts varying the combination ratio of Phyllostachys pubescens leaf extract and Scutellaria baicalensis root extract. *Evidence-Based Complementary and Alternative Medicine,* 2016: 1–11. DOI: org/10.1155/2016/9735276

Kim, E.Y., Jung, E.Y., Lim, H.S. and Heo, Y.R. 2007b. The effects of the *Sasa borealis* leaves extract on plasma adiponectin, resistin, C-reactive protein and homocysteine levels in high fat diet-induced obese C57/BL6J mice. *Korean Journal of Nutrition* 40(4):303–311.

Kim, J.S., Nam, J.B. and Yang, J.K. 2013. Antioxidant activity and inhibition of PC-3 prostate cancer cell growth by volatile extracts from bamboo. *Korea Society of Wood Science and Technology Conference* 27(4):224–225.

Kim, K.M., Kim, Y.S., Lim, J.Y. et al. 2015. Intestinal anti-inflammatory activity of Sasa quelpaertensis leaf extract by suppressing lipopolysaccharide-stimulated inflammatory mediators in intestinal epithelial Caco-2 cells co-cultured with RAW 264.7 macrophage cells. *Nutrition Research and Practice* 9(1):3–10.

Kim, Y.N., Giraud, D.W. and Driskell, J.A. 2007a. Tocopherol and carotenoid contents of selected Korean fruits and vegetables. *Journal of Food Composition and Analysis* 20(6):458–465.

Kiruba, S., Jeeva, S., Das, S.S.M. and Kannan, D. 2007. Bamboo seeds as a mean to sustenance of the indigenous community. *Indian Journal of Traditional Knowledge* 6(1):199–203.

Kiruba, S., Jeeva, S., Dhas, S.S.M. and Kannan, D. 2007. Bamboo seeds as a mean to substance of the indigenous community. *Indian Journal of Traditional Knowledge* 6:199–203.

Kleinhenz, V., Gosbee, M., Elsmore, S. et al. 2000. Storage methods for extending the shelf-life of fresh, edible bamboo shoots [Bambusa oldhamii (Munro)]. *Postharvest Biology and Technology* 19(3):253–264.

Ko, B.S., Jun, D.W., Jang, J.S., Kim, J.H. and Park, S. 2006. Effect of Sasa borealis and white lotus root and leaves on insulin action and secretion in vitro. *Korean Journal of Food Science and Technology* 38:114–120.

Koide, C.L., Collier, A.C., Berry, M.J. and Panee, J. 2011. The effect of bamboo extract on hepatic biotransforming enzymes–findings from an obese–diabetic mouse model. *Journal of Ethnopharmacology* 133(1):37–45.

Kornsteiner, M., Wagner, K. and Elmadfa, I. 2006. Tocopherols and total phenolics in 10 different nut types. *Food Chemistry* 98(2):381–387.

Kozukue, E., Kozukue, N. and Kurosaki, T. 1983. Organic acid, sugar and amino acid composition of bamboo shoots. *Journal of Food Science* 48(3):935–938.

Kozukue, E., Kozukue, N. and Tsuchida, H. 1998. Identification and changes of phenolic compounds in bamboo [Gramineae] shoots during storage at 20 degree centigrade. *Journal of the Japanese Society for Horticultural Science (Japan)* 67(5):805–811.

Kozukue, E., Kozukue, N. and Tsuchida, H. 1999. Changes in several enzyme activities accompanying the pulp browning of bamboo shoots during storage. *Journal of the Japanese Society for Horticultural Science* 68(3):689–693.

Kumar, P.S., Kanwat, M. and Choudhary, V.K. 2012. Mathematical modeling and thin-layer drying kinetics of bamboo slices on convective tray drying at varying temperature. *Journal of Food Processing and Preservation* 37(5):914–923.

Kumbhare, V. and Bhargava, A. 2007. Effect of processing on nutritional value of central Indian bamboo shoots. Part I. *Journal of Food Science and Technology* 44(1):29–31.

Kumbhare, V. and Bhargava, A. 2007. Effect of processing on nutritional value of central Indian bamboo shoots. *Journal of Food Science and Technology* 44(1):29–31.

Kumbhare, V.R. 2003. *Studies on Some Indian Bamboos for Their Nutritional Values.* A thesis-Tropical Forest Research Institute (TFRI), Jabalpur (India).

Kynes, S. 2006. *Whispers from the Woods: The Lore and Magic of Trees.* Llewellyn Worldwide: Woodbury, MN

Lachance, P.A. and He, Y.H. 1998. Hypocholesterolemic compositions from bamboo shoots, PCT. International Patent, PCT/US98/12556.

Ladio, A.H. and Lozada, M. 2000. Edible wild plant use in a Mapuche community of Northwestern Patagonia. *Human Ecology* 28(1):53–71.

Landete, J.M. 2012. Updated knowledge about polyphenols: Functions, bioavailability, metabolism and health. *Critical Reviews in Food Science and Nutrition* 52(10):936–948.

Lantican, C.B., Armando, M.P. and Carmen, G.S. 1985. Bamboo research in Philippines .recent research on Bamboos. In: *Proceedings of the International Bamboo Workshop*, Chinese Academy of Forestry (CAF), Hangzhou, People's Republic of China.

Laura, A., Moreno-Escamilla, J.O., Rodrigo-García, J. and Alvarez-Parrilla, E. 2019. *Phenolic Compounds in Postharvest Physiology and Biochemistry of Fruits and Vegetables*. In Elhadi Yahia and Armando Carillo-Lopez (Eds) *Postharvest Physiology and Biochemistry of Fruits and Vegetables*, Woodhead Publishing: London, United Kingdom, pp. 253–271.

Li, X., Guo, J., Ji, K. and Zhang, P. 2016. Bamboo shoot fiber prevents obesity in mice by modulating the gut microbiota. *Scientific Reports* 6:32953.

Li, Z.H. and Kobayashi, M. 2004. Plantation future of bamboo in China. *Journal of Forestry Research* 15(3):233–242.

Liu, L., Liu, L., Lu, B., Chen, M. and Zhang, Y. 2013. Evaluation of bamboo shoot peptide preparation with angiotensin converting enzyme inhibitory and antioxidant abilities from by-products of canned bamboo shoots. *Journal of Agricultural and Food Chemistry* 61(23):5526–5533.

Liu, L., Liu, L., Lu, B., Xia, D. and Zhang, Y. 2012. Evaluation of antihypertensive and anti-hyperlipidemic effects of bamboo shoot angiotensin converting enzyme inhibitory peptide in vivo. *Journal of Agricultural and Food Chemistry* 60(45):11351–11358.

Liu, M.H., Ko, C.H., Ma, N., Tan, P.W., Fu, W.M. and He, J.Y. 2016. Chemical profiles, antioxidant and anti-obesity effects of extract of Bambusa textilis McClure leaves. *Journal of Functional Foods* 22:533–546.

Liu, M.S. 1992. Bamboo shoot. In: Y.H. Hui (Ed.) *Encyclopedia of Food Science and Technology* (Vol. 3). Wiley, New York, pp. 177–180.

Liu, T. 2011. Surveys of harvest technology of winter bamboo shoots. *Journal of Forestry Research* 22(3):487–490.

Liu, Z.Y. and Jiang, W.B. 2006. Lignin deposition and effect of postharvest treatment on lignification of green asparagus (Asparagus officinalis L.). *Plant Growth Regulators* 48(2):187–193.

Lobovikov, M., Paudel, S., Piazza, M., Ren, H. and Wu, J. 2007. *World Bamboo Resources*, ed. INBAR and FAO (Vol. 18, no. 1), pp. 7–8.

Londoño, X. 2001. *Evaluation of Bamboo Resources in Latin America. Summary of the Final Report of Project 96-8300-01-4*. INBAR, Beijing.

Londoño, X. and Peterson, P.M. 1991. Guadua sarcocarpa (Poaceae: Bambuseae), a new species of Amazonian bamboo with fleshy fruits. *Systematic Botany* 16(4):630–638.

Lowrie, A.G. 1900. Effects of the late drought in the Chanda district. *Indian Forester* 26(10):504–506.

Lu, B.Y., Bao, J.F., Shan, L. and Zhang, Y. 2009a. Technology for supercritical CO_2 extraction of bamboo shoot oil and components of product. *Transactions of the Chinese Society of Agricultural Engineering* 25(8):312–316.

Lu, B., Cai, H., Huang, W., Wu, X., Luo, Y., Liu, L. and Zhang, Y. 2011. Protective effect of bamboo shoot oil on experimental nonbacterial prostatitis in rats. *Food Chemistry* 124(3):1017–1023.

Lu, B., Ren, Y., Zhang, Y. and Gong, J. 2009b. Effects of genetic variability, parts and seasons on the sterol content and composition in bamboo shoots. *Food Chemistry* 112(4):1016–1021.

Lu, B., Wu, X., Shi, J., Dong, Y. and Zhang, Y. 2006. Toxicology and safety of antioxidant of bamboo leaves. Part 2: Developmental toxicity test in rats with antioxidant of bamboo leaves. *Food and Chemical Toxicology* 44(10):1739–1743.

Lu, B., Wu, X., Tie, X., Zhang, Y. and Zhang, Y. 2005. Toxicology and safety of antioxidant of bamboo leaves. Part I: Acute and sub chronic toxicity studies on antioxidant of bamboo leaves. *Food and Chemical Toxicology* 43(5):783–792.

Lu, B., Xia, D., Huang, W., Wu, X., Zhang, Y. and Yao, Y. 2010. Hypolipidemic effect of bamboo shoot oil (P. pubescens) in Sprague–Dawley rats. *Journal of Food Science* 75(6):205–211.

Lu, S.M. and Xu, Y.G. 2004. Physiological and biochemical changes of fresh-cut bamboo shoot (Phyllostachys heterocycla var pubescens) during cold storage. *Journal of the Science of Food and Agriculture* 84(8):772–776.

Luo, Z., Wu, X., Xie, Y. and Chen, C. 2012. Alleviation of chilling injury and browning of postharvest bamboo shoot by salicylic acid treatment. *Food Chemistry* 131(2):456–461.

Luo, Z., Xu, X., Cai, Z. and Yan, B. 2007. Effect of ethylene and 1-Methylcyclopropene (1-MPC) on lignifications of post harvest bamboo shoot. *Food Chemistry* 105(2):521–527.

Luo, Z.S., Xu, X.L. and Yan, B.F. 2008. Accumulation of lignin and involvement of enzymes inbamboo shoot during storage. *European Food Research and Technology* 226(4):635–640.

Madamba, P.S. 2003. Physical changes in bamboo (Bambusa Phyllostachys) shoot during hot air drying: Shrinkage, density, and porosity. *Drying Technology* 21(3):555–568.

Mahayotpanya, C. and Phoungchandang, S. 2016. Drying characteristics, quality and safety aspects of bamboo shoots using difference drying methods. *Agricultural Engineering International: CIGR Journal* 18(3):205–219.

Mainka, S.A., Guanlu, Z. and Mao, L. 1989. Utilization of a bamboo, sugar cane, and gruel diet by two juvenile giant pandas (Ailuropoda melanoleuca). *Journal of Zoo and Wildlife Medicine* 20(1):39–44.

Malla, S., Hobbs, J.E. and Sogah, E.K. 2014. Functional foods, health benefits and health claims. *Athens Journal of Health* 1(1):37–46.

Maoyi, F. 1998. Bamboo resources and utilization in China. In: A.N. Rao and V.R. Rao (Eds.) *Bamboo-conservation, Diversity, Ecogeography, Germplasm, Resource Utilization, and Taxonomy. Proceeding of a Training Course Cum Workshop*, May 10–17, 1998, Kunming and Xishaungbanna, Yunnan, China, IPGRI-ARO, Serdang, Malaysia.

Marden, L. 1980. Bamboo, the giant grass. *National Geographic Society* 158(4):502–528.

Maroma, D.P. 2015. Utilization of bamboo shoots (Bambusa vulgaris) in chips production. *Open Access Library Journal* 2(05):1.

Mattioli, R., Mosca, L., Sánchez-Lamar, A., Tempera, I. and Hausmann, R. 2018. Natural bioactive compounds acting against oxidative stress in chronic, degenerative, and infectious diseases. *Oxidative Medicine and Cellular Longevity*. DOI: 10.1155/2018/3894381.

McClure, F.A. 1934. Inflorescence in Schizostachyum Nees. *Journal of the Washington Academy of Sciences* 24:541–548.

McClure, F.A. 1966. *The Bamboos: A Fresh Perspective*. Harvard University Press, Cambridge.

Medhi, P., Sarma, A. and Borthakur, S.K. 2014. Wild edible plants from the DimaHasao District of Assam, India. *Pleione* 8(1):133–148.

Meija, L.A. 1994. Fortification of foods: Historical development and current practices. *Food and Nutrition Bulletin* 15(4):1–4.

Merchant, A.T., Hu, F.B., Spiegelman, D., Willett, W.C., Rimm, E.B. and Ascherio, A. 2003. Dietary fiber reduces peripheral arterial disease risk in men. *The Journal of Nutrition* 133(11):3658–3663.

Menghao, D., Jinping, Z., Jingwen, W., Lisong, H. and Weifang, S. 2012. Evaluation of silicon extract from leaves of Phyllostachys edulis for topical anti-osteoporosis activity. In: *World Automation Congress 2012*, June 24. IEEE, pp. 1–4.

Middha, S.K. and Usha, T. 2012. An in vitro new vista to identify hypoglycemic activity. *International Journal of Fundamental and Applied Science* 1(2):27–29.

Mina, T., Giri, S. and Shantibala 2014. Contents of anti-nutritional substances of bamboo shoots and relation of these to sensory characters of their intact and fermented forms. *The Bioscan* 9 (3):1123–1126.

Mitra, G.N. and Nayak, Y. 1972. Chemical composition of bamboo seeds (Bambusa arundinacea Willd.). *Indian Forester* 98(8):479–481.

Miura, M., Watanabe, I., Shimotori, Y., Aoyama, M., Kojima, Y. and Kato, Y. 2013. Microbial conversion of bamboo hemicellulose hydrolysate to xylitol. *Wood Science and Technology* 47(3):515–522.

Møller, B.L. and Seigler, D.S. 1998. Biosynthesis of cyanogenic glycosides, cyanolipids, and related compounds. In: *Plant Amino Acids: Biochemistry and Biotechnology*. Marcel Dekker, pp. 563-609.

Moreau, R.A., Nyström, L., Whitaker, B.D., Winkler-Moser, J.K., Baer, D.J., Gebauer, S.K. and Hicks, K.B. 2018. Phytosterols and their derivatives: Structural diversity, distribution, metabolism, analysis, and health-promoting uses. *Progress in Lipid Research* 70:35–61.

Muchtadi, T.R. and Adawiyah, D.R. 1996. Bamboo shoot drying technology. In: P.M. Ganapathy, J.A. Janssen and C.B. Sastry (Eds.), *Engineering and Utilization*, pp. 239–245. Ubud, Bali, Indonesia.

Mulyono, N., Lay, B.W., Rahayu, S. and Yaprianti, I. 2012. Antibacterial activity of Petung bamboo (Dendrocalamus asper) leaf extract against pathogenic Escherichia coli and their chemical identification. *International Journal of Pharmaceutical & Biological Archive* 3(4):770–778.

Muniappan, M. and Sundararaj, T. 2003. Anti-inflammatory and antiulcer activities of Bambusa arundinacea. *Journal of Ethnopharmacology* 88(2-3):161–167.

Munro, W. 1868. Monograph of the Bambusaceae. *Transactions of the Linnean Society of London, Botany* 26:1–157.

Murphy, M.E. 1996. Nutrition and metabolism. In: C. Carey (Ed.) *Avian Energetics and Nutritional Ecology*. Springer, Boston, MA, pp. 31–60.

Mustafa, U., Naeem, N., Masood, S. and Farooq, Z. 2016. Effect of bamboo powder supplementation on physicochemical and organoleptic characteristics of fortified cookies. *Food Science and Technology* 4(1):7–13.

Naito, R., Shiino, S. and Inahara, H. 1980. The Green Cross Corporation. Powdered water-swellable fiber bundle of bamboo shoots. U.S. Patent 4,201,776.

Nam, J.S., Chung, H.J., Jang, M.K., Jung, I.A., Park, S.H., Cho, S.I. and Jung, M.H. 2013. Sasa borealis extract exerts an antidiabetic effect via activation of the AMP-activated protein kinase. *Nutrition Research and Practice* 7(1):15–21.

Nayak, L. and Mishra, S.P. 2016. Prospect of bamboo as a renewable textile fiber, historical overview, labeling, controversies and regulation. *Fashion and Textiles* 3(1):2.

Nemenyi, A., Stefanovitsne-Banyai, E., Zoltán, P.E.K. et al. 2015. Total antioxidant capacity and total phenolics content of Phyllostachys taxa shoots. *Notulae Botanicae Horti Agrobotanici Cluj-Napoca* 43(1):64–69.

Nicoli, M.C., Anese, M., Manzocco, L. and Lerici, C.R. 1997. Antioxidant properties of coffee brews in relation to the roasting degree. *LWT- Food Science and Technology* 30(3):292–297.

Nimisha, S.M., Chauhan, A.S., Rekha, M.N., Negi, P.S., Nusrath, N. and Asha, M.R. 2015. Composition of edible portion of tender bamboo shoot (tbs) and development of various candies with and without incorporation of ginger and pineapple flavors. *American Journal of Nutrition and Food Science* 2(1):7–15.

Ningtyas, F.W., Asdie, A.H., Julia, M. and Prabandari, Y.S. 2014. Local wisdom exploration of community in goitrogenic food consumption to yodium deficiency disorder. *Kesmas, National Public Health Journal* 8(7):306–312.

Nishina, A., Hasegawa, K., Uchibori, T., Seino, H. and Osawa, T. 1991. 2,6-Dimethoxy-P-benzoquinone as an antibacterial substance in the bark of Phyllostachys heterocycla var. pubescens, a species of thick-stemmed bamboo. *Journal of Agricultural and Food Chemistry* 39(2):266–269.

NMBA 2009. *Bamboo Shoot Composition. National Mission on Bamboo Application, India. No. 379:1-20.* United States Department of Agriculture, Washington, DC.

Noltie, H.J. 2000. *Flora of Bhutan, Vol. 3 Part 2.* Royal Botanic Garden Edinburgh.

Numata, M. 1970. Conservational implications of bamboo flowering and death in Japan. *Biological Conservation* 2(3):227–229.

Obafaye, O. and Omoba, O. 2018. Orange Peel Flour: A potential source of antioxidant and dietary fiber in pearl-millet biscuit. *Journal of Food Biochemistry* 42(1):12523.

Ogbadoyi, E.O., Makun, H.A., Bamigbade, R.O., Oyewale, A.O. and Oladiran, J.A. 2006. The effect of processing and preservation methods on the oxalate levels of some Nigerian leafy vegetables. *Biokemistri* 18(2):121–125.

Ogunjinmi, A.A., Ijeomah, H.M. and Aiyeloja, A.A. 2009. Socio-economic importance of bamboo (Bambusa vulgaris) in Borgu local government area of Niger State, Nigeria. *Journal of Sustainable Development in Africa* 10(4):284–289.

Ogunlesi, M., Okiei, W., Azeez, L., Obakachi, V., Osunsanmi, M. and Nkenchor, G. 2010. Vitamin C contents of tropical vegetables and foods determined by voltammetric and titrimetric methods and their relevance to the medicinal uses of the plants. *International Journal of Electrochemical Science* 5:05–115.

Oh, H.K. and Lim, H.S. 2009. Effects of hamburger patties with bamboo leaf (Sasa borealis) extract or sea tangle (Laminaria japonica) powder on plasma glucose and lipid profiles. *The FASEB Journal* 23:563–517.

Ohrnberger, D. 1999. *The Bamboos of the World: Annotated Nomenclature and Literature of the Species and the Higher and Lower Taxa.* Elsevier.

Ohtsuka, H., Fujiwara, H., Nishio, A. et al. 2014. Effect of oral supplementation of bamboo grass leaves extract on cellular immune function in dairy cows. *Acta Veterinaria Brno* 83(3):213–218.

Okeyo, D.O. 2019. Impact of food fortification on child growth and development during complementary feeding. *Annals of Nutrition and Metabolism* 73(1):7–13.

Ottaway, P.B. 2008. *Food Fortification and Sup-Plementation: Technological, Safety and Regulatory Aspects.* Woodhead Publishing Ltd, Cambridge.

Owokotomo, I.A. and Owoeye, G. 2011. Proximate analysis and antimicrobial activities of Bambusa vulgaris L. leaves' beverage. *African Journal of Agricultural Research* 6(21):5030–5032.

Owolabi, M.S. and Lajide, L. 2015. Preliminary phytochemical screening and antimicrobial activity of crude extracts of Bambusa vulgaris Schrad. Ex JC Wendl.(Poaceae) from southwestern Nigeria. *American Journal of Essential Oils and Natural Products* 3(1):42–45.

Pan, C. 1995. *Market Opportunities for Fresh and Processed Asian Vegetables: A Report for RIRDC.* Rural Industries Research and Development Corporation.

Panda, T. and Padhy, R.N. 2007. Sustainable food habits of the hill-dwelling Kandha Tribe in Kalahandi District of Orissa. *Indian Journal of Traditional Knowledge* 6(1):103–105.

Pandey, A.K. and Ojha, V. 2013. Standardization of harvesting age of bamboo shoots with respect to nutritional and anti-nutritional components. *Journal of Forestry Research* 24(1):83–90.

Pandey, A.K. and Ojha, V. 2014. Precooking processing of bamboo shoots for removal of antinutrients. *Journal of Food Science and Technology* 51(1):43–50.

Pandey, A.K., Ojha, V. and Choubey, S.K. 2012. Development and shelf-life evaluation of value-added edible products from bamboo shoots. *American Journal of Food Technology* 7(3):363–371.

Panee, J. 2009. *Bamboo Extract in the Prevention of Diabetes and Breast Cancer. Complementary and Alternative Therapies and the Aging Population*. Academic Press, pp. 159–177.

Panee, J. 2015. Potential medicinal application and toxicity evaluation of extracts from bamboo plants. *Journal of Medicinal Plant Research* 9(23):681–692.

Park, E. and Jhon, D. 2009. Effects of bamboo shoot consumption on lipid profiles and bowel function in healthy young women. *Nutrition* 25(7):723–728.

Park, E.J. and Jhon, D.Y. 2010. The Antioxidant, angiotensin converting enzyme inhibition activity, and phenolic compounds of bamboo shoot extracts. *LWT-Food Science and Technology* 43(4):655–659.

Park, E.J. and Jhon, D.Y. 2013. The nutritional composition of bamboo shoots and the effects of its fiber on intestinal microorganisms. *Korean Journal of Food Culture* 28(5):502–511.

Park, K.Y., Ju, J.H., Song, J.L. and Moon, S.H. 2014. Anti-obesity effect of bamboo salt on -diet-induced obesity in C57BL/6 Mice. *The FASEB Journal* 28(1):811–812.

Park, K.Y., Zhao, X. and Mun, S.H. 2013. Anticancer effects of bamboo salt on human cancer cells and on buccal mucosa cancer in mice. *The FASEB Journal* 27(1).

Pasqualone, A., Bianco, A.M., Paradiso, V.M., Summo, C., Gambacorta, G., Caponio, F. and Blanco, A. 2015. Production and characterization of functional biscuits obtained from purple wheat. *Food Chemistry* 180:64–70.

Patil, A.S.S., Hoskeri, H.J., Rajeev, P. et al. 2018. Hepatoprotective activity of methanolic shoot extract of Bambusa bambos against carbon tetrachloride induce acute liver toxicity in Wistar rats. *Journal of Applied Biology and Biotechnology* 6(04):37–40.

Patil, M.P., Palma, J., Simeon, N.C. et al. 2017. Sasa borealis leaf extract-mediated green synthesis of silver-silver chloride nanoparticles and their antibacterial and anticancer activities. *New Journal of Chemistry* 41(3):1363–1371.

Patil, R.N. and Rothe, S.P. 2016. Antifungal activity of some fodder plants leaf extract. *International Advanced Research Journal in Science and Engineering* 3(11):205–208.

Peng, H., Wang, N., Zhengrong, Y., Liu, Y., Zahng, J. and, Ruan, R. 2012. Physiochemical characterization of hemicelluloses from bamboo (Phyllostachys pubescens Mazel) stem. *Industrial Crops and Products* 37(1):41–50.

Phithakpol, B., Varanyanond, W., Reungmaneepaitoon, S. and Wood, H. 1995. *The Traditional Fermented Foods of Thailand. Institute of Food Research and Development*. Kasetsart University, Bangkok, Thailand.

Piironen, V., Toivo, J., Puupponen-Pimiä, R. and Lampi, A.M. 2003. Plant sterols in vegetables, fruits and berries. *Journal of the Science of Food and Agriculture* 83(4):330–337.

Piwsaoad, J. and Pusumpao, C. 2015. Experimental performance and neural network modeling of solar dryer for drying bamboo shoot strips in Thailand. *International Journal of Scientific and Engineering Research* 6(6):1306–1310.

Plat, J. and Mensink, R.P. 2005. Plant stanol and sterol esters in the control of blood cholesterol levels: Mechanism and safety aspects. *The American Journal of Cardiology* 96(1A):15D–22D.

Pongprasert, N., Wongs-Aree, C., Srilaong, V. and Kanlayanarat, S. 2007. Alleviation of browning and lignification in minimally processed sweet bamboo (Dendrocalamus asper) shoots by packaging. *New Zealand Journal of Crop and Horticultural Science* 35(2):253–257.

Poudyal, P.P. 2006. *Bamboos of Sikkim (India), Bhutan, and Nepal.*.New Hira Books Enterprises: Kathmandu, Nepal.

Prakash, G., Varma, A.J., Prabhune, A., Shouche, Y. and Rao, M. 2011. Microbial production of xylitol from d-xylose and sugarcane bagasse hemicellulose using newly isolated thermotolerant yeast Debaryomyces hansenii. *Bioresource Technology* 102(3):3304–3308.

Premlata, T., Saini, N., Chongtham, N. and Bisht, M.S. 2015. Nutrient components in young shoots of edible bamboos of Manipur, India. In: *Proceedings of the 10th World Bamboo Congress*, Damyang, South Korea.

Puupponen-Pimiä, R., Nohynek, L., Meier, C., Kähkönen, M., Heinonen, M., Hopia, A. and Oksman-Caldentey, K.M. 2001. Antimicrobial properties of phenolic compounds from berries. *Journal of Applied Microbiology* 90(4):494–507.

Qing, Y., Zhu, B.D., Zheng, L.W., Kai, H.H., Qi, X.S. and Zhen, H.P. 2008. Bamboo resources, utilization and ex-situ conservation in Xishuangbanna, South-Eastern China. *Journal of Forestry Research* 19(1):79–83.

Qiu, F.G. 1992. The recent development of bamboo foods. In: *Proceedings of the International Symposium on Industrial Use of Bamboo,* International Timber Organization and Chinese Academy of Forestry, Beijing, China, Bamboo and Its Use, pp. 333–337.

Qiu, Y.H., Shao, X.G., Zhang, F.G., Hua, W.L. and Bao, L.W. 1999. Analysis of physical behaviours and nutrition constituents of Phyllostachys heteroclada bamboo shoots. *Journal of Zhejiang Forestry College* 16(2):200–202.

Rajyalakshmi, P. and Geervani, P. 1994. Nutritive value of the foods cultivated and consumed by the tribals of South India. *Plant Foods for Human Nutrition* 46(1):53–61.

Ramakrishnappa, K. 2002. Biodiversity and the ecosystem approach in agriculture, forestry and fisheries. In: *Satellite Event on the Occasion of the Ninth Regular Session of the Commission on Genetic Resources for Food and Agriculture*, October 12–13, 2002, Rome. Inter-departmental working group on biological diversity for food and agriculture.

Rana, B., Awasthi, P. and Kumbhar, B.K. 2012. Optimization of processing conditions for cyanide content reduction in fresh bamboo shoot during NaCl treatment by response surface methodology. *Journal of Food Science and Technology* 49(1):103–109.

Ranilla, L.G., Kwon, Y.I., Genovese, M.I., Lajolo, F.M. and Shetty, K. 2010. Effect of thermal treatment on phenolic compounds and functionality linked to Type 2 Diabetes and hypertension management of Peruvian and Brazilian bean cultivars (Phaseolus vulgaris L.) using in vitro methods. *Journal of Food Biochemistry* 34(2):329–355.

Rathod, J.D., Pathak, N.L., Patel, R.G., Jivani, N.P. and Bhatt, N.M. 2011. Phytopharmacological properties of Bambusa arundinacea as a potential medicinal tree: An overview. *Journal of Applied Pharmaceutical Science* 1(10):27–31.

Rawat. 2017. *Effect of Various Processing Techniques on the Nutrient Content of Juvenile Edible Shoots of Some Commercially Important Bamboo.* A thesis submitted to Panjab University, Chandigarh, India.

Rawat, K., Chongtham, N. and Bisht, M.S. 2015. Processing techniques for reduction of cyanogenic glycosides from bamboo shoots. In: *10th World Bamboo Congress*, Korea.

Rawat, K., Chongtham, N. and Bisht, M.S. 2018. Quantitative assessment of silicon in fresh and processed bamboo shoots and its potential as functional element in food, nutraceuticals and cosmeceuticals. In: *11th World Bamboo Congress*, Mexico.

Rawat, K., Sharma, V., Saini, N., Chongtham, N. and Bisht, M.S. 2016. Impact of different boiling and soaking treatments on the release and retention of antinutrients and nutrients from the edible shoots of three bamboo species. *American Journal of Food Science and Nutrition Research* 3(3):31–41.

Ribas-Agustí, A., Martín-Belloso, O., Soliva-fortuny, R. and Elez-Martínez, P. 2018. Food processing strategies to enhance phenolic compounds bioaccessibility and bioavailability in plant-based foods. *Critical Reviews in Food Science and Nutrition* 58(15):2531–2548.

Rosales, S.L.O., Anog, B.F.A., Blanza, R.M. et al. 2013. Cardio protective activity of Bambusa blumeana Schultes leaf crude extract against isoproterenol-induced myocardial infarction in Sprague-Dawley rats.

Rosalki, S.B. and Mcintyre, N.I. 1999. Biochemical Investigations in the Management of Liver Disease. In: *Oxford Textbook of Clinical Hepatology* (Vol. 2). pp. 506–507.

Rosen, H.R. and Keeffe, E.B. 2000. *Evaluation of Abnormal Liver Enzymes, Use of Liver Test, and the Serology of Viral Hepatitis, Liver Disease Diagnosis and Management.* Churchill, New York.

Ruan, Q.Y., Zheng, X.Q., Chen, B.L., Xiao, Y., Peng, X., Leung, D.W.M. and Liu, E. 2013. Determination of total oxalate contents of a great variety of foods commonly available in southern China using an oxalate oxidase prepared from wheat bran. *Journal of Food Composition and Analysis* 32(1):6–11.

Ruenkaew, P. 2009. Towards the formation of a community: Thai migrants in Japan. In: R.G. Abad (Ed.) *Part III: Outcomes of Globalisation (The Papers of the 2001 API Fellows).* The Nippon Foundation, Tokyo, pp. 36–55.

Rui, L. and Liangru, W. 2008. Bamboo shoots as natural resources of high-zinc vegetables. *Journal of Bamboo Research* 27:4.

Ruiz-Ozeda, L.M. and Penas, F.J. 2013. Comparison study of conventional hot-water and microwave blanching on quality of green beans. *Innovative Food Science and Emerging Technologies* 20:191–197.

Rukaguer, M., Neugebauer, R.J. and Plecko, T. 2001. The relation between selenium, zinc and copper concentration and trace element dependent antioxidative status. *Journal of Trace Elements in Medicine and Biology* 15:73–78.

Saini 2019. *Shelf-Life Enhancement of Juvenile Shoots of Edible Bamboos through Different Processing and Preservation Techniques, and Evaluation of Their Phytochemicals.* A thesis submitted to Panjab University, Chandigarh, India.

Saini, N., Chongtham, N. and Bisht, M.S. 2015. Bamboo resource of Himachal Pradesh (India) and potential of shoots in socio-economic development of the state. In: *Proceedings of the 10th World Bamboo Congress*, Damyang, Korea.

Saini, N., Rawat, K., Bisht, M.S. and Chongtham, N. 2017. Qualitative and quantitative mineral element variances in shoots of two edible bamboo species after processing and storage evaluated by Wavelength Dispersion X-ray fluorescence Spectrometry. *International Journal of Innovative Research in Science, Engineering and Technology* 6(5):8265–8270.

Sakai, S., Saito, G., Sugayama, J., Kamasuka, T., Takada, S. and Takano, T. 1963. On the anticancer action of bamboo extract. *The Journal of Antibiotics.Series B* 16:387.

Saliu, J.A., Ademiluyi, A.O., Akinyemi, A.J. and Oboh, G. 2012. In vitro antidiabetes and antihypertension properties of phenolic extracts from bitter leaf (Vernonia amygdalina Del.). *Journal of Food Biochemistry* 36(5):569–576.

Sandhiya, S., Subhasree, N., Shivapriya, S., Agrawal, A. and Dubey, G.P. 2013. In vitro antioxidant and antimicrobial potential of Bambusa arundinacea (Retz.) wild. *International Journal of Pharmacy and Pharmaceutical Sciences* 5(2):359–362.

Sanlier, N., Gokcen, B.B. and Sezgin, A. 2019. Health benefits of fermented foods. *Critical Reviews in Food Science and Nutrition* 59(3):506–527.

Santosh, O., Bajwa, H.K. and Bisht, M.S. 2018. Freeze-dried bamboo shoot powder for food fortification: Enrichment of nutritional content and organoleptic qualities of fortified biscuits. *MOJ Food Processing and Technology* 6(4):342–348.

Santosh, O., Bajwa, H.K., Bisht, M.S. and Chongtham, N. 2019. Functional biscuits from bamboo shoots: Enrichment of nutrients, bioactive compounds and minerals in bamboo shoot paste fortified biscuits. *International Journal of Food Science and Nutrition* 4(1):89–94.

Sarangthem, K. and Singh, T. 2013. Fermentation decreases the antinutritional content in bamboo shoots. *International Journal of Current Microbiology and Applied Sciences* 2(11):361–369.

Sarangthem, K. and Singh, T.N. 2003a. Microbial bioconversion of metabolites from fermented succulent bamboo shoots into phytosterols. *Current Science* 84:1544–1547.

Sarangthem, K. and Singh, T.N. 2003b. biosynthesis of succulent bamboo shoots of Bambusa balcooa into phytosterols and its biotransformation into ADD. *Acta Botanica Sinica* 45(1):114–117.

Sarangthem, K. and Singh, T.N. 2003c. Transformation of fermented bamboo (Dendrocalamus hamiltonii) shoots into phytosterols by microorganisms. *Journal of Food Science and Technology* 40:622–625.

Sarangthem, K., Singh, L.J. and Srivastava, R.C. 2003. Isolation of phytosterols from fresh and fermented succulent bamboo shoots grown in Manipur and their bioconversion into androsta-1, 4-diene-3, 17-dione. In: P. Shanmughavel, R.S. Peddappaiah and W. Liese (Eds.) *Recent Advances in Bamboo Research*, Scientific Publishers: Jodhpur, India. pp. 121–130.

Sastry, C.B. 2008. A 2020 Vision for bamboos in India: Opportunities and challenges. In: *Proceedings of the International Conference. Improvement of Bamboo Productivity and Marketing for Sustainable Livelihood*, April 15–17, New Delhi, pp. 6–15.

Satya, S., Singhal, P., Prabhu, V.G., Bal, L.M. and Sudhakar, P. 2009. Exploring the nutraceutical potential and food safety aspect of bamboo shoot of some Indian species. In: *VIII World Bamboo Conference*, Bangkok, Thailand.

Schillaci, C., Nepravishta, R. and Bellomaria, A. 2013. Antioxidants in food and pharmaceutical research. *Albanian Journal of Pharmaceutical Sciences* 1(1):9–15.

Schulz, H., Engelharat, U.H., Wegent, A., Drews, H.H. and Lapezynski, S. 1999. Application of near infrared reflectance spectroscopy to the simultaneous prediction of alkaloids and phenolic substances in green tea leaves. *Journal of Agricultural and Food Chemistry* 47(12):5064–5067.

Scurlock, J.M.O., Dayton, D.C. and Hames, B. 2000. Bamboo: An overlooked biomass resource? *Biomass and Bioenergy* 19(4):229–244.

Seethalakshmi, K.K. and Kumar, M.S.M. 1998. *Bamboos of India: A Compendium*. Kerala Forest Research Institute, Kerala, India and INBAR, China.

Seki, T., Kida, K. and Maeda, H. 2010. Immunostimulation-mediated anti-tumor activity of bamboo (Sasa senanensis) leaf extracts obtained under 'vigorous' condition. *Evidence-Based Complementary and Alternative Medicine* 7(4):447–457.

Seki, T. and Maeda, H. 2010. Cancer preventive effect of Kumaizasa bamboo leaf extracts administered prior to carcinogenesis or cancer inoculation. *Anticancer Research* 30(1):111–118.

Senthilkumar, M.K., Sivakumar, P., Changanakkattil, F., Rajesh, V. and Perumal, P. 2011. Evaluation of anti-diabetic activity of Bambusa vulgaris leaves in streptozotocin induced diabetic rats. *International Journal of Pharmaceutical Sciences and Drug Research* 3(3):208–210.

Shanmugam, S., Bora, A., Raju, A., Asokapandian, S., Gabriela John, S. and Maharaja Sundari, K. 2016. Application of antioxidant from bamboo shoot (Bambusa balcooa) as an effective way to reduce the formation of acrylamide in fried potato chips. *Current Nutrition and Food Science* 12(4):256–263.

Shanmughavel, P. 2004. Cultivation potential of culinary bamboos in Southern India. *Natural Product Radiance* 3(4):237–239.

Shapiro, T.A., Fahey, J.W., Dinkova-Kostova, A.T. et al. 2006. Safety, tolerance, and metabolism of Broccoli Sprout glucosinolates and isothiocyanates: A clinical phase I study. *Nutrition and Cancer* 55(1):53–62.

Shapiro, T.A., Fahey, J.W., Wade, K.L., Stephenson, K.K. and Talalay, P. 2001. Chemoprotective glucosinolates and isothiocyanates of Broccoli sprouts: Metabolism and excretion in humans. *Cancer Epidemiology, Biomarkers and Prevention* 10(5):501–508.

Sharma, M.L. and Chongtham, N. 2015. Bamboo diversity of India: An update. In: *Proceedings of the 10th World Bamboo Congress*, Damyang, Korea.

Sharma, M.L., Chongtham, N., Richa and David, E. 2004. Variations in nutrient and nutritional components of juvenile bamboo shoots. *Panjab University Research Journal (Sci)* 54:101–104.

Sharma, N. and Barooah, M. 2017. Microbiology of khorisa, its proximate composition and probiotic potential of lactic acid bacteria present in khorisa, a traditional fermented bamboo shoot product of Assam. *Indian Journal of Natural Products and Resources (IJNPR) [formerly Natural Product Radiance (NPR)]* 8(1):78–88.

Sharma, U.K. and Pegu, S. 2011. Ethnobotany of religious and supernatural beliefs of the Mising tribes of Assam with special reference to the 'Dobur Uie'. *Journal of Ethnobiology and Ethnomedicine* 7(1):16.

Sharma, V. 2018. *Changes in Bioactive Components and Anti-Nutrients during Processing of Bamboo Shoots*. Ph.D. Thesis, Panjab University, Chandigarh, India.

Shen, Q., Kong, F. and Wang, Q. 2006. Effect of modified atmosphere packaging on the browning and lignification of bamboo shoots. *Journal of Food Engineering* 77(2):348–354.

Shi, Q.T. and Yang, K.S. 1992. Study on relationship between nutrients in bamboo shoots and human health. In: *Bamboo and Its Use. Proceedings of the International Symposium on Industrial Use of Bamboo. International Tropical Timber Organization and Chinese Academy*, Beijing, China, pp. 338–346.

Shimizu, J., Yamada, N., Nakamura, K., Takita, T. and Innami, S. 1996. Effects of different types of dietary fibre preparations isolated from bamboo shoots, edible burdock, apple and corn on fecal steroid profiles of rats. *Journal of Nutritional Science and Vitaminology* 42(6):527–539.

Shin, H.Y., Lee, E.H., Kim, C.Y. et al. 2003. Anti-inflammatory activity of Korean folk medicine purple bamboo salt. *Immunopharmacology and Immunotoxicology* 25(3):377–384.

Singh, B., Singh, J.P., Kaur, A. and Singh, N. 2016. Bioactive compounds in banana and their associated health benefits–A review. *Food Chemistry* 206:1–11.

Singh, H.B., Kumar, B. and Singh, R.S. 2003. Bamboo resources of Manipur: An overview for management and conservation. *Journal of Bamboo and Rattan* 2(1):43–55.

Singh, S.A., Bora, T.C. and Singh, N.R. 2012. Preliminary phytochemical analysis and antimicrobial potential of fermented bambusa balcooa shoots. *The Bioscan* 7(3):391–394.

Singh, V.K., Rahul, S., Satish, V., Shankul, K., Sumit, G. and Ashutosh, M. 2010. Antibacterial activity of leaves of bamboo. *International Journal of Pharmacy and Biological Sciences* 1(2):33.

Soesanto, E. 2016. Antioxidant activity of extracts from Bambusa vulgaris and Gigantochloa apus Kurz bamboo shoots. *Pakistan Journal of Nutrition* 15(6):580.

Song, L., Chen, H., Gao, H. et al. 2013. Combined modified atmosphere packaging and low temperature storage delay lignification and improve the defence response of minimally processed water bamboo shoot. *Chemistry Central Journal* 7(1):147.

Song, L.L., Gao, H.Y., Chen, W.X. et al. 2011. The role of 1-Methylcyclopropene in lignification and expansin gene expression in peeled water bamboo shoot (Zizania caduciflora L.). *Journal of the Science of Food and Agriculture* 91(14):2679–2683.

Soni, V., Jha, A.K., Dwivedi, J. and Soni, P. 2013. Traditional uses, phytochemistry and pharmacological profile of Bambusa arudinacea Retz. *TANG [Humanitas Medicine]* 3(3):6.

Sood, S., Walia, S., Gupta, M. and Sood, A. 2013. Nutritional characterization of shoots and other edible products of an edible bamboo–Dendrocalamus hamiltonii. *Current Research in Nutrition and Food Science Journal* 1(2):169–176.

Sood, S., Walia, S. and Sood, A. 2017. Quality evaluation of different species of edible bamboo shoots. *ARC Journal of Nutrition and Growth* 3(1):1–6.

Srivastava, R.C. 1990. Bamboo: New raw materials for phytosterols. *Current Science* 59:1333–1334.

Srivastava, G., Su, T., Mehrotra, R.C., Kumari, P. and Shankar, U. 2019. Bamboo fossils from Oligo–Pliocene sediments of northeast India with implications on their evolutionary ecology and biogeography in Asia. *Review of Palaeobotany and Palynology* 262:17–27.

Stapleton, C.M.A. 1994. The bamboos of Nepal and Bhutan. Part I: Bambusa, Dendrocalamus, Melocanna, Cephalostachyum, Teinostachyum, and Pseudostachyum (Gramineae: Poaceae, Bambusoideae). *Edinburgh Journal of Botany* 51(1):1–32.

Sukenti, K. 2014. Gastronomy tourism in several neighbour countries of Indonesia: A Brief Review. *Journal of Indonesian Tourism and Development Studies* 2(2):55–63.

Sukmaningsih, A.A.S.A., Gunam, I.B.W., Antara, N.S., Kencana, P.K.D. and Widia, I.W. 2017. Potential aphrodisiac activity of tabah bamboo shoots (Gigantochloa nigrociliata) in male mouse. *Jurnal Veteriner* 18(3):393–402.

Sun, J., Chu, Y.F., Wu, X. and Liu, R.H. 2002a. Antioxidant and antiproliferative activities of common fruits. *Journal of Agricultural and Food Chemistry* 50(25):7449–7454.

Sun, J., Ding, Z.Q., Gao, Q., Xun, H., Tang, F. and Xia, E.D. 2015. Major chemical constituents of bamboo shoots (Phyllostachys pubescens): Qualitative and quantitative research. *The Journal of Agricultural and Food Chemistry* 64(12):2498–2505.

Sun, R.C., Sun, X.F. and Ma, X.H. 2002b. Effect of ultrasound on the structural and physiochemical properties of organosolv soluble hemicelluloses from wheat straw. *Ultrasonics Sonochemistry* 9(2):95–101.

Sundriyal, M. and Sundriyal, R.C. 2001. Wild edible plants of the Sikkim Himalaya: Nutritive values of selected species. *Economic Botany* 55(3):377–390.

Svanberg, U., Lorri, W. and Sandberg, A.S. 1993. Lactic fermentation of non-tannin and high-tannin cereals: Effect on *in vitro* estimation of iron availability and phytate hydrolysis. *Journal of Food Science* 58(2):408–412.

Tabet, R.B., Oftedal, O.T. and Allen, M.E. 2004. Seasonal differences in composition of bamboo fed to giant pandas (*Ailuropoda malanoleuca*) at the National Zoo. In: *Proceedings of the Fifth Comparative Nutrition Society Symposium*, pp. 176–180.

Tamang, B. and Tamang, J.P. 2009. Traditional knowledge of biopreservation of perishable vegetable and bamboo shoots in Northeast India as food resources. *Indian Journal of Traditional Knowledge* 8(1):89–95.

Tamang, B., Tamang, J.P., Schillinger, U., Franz, C.M.A.P., Gores, M. and Holzapfel, W.H. 2008. Phenotypic and genotypic identification of lactic acid bacteria isolated from ethnic fermented bamboo tender shoots of north east India. *International Journal of Food Microbiology* 121(1):35–40.

Tanabe, C., Furuta, K., Maeda, M. and Kimura, Y. 2017. Structural feature of N-glycans of bamboo shoot glycoproteins: Useful source of plant antigenic N-glycans. *Bioscience, Biotechnology, and Biochemistry* 81(7):1405–1408.

Tanaka, A., Kim, H.J., Oda, S., Shimizu, K. and Kondo, R. 2011. Antibacterial activity of Moso bamboo shoot skin (Phyllostachys pubescens) against Staphylococcus aureus. *Journal of Wood Science* 57(6):542–544.

Tanaka, A., Shimizu, K. and Kondo, R. 2013. Antibacterial compounds from shoot skins of Moso bamboo (Phyllostachys pubescens). *Journal of Wood Science* 59(2):155–159.

Tandug, L.M. and Torres, F.G. 1985. Mensurational attributes of five Philippine erect bamboos. In recent research on bamboos. In: *Proceedings of the International Bamboo Workshop*, Chinese Academy of Forestry (CAF), Hangzhou, People's Republic of China.

Tao, C., Wang, Y., Zhang, X. et al. 2019. Mechanism of action of essential oils extracted from bamboo (Phyllostachys heterocycla cv. pubescens) leaves: Chemical composition and antimicrobial activity against four food-related microorganisms. *BioResources* 14(1):1419–1434.

Tao, C., Wu, J., Liu, Y., Liu, M., Yang, R. and Lv, Z. 2018.Antimicrobial activities of bamboo (Phyllostachys heterocycla cv. *Pubescens*) leaf essential oil and its major components. *European Food Research and Technology* 244(5):881–891.

Taylor, E.N. and Curhan, G.C. 2008. Determinants of 24-hour urinary oxalate excretion. *Clinical Journal of the American Society of Nephrology: CJASN* 3(5):1453–1460.

Teron, R. and Borthakur, S.K. 2012. Traditional uses of bamboos among the Karbis, a hill tribe of India. *Bamboo Science and Culture* 25(1):43–49.

Tewari, D.N. 1992. *A Monograph on Bamboo.* International Book Distributors, Dehradun, Uttaranchal, India.

Thamizharasan, S., Umamaheswari, S., HARI, R. and Monisha, S. 2015. Antimicrobial activity of Bambusa arundinacea seeds. *International Journal of Pharmacy and Biological Sciences* 6(4):540–546.

Thomas, R., Jebin, N., Barman, K. and Das, A. 2014. Quality and shelf life evaluation of pork nuggets incorporated with fermented bamboo shoot (Bambusa polymorpha) mince. *Meat Science* 96(3):1210–1218.

Thomas, R., Jebin, N., Saha, R. and Sarma, D.K. 2016. Antioxidant and antimicrobial effects of kordoi (Averrhoa carambola) fruit juice and bamboo (Bambusa polymorpha) shoot extract in pork nuggets. *Food Chemistry* 190:41–49.

Toan, N., Xuan, T., Thu Ha, P., Tu Anh, T. and Khanh, T. 2018. Inhibitory effects of bamboo leaf on the growth of Pyricularia grisea fungus. *Agriculture* 8(7):92.

Tom, K.S. 1989. *Echoes from Old China: Life, Legends, and Lore of the Middle Kingdom.* University of Hawaii Press, Honolulu, HI. pp. 108.

Tripathi, Y.C. 1998. Food and nutrition potential of bamboo. *MFP News* 8(1):10–11.

Triplett, J.K., Weakley, A.S. and Clark, L.G. 2006. Hill Cane. (Arundinaria appalachiana) A new species of bamboo from the southern appalachian mountains. *Sida* 22:79–85.

Tsunoda, S., Yamamoto, K., Sakamoto, S., Inoue, H. and Nagasawa, H. 1998. Effects of Sasa health, extract of bamboo grass leaves, on spontaneous mammary tumourigenesis in SHN Mice. *Anticancer Research* 18(1A):153–158.

Valkosen. 2001. Efficacy of garlic fruits and bamboo shoots in deworming Swine. In: *Proceedings of the 26th Annual Conference of the Nigerian Society of Animal Production*, NAPRI, Zaria, Nigeria, pp. 50–51.

Velioglu, Y.S., Mazza, G., Gao, L. and Oomah, B.D. 1998. Antioxidant activity and total phenolics in selected fruits, vegetables and grain production. *Journal of Agricultural and Food Chemistry* 46(10):4113–4117.

Velmurugan, R. and Muthukumar, K. 2011. Utilization of sugarcane bagasse for bioethanol production: Sono-assisted acid hydrolysis approach. *Bioresource Technology* 102(14):7119–7123.

Vilahur, G., Ben-Aicha, S., Diaz, E., Badimon, L. and Padró, T. 2019. Phytosterols and inflammation. *Current Medicinal Chemistry.* DOI: 10.2174/0929867325 666180622151438.

Visuphaka, K. 1985. The role of bamboo as a potential food source in Thailand. In: *Proceedings of the International Bamboo Workshop, October 6–14, 1985*, Hangzhou, China. Recent Research on Bamboos, pp. 301–303.

Viswanath, S., Geeta, J., Somashekar, P.V., Jagadish, M.R. and Joshi, S.C. 2012. *Guadua angustifolia Kunth: Potential Bamboo Species for Humid Tropics of Peninsular India.* IWST Publication, Bangalore.

Vivekanandan, K. 1985. Bamboo research in Sri Lanka. Recent research on bamboos. In: *Proceedings of the International Bamboo Workshop*, Chinese Academy of Forestry (CAF), Hangzhou, People's Republic of China, p. 61.

Waikhom, S.D., Louis, B., Sharma, C.K., Kumari, P., Somkuwar, B.G., Singh, M.W. and Talukdar, N.C. 2013. Grappling the high altitude for safe edible bamboo shoots with rich nutritional attributes and escaping cyanogenic toxicity. *BioMed Research International* 2013:1–11. Article ID 289285. DOI: org/10.1155/2013/289285.

Wang, C.H., Ma, Y.L., Zhu, D.Y. et al. 2017. Physicochemical and functional properties of dietary fiber from bamboo shoots (Phyllostachys praecox). *Emirates Journal of Food and Agriculture* 29(7):509–517.

Wang, C.H., Ni, Z.J., Ma, Y.L. et al. 2019. Antioxidant and hypolipidemic potential of soluble dietary fiber extracts derived from bamboo shoots (Phyllostachys praecox). *Current Topics in Nutraceutical Research* 17(2).

Wang, J., Yue, Y.D., Jiang, H. and Tang, F. 2012. Rapid screening for flavone C-glycosides in the leaves of different species of bamboo and simultaneous quantitation of four marker compounds by HPLC-UV/DAD. *International Journal of Analytical Chemistry.* 2012:205101. DOI: 10.1155/2012/205101

Wang, K.H. and He, Y.F. 1989. Study on physiological characters of bamboo shoots in storage. *Journal of Zhejiang Forestry Science and Technology* 5:19–25.

Wani, M.A., Prasad, S. and Prakash, O. 2019. Qualitative phytochemical analysis of various parts of bamboo (*Bambusa balcooa*) for possible therapeutic usages in bovine reproductive disorders. *Journal of Pharmacognosy and Phytochemistry* 8(1):217–221.

Wasnik, D.D. and Tumane, P.M. 2014. Antibacterial activity of Bambusa bambose L. against multiple drug resistant bacteria isolated from clinical specimen. *International Journal of Pharmaceutical Sciences Review and Research* 25:215–218.

Wedler, J., Daubitz, T., Schlotterbeck, G. and Butterweck, V. 2014. In vitro anti-inflammatory and wound-healing potential of a Phyllostachys edulis leaf extract–identification of isoorientin as an active compound. *Planta Medica* 80(18):1678–1684.

Weihrauch, J.L. and Gardner, J.M. 1978. Sterol content of foods of plant origin. *Journal of the American Dietetic Association* 73(1):39–47.

Weiner, I.D., Linas, S.L. and Wingo, C.S. 2018. Disorders of potassium metabolism. In: R. Johnson, J. Fluege, J. Feehally and T. Marcello (Eds.) *Comprehensive Clinical Nephrology*, 4th ed. Elsevier Saunders, Philadelphia, PA, pp. 111–124.

WHO. 2015. *The Global Prevalence of Anaemia in 2011.* World Health Organization, Geneva.

WHO. 2019. Global Spending on Health: A World in Transition, Global Report 2019.

Wongsakpairod, T. 2000. *Bamboo Shoot Drying Using Superheated Steam.* Meng Thesis. King Mongkut's University of Technology, Thonburi, Bangkok, Thailand.

Woyengo, T.A., Ramprasath, V.R. and Jones, P.J.H. 2009. Anticancer effects of phytosterols. *European Journal of Clinical Nutrition* 63(7):813–820.

Wróblewska, K.B., Baby, A.R., Guaratini, M.T.G. and Moreno, P.R.H. 2019. *In vitro* antioxidant and photoprotective activity of five native Brazilian bamboo species. *Industrial Crops and Products* 130:208–215.

Wu, G. 2013. *Amino Acids: Biochemistry and Nutrition*. CRC Press, Boca Raton, FL.

Xia, N.H. 1989. Analysis of nutritive constituents of bamboo shoots in Guangdong. *Acta Botanica Austro Sinica* 4:199–206.

Xia, Y., Hill, K.E. and Burk, R.F. 1985. Effect of selenium deficiency on hydroperoxide-induced glutathione release from the isolated perfused rat heart. *The Journal of Nutrition* 115(6):733–742.

Xu, S., Cao, W., Song, Y. and Fang, L. 2005. Analysis and evaluation of protein and amino acid nutritional components of different species of bamboo shoots. *Food Science* 26:222–227.

Xu, X.B., Tang, F., Guo, X.F. et al. 2015. Isolation, identification and determination of six nucleosides and two amino acids from bamboo shoots of Gramineae Phyllostachys prominens (WY Xiong). *Tropical Journal of Pharmaceutical Research* 14(12): 2239–2246.

Xu, Y., Zhang, M., Tu, D., Sun, J., Zhou, L. and Mujumdar, A.S. 2005. A two-stage convective air and vacuum freeze drying technique for bamboo shoots. *International Journal of Food Science and Technology* 40(6):589–595.

Yamaguchi, M. 1983. Other succulent vegetables. In: *World Vegetables*. Springer, Netherlands, pp. 356–380.

Yamaguchi, T., Katsuda, M., Oda, Y. et al. 2003. Influence of polyphenol and ascorbate oxidases during cooking process on the radical scavenging activity of vegetables. *Food Science and Technology Research* 9(1):79–83.

Yang, G.Q., Wang, S.Z., Zhou, R.H. and Sun, S.Z. 1983. Endemic selenium intoxication of humans in China. *The American Journal of Clinical Nutrition* 37(5):872–881.

Yang, H., Zheng, J., Huang, C., Zhao, X., Chen, H. and Sun, Z. 2015. Effects of combined aqueous chlorine dioxide and chitosan coatings on microbial growth and quality maintenance of fresh-cut bamboo shoots (Phyllostachys praecox F. prevernalis.) during Storage. *Food and Bioprocess Technology* 8(5):1011–1019.

Yang, H., Zhou, C., Wu, F. and Cheng, J. 2010. Effect of nitric oxide on browning and lignification of peeled bamboo shoots. *Postharvest Biology and Technology* 57(1):72–76.

Yang, J.H., Choi, M.H., Yang, S.H., Cho, S.S., Park, S.J., Shin, H.J. and Ki, S.H. 2017. Potent anti-inflammatory and antiadipogenic properties of bamboo (Sasa coreana Nakai) leaves extract and its major constituent flavonoids. *Journal of Agricultural and Food Chemistry* 65(31):6665–6673.

Yang, J.H., Lim, H.S. and Heo, Y.R. 2010. Sasa borealis leaves extract improves insulin resistance by modulating inflammatory cytokine secretion in high fat diet-induced obese C57/BL6J Mice. *Nutrition Research and Practice* 4(2):99–105.

Yang, Q., Duan, Z., Wang, Z., He, K., Sun, Q. and Peng, Z. 2008. Bamboo resources, utilization and ex-situ conservation in Xishuangbanna, South-Eastern China. *Journal of Forestry Research* 19(1):79–83.

Yang, R.Y., Tsou, S.C.S., Lee, T.C., Hanson, P.M. and Lai, P.Y. 2005. Antioxidant capacities and daily antioxidant intake from vegetables consumed in Taiwan. In: *Symposium on Taiwan-America Agricultural Cooperative Projects*, National Taiwan University, Taipei, Taiwan.

Yang, Y. 2002. *Chinese Herbal Medicines Comparisons and Characteristics*. Churchill Livingstone, London.

Yasin, S., Liu, L. and Yao, J. 2013. Biosynthesis of silver nanoparticles by bamboo leaves extract and their antimicrobial activity. *Journal of Fiber and Bioengineering and Informatics* 6(6):77–84.

Yaun, J.X. 1983. Research on the production and botanical origin of bamboo juice in Eastern China. *Zhong Yao Tong Bao (Beijing, China: 1981)* 8(2):10–12.

Ying, C., Mao, Y., Chen, L., Wang, S., Ling, H., Li, W. and Zhou, X. 2017. Bamboo leaf extract ameliorates diabetic nephropathy through activating the AKT signalling pathway in rats. *International Journal of Biological Macromolecules* 105(3):1587–1594.

Yiping, L., Yanxia, L., Buckingham, K., Henley, G. and Guomo, Z. 2010. Bamboo and climate change mitigation. *International Network Bamboo and Rattan* 32.

Yoon, K.Y., Woodams, E.E. and Hang, Y.D. 2006. Enzymatic production of pentoses from the hemicellulose fraction of corn residues. *LWT-Food Science and Technology* 39(4):388–392.

Yoshioka, H., Mori, M., Yoshikawa, M., Fujii, H., Nagatsu, A. and Nonogaki, T. 2017b. Suppressive effect of Sasa veitchii extract on obesity induced by a high-fat diet through modulation of adipose differentiation in mice. *Fundamental Toxicological Sciences* 4(6):261–268.

Yoshioka, H., Usuda, H., Fujii, H. and Nonogaki, T. 2017a. Sasa veitchii extracts suppress acetaminophen-induced hepatotoxicity in mice. *Environmental Health and Preventive Medicine* 22(1):54.

You, Y., Kim, K., Heo, H., Lee, K., Lee, J., Shim, S. and Jun, W. 2006. Stimulatory effects of Pseudosasa japonica leaves on exercise performance. *Bioscience, Biotechnology and Biochemistry* 70(10):2532–2535.

You, Y., Kim, K., Yoon, H.G., Choi, K.C., Lee, Y.H., Lee, J. and Jun, W. 2015. Sasa borealis extract efficiently enhanced swimming capacity by improving energy metabolism and the antioxidant defense system in mice. *Journal of Nutritional Science and Vitaminology* 61(6):488–496.

Yudodibroto, H. 1985. Bamboo research in Indonesia. In: *Recent Research on Bamboos. Proceedings of the International Bamboo Workshop*, Chinese Academy of Forestry (CAF), Hangzhou, People's Republic of China, pp. 33–44.

Yuming, Y. and Jiru, X. 1998. Bamboo resources and their utilization in China. In: *Proceedings of the Workshop 'Bamboo Conservation, Diversity, Eco-Geography, Germplasm, Resource Utilization and Taxonomy'*. Kunming and Xishaungbanna, Yunnan, China, pp. 10–17.

Yuming, Y., Kanglin, W., Shengji, P. and Jiming, H. 2004. Bamboo diversity and traditional uses in Yunnan, China. *Mountain Research and Development* 24(2):157–165.

Zeng, F., Luo, Z., Xie, J. and Feng, S. 2015. Gamma radiation control quality and lignification of bamboo shoots (Phyllostachys praecox F. prevernalis.) stored at low temperature. *Postharvest Biology and Technology* 102:17–24.

Zeng, H., Chen, J., Zhai, J., Wang, H., Xia, W. and Xiong, Y.L. 2016. Reduction of the fat content of battered and breaded fish balls during deep-fat frying using fermented bamboo shoot dietary fiber. *LWT – Food Science and Technology* 73:425–431.

Zhang, H., Zhang, Y., Wang, X., Xiang, Q., Bai, Y., Li, S. and Yang, L. 2017. Effects of bamboo shoot dietary fiber on mechanical properties, moisture distribution, and microstructure of frozen dough. *Journal of Chemistry*. 2017: 1–7. DOI: org/10.1155/2017/4513410.

Zhang, J., Gong, J., Ding, Y., Lu, B., Wu, X. and Zhang, Y. 2010. Antibacterial activity of water-phase extracts from bamboo shavings against food spoilage microorganisms. *African Journal of Biotechnology* 9(45):7710–7717.

Zhang, J.J., Ji, R., Hu, Y.Q., Chen, J.C. and Ye, X.Q. 2011. Effect of three cooking methods on nutrient components and antioxidant capacities of bamboo shoot (Phyllostachys praecox C.D. Chu et C.S. Chao). *Journal of Zhejiang University. Science. B* 12(9):752–759.

Zhang, S., Chen, J., Sun, A. and Zhao, L. 2014. Protective effects and antioxidant mechanism of bamboo leaf flavonoids on hepatocytes injured by CCl_4. *Food and Agricultural Immunology* 25(3):386–396.

Zhang, X.Y., Peng, Y., Su, R., Chen, Q.H., Ruan, H. and He, G.Q. 2013. Optimization of biotransformation from phytosterol to androstenedione by a mutant Mycobacterium neoaurum ZJUVN-08. *Journal of Zhejiang University – Science B* 14(2):132–143.

Zhang, Y. and Tang, L. 1997. Experimental studies on anti-aging effect of the leaf-extract of P. nigra var. henonis. *Journal of Bamboo Research* 16(4):62–67.

Zhang, Y., Yao, X., Bao, B. and Zhang, Y. 2006. Anti-fatigue activity of atriterpenoid-rich extract from Chinese bamboo shavings (Caulis Bamfusae in Taeniam). *Phytotherapy Research* 20(10):872–876.

Zhanwang, H., Shuangshuang, Z. and Shuibo, X. 2005. A study on antibacterial properties of bamboo leaf extracts from Phyllostachys pubescens. *Acta Agriculturae Universitatis Jiangxiensis* 27(6):960–963.

Zhao, X., Song, J.L., Kil, J.H. and Park, K.Y. 2013. Bamboo salt attenuates CCl_4-induced hepatic damage in Sprague-Dawley rats. *Nutrition Research and Practice* 7(4):273–280.

Zhaohua, Z. and Wei, J. 2018. *Sustainable Bamboo Development*. CABI. CPI Group UK (Ltd): Croydon, UK. ISBN-13: 9781786394019.

Zheng, J., Wu, J., Dai, Y., Kan, J. and Zhang, F. 2017. Influence of bamboo shoot dietary fiber on the rheological and textural properties of milk pudding. *LWT-Food Science and Technology* 84:364–369.

Zheng, J., Zhang, F., Zhou, C., Chen, G., Lin, M. and Kan, J. 2013. Changes in amino acid contents, texture and microstructure of bamboo shoots during pickling process. *International Journal of Food Science and Technology* 48(9):1847–1853.

Zheng, X.X., Chen, R.S., Shen, Y. and Yin, Z.Y. 2014. phytosterols elevation in bamboo shoot residue through laboratorial scale solid-state fermentation using isolated Aspergillus niger CTBU. *Applied Biochemistry and Biotechnology* 172(8):4078–4083.

Zhou, F. 1998. *Bamboo Forest Cultivation*. China Forestry Publishing House, Beijing.

Zhu, S.L., Ma, N.N. and Fu, M.Y. 1994. *A Compendium of Chinese Bamboo*. China Forestry Publishing House, Beijing.

Index

A

ACE, *see* Angiotensin converting enzyme
Acid detergent fibre (ADF), 98, 104, 183
ADF, *see* Acid detergent fibre
Alu-tama, 51
Amino acids, 76–78
AMP-activated protein kinase (AMPK), 60
AMPK, *see* AMP-activated protein kinase
Angiotensin converting enzyme (ACE), 67, 93
Anti-cancer properties, 58–59
Anti-diabetic properties, 60–61
Anti-fatigue properties, 61
Anti-inflammatory effect, 66
Anti-microbial activity, 63–65
Anti-nutrient compounds, 107, 112, 137–138, 144–145
  chemical structure, 114
  cyanogenic glycoside, 107–111, 133–135
  glucosinolates, 112–113
  oxalates, 110–112
  phytates, 113–114
  removal process, 133, 134
  saponins, 114–115
  tannins, 115
Anti-obesity properties, 61–63
Anti-oxidant activity, 192, 194–196
Anti-oxidant defense system, 197

B

Bamboo
  acreage, Asian countries, 14
  China, 5–6
  culms, 19–21
  culturally/economically important, 5–10
  diversity and distribution, 9–15
  flowers, 22–23
  food
    leaves, 30–31
    seeds, 30
    shoots, 31–32
  global regions, 12
  health benefits
    anti-cancer properties, 58–59
    anti-diabetic properties, 60–61
    anti-fatigue properties, 61
    anti-inflammatory effect, 66
    anti-microbial activity, 63–65
    anti-obesity properties, 61–63
    cardioprotective properties, 66–68
    hepatoprotective activity, 68–69
    immunomodulatory activity, 69
    prebiotics, 69–70
  lateral branching, 18
  leaves, 21
  medicine, 52–57
  nutraceutical products, 188–191
  origin, 4–5
  rhizome, 17–19
  rituals, 7–9
  roots, 19
  shoots, 21 (*see also* Bamboo shoots)
  south-east Asian countries, 6–10
  tribes, 11
  uses, 6–7, 23–25
    beer, 35
    biofuel, 29
    charcoal, 28–29
    cycle, 35
    decor/ornamental landscapes, 33
    fibre/fabric, 26–27
    fuel, 27
    gas, 29
    housing/building, 25–26
    leaf tea, 34
    medicine, 32
    paper/pulp industries, 26
    salt, 33
    toys, 34
Bamboo housing, 25
Bamboo linen, 27
Bamboo-manna/silica, 55, 56
Bamboo rayon, 27
Bamboo shoot dietary fibre (BSDF), 102, 103, 179, 180, 189
Bamboo shoot oil (BSO), 97
Bamboo shoot powder, 102, 105, 182, 183, 191, 205
Bamboo shoots
  aphrodisiac activity, 106
  vs. bacterial/fungal strains, 93
  consumption
    dish, Manipur, 49
    fermented, 49–51, 54
    fresh shoots, 47, 49
    recipes, 50–53, 55
  dietary fibre, 157–161
  extract preparation, 196
  food processing, 117 (*see also* Food fortification)
  GC-MS spectra, 192

health-enhancing properties, 71
morphology, 40, 46
names, 47
nutraceuticals, 188–189, 191 (*see also* Nutraceuticals)
nutrient content, processing, 137–138
ash, 148
carbohydrate, 139, 142, 143
fat, 146–147
free amino acid, 142, 143, 146
macronutrients, 140–141
moisture, 148, 149
protein, 139, 142
starch, 146, 147
vitamins, 148–150
nutrients (*see* Macro-minerals; Macro-nutrients; Micro-mineral elements; Micro-nutrients)
package, 165–166
atmospheric, 174
edible film/coatings, 174–175
effect, 167
material, 167
mode, 167
polyethylene, 168–171
polyvinyl chloride film, 171–173
vacuum, 173
phenol, 154–156
phytosterols, 157
processing unit, Korea, 118
species, 72
traditional practices/approaches, 57–58
Bambusa balcooa, 31, 86, 91, 119, 155, 175, 182
Banslochan, 4–5, 32, 55, 84, 203
Bansuri, 5, 8–9
Bas-tenga, 49
Bashchuri, 49
Bioactive compounds, 89
dietary fibre, 157–161
phenol, 154–156
phytosterols, 157
Biofuel, 29
Biscuits/cookies, 180, 182, 183
Black diamond, 28
Blanching, 124–125
Blood urea nitrogen (BUN), 201
Boiling, 125, 134, 139, 142, 146, 155, 159, 185
Bradford reagent, 76
BSDF, *see* Bamboo shoot dietary fibre
BSO, *see* Bamboo shoot oil
BUN, *see* Blood urea nitrogen

C

CAD, *see* Cinnamyl alcohol dehydrogenase
Candies, 184–185
Canning process, 133
Calcium, 80, 82
Carbohydrates, 78
Carbon sequestration, 3
Carboxymethyl cellulose (CMC), 175
Cardioprotective properties, 66–68
Cardiovascular disease (CVD), 66–68, 89, 194, 204
Caustic soda/lye, 27
Chanduwa, 7
Chimaki, 31
Chips, 185
Chyawanprash, 4–5, 32, 54–55
Cinnamyl alcohol dehydrogenase (CAD), 122
CMC, *see* Carboxymethyl cellulose
Convective tray-drying, 130–131
Copper, 85
Cornstarch, 185
Crackers, 186
Crude fibre content, 101, 102
Culm leaves, 17
Culm sheaths, 17, 21, 32, 64, 119, 133
CVD, *see* Cardiovascular disease
Cyanogenic glycosides, 133–135
animals, 108
content, 110, 111
enzymatic breakdown pathways, 109
freezing/maceration, 108
intact cells, 108
picrate paper, 109
plants, 107–108
species, 108–109
toxicity, 108

D

Dehydration, 126
Dietary fibre, 157–161
bamboo shoot powder, 102
blood biochemical parameters, 103–104
components, 103, 105
crude fibre content, 101, 102
definition, 98
forms, 98
functional properties, 98
heat digestion, ADF, 104
hemicelluloses, 101
ignition, NDF, 105
species, 101–102
water-soluble hemicelluloses, 104
Dobur Uie, 10
Domestic health expenditure, 90
Drying process, 125–126

E

EBS, *see* Extract from bamboo shavings
Eco-guardians, 3
Edible shoots, 39–45
Enzymatic breakdown pathways, 109

Epan thaba, 7
Ethylene treatment, 122
Extract from bamboo shavings (EBS), 61

F

FBS, *see* Fermented bamboo shoot
FBSM, *see* Fermented bamboo shoot mince
Female bamboos, 20
Fermentation, 49–50, 127–128
Fermented bamboo shoot (FBS), 49, 50, 95, 105, 128, 157, 184, 186
Fermented bamboo shoot mince (FBSM), 184
Flowering cycle, 22
Folin-Ciocalteu reagent, 91
Food fortification, 178–179
  biscuits/cookies, 180, 182, 183
  BSDF, 180
  candies, 184–185
  chips, 185
  crackers, 186
  dietary fibre, 179
  healthy diets, 179
  nuggets, 183–184
  pickles, 186–187
  XOS, 180
Fortification, 178
Fortified biscuits/cookies, 180, 182, 183
Freeze-drying, 131–132, 138
Freezing/maceration, 108
Fresh shoot extract, 199–201
Fuel
  biofuel, 29
  charcoal, 28–29
  gas, 29
Functional foods, 178

G

Gas chromatography combined with mass spectrometry (GC-MS), 97
GC-MS, *see* Gas chromatography combined with mass spectrometry
GFR, *see* Glomerular filtration rate
Gigantochloa atroviolacea, 14
Global environmental services, 3
Glomerular filtration rate (GFR), 202
Glucosinolates, 112–113, 135–136

H

Harvesting, 118–120
HDL, *see* High-density lipoproteins
HDPE, *see* High density polyethylene
Health benefits
  anti-cancer properties, 58–59
  anti-diabetic properties, 60–61
  anti-fatigue properties, 61
  anti-inflammatory effect, 66
  anti-microbial activity, 63–65
  anti-obesity properties, 61–63
  cardioprotective properties, 66–68
  hepatoprotective activity, 68–69
  immunomodulatory activity, 69
  prebiotics, 69–70
Healthy diets, 179
Hemicelluloses, 101
Hendua, 51
Hepatoprotective activity, 68–69, 94
High density polyethylene (HDPE), 168
High-density lipoproteins (HDL), 67, 199
Hot air-drying, 130–131
Hypocholesterolemic formulation, 95

I

IDF, *see* Insoluble dietary fibre
Immunomodulatory activity, 69
Incense bamboo, 20
Insoluble dietary fibre (IDF), 98, 105
Iron, 84–85

J

Jiang-sun, 47, 128, 130
Jukyeom, 33

K

Kalpavirksha, 5
Karbis, 7
Khorisa, 105
'King of Forest Vegetables,' 38
Kumaizasa bamboo, 59, 69

L

LAB, *see* Lactic Acid Bacteria
Lactic Acid Bacteria (LAB), 106, 128
LDL, *see* Low-density lipoprotein
LDL-C, *see* Low-density lipoprotein cholesterol
LDPE, *see* Low density polyethylene
Lignification process, 122
Low-density lipoprotein (LDL), 66, 95, 104, 189, 199
Low-density lipoprotein cholesterol (LDL-C), 67
Low density polyethylene (LDPE), 168
Lumpia wrapper, 52
Lyophilization, *see* Freeze-drying

M

Macro-minerals
  calcium, 80, 82
  magnesium, 83
  phosphorous, 82
  potassium, 80

silicon, 83–84
sodium, 82–83
sulphur, 83
X-ray fluorescence spectrometry, 81, 82
Macro-nutrients
amino acids, 76–78
carbohydrates, 78
protein, 72–76
starch, 73–75, 140–141
Magnesium, 83
Manganese, 85–86
Mesu, 50–51
Micro-mineral elements
copper, 85
iron, 84–85
manganese, 85–86
selenium, 86
zinc, 85
Micro-nutrients
extraction, 78–79
minerals, 79–80
Microwave drying, 130
Minerals, processing on, 150, 154
methods, 151–153
Modern methods
canning, 133
convective tray-drying, 130–131
freeze-drying, 131–132
hot air-drying, 130–131
microwave drying, 130
osmotic dehydration, 132
solar-drying, 130
Modified atmospheric packaging, 174
Moiya-koshak, 50
Monopodial bamboo, 16
Mungil-arisee, 30

N

Naw-mai-dong, 51
NBS, *see* Non-bacterial prostatitis
NDF, *see* Neutral detergent fibre
Neutral detergent fibre (NDF), 98, 105, 183
9-point Hedonic scale, 162, 163
No-mai, 47
Non-bacterial prostatitis (NBS), 97
Non-Steroidal Anti-inflammatory Agent (NSAIA), 66
Nongseij, 6
Nor-mai-dorng, 51
NSAIA, *see* Non-Steroidal Anti-inflammatory Agent
Nuggets, 183–184
Nutraceuticals, 177, 187–188
anti-oxidant activity, 192, 194–196
anti-oxidant defense system, 197
aqueous extract, 198
body/organ weight, 196, 197
fresh shoot extract, 199–201
glucose/lipid profile, 197, 199
in-vivo studies in Balb/c mice, 196
kidney function, 201–202
liver function, 199–201
phytochemicals, 193
Nutrient content, processing, 137–138
ash, 148
carbohydrate, 139, 142, 143
fat, 146–147
free amino acid, 142, 143, 146
macronutrients, 140–141
moisture, 148, 149
protein, 139, 142
starch, 146, 147
vitamins, 148–150
Nutrient-rich food, 38
edible shoots, 39–45
exporters/importers, 39

O

Organoleptic properties, 159, 162
Osmotic dehydration, 132
Oven-drying, 127, 138
Oxalates, 110–112, 135–136

P

Packaging
distribution/marketability, 165
edible coating, 174–175
enzymatic/microbial activities, 166
MAP, 174
materials/modes, 167, 168
polyethylene packaging, 168–169, 171
preservation materials, 172
PVC film, 171, 173
storage, 170
vacuum, 173
PAL, *see* Phenylalanine ammonia-lyase
Phenol, 154–156
Phenolic compounds
bamboo shoots *vs.* bacterial/fungal strains, 93
content, 99, 100
estimation, 91–92
flavonoid content, 94
GC-MS analysis, 93
health benefits, 90
hepatoprotective activity, 94
phenolic content *vs.* anti-oxidant activity, 91
plant, 90
significance, 90
structure, 90
types, 94
young shoots, 94

Phenolic content *vs.* anti-oxidant activity, 91
Phenylalanine ammonia-lyase (PAL), 122, 131, 166
Phiruk/Phingaruk, 8, 9
Phosphorous, 82
Phyllostachys edulis, 14, 21, 40, 60, 84, 95
Physiological cycle, 22
Phytate, 113–114, 135–136
Phytic acid, *see* Phytate
Phytochemicals, 193
Phytosterol oxidation products (POPs), 157
Phytosterols, 157
 chemical structures, 96
 content, 92, 97, 99–101
 fermented shoots, 97
 GC-MS chromatogram, 98
 genetic variability, 95
 hypocholesterolemic formulation, 95
 species, 95, 97
 steroid products, 96
Pickles, 186–187
Picrate paper, 109
Plant sterols, *see* Phytosterols
Polyethylene packaging, 168–169, 171
Polyvinyl chloride (PVC), 171, 173
POP, *see* Phytosterol oxidation products
Potassium, 80
Pre-cooking processing
 decolouration, 121
 ethylene treatment, 122
 lignification process, 122
 shapes, 121
 techniques, 121
Protein, 72–76, 139, 142
Purple bamboo salt, 33

R

Rebung, 47
Renewable grass, 4

S

Saccar Mambu, 4
Sandhana, 49
Saponins, 114–115, 135–136
Sasa borealis leaves (SBE), 61
SBE, *see Sasa borealis* leaves
SDF, *see* Soluble dietary fibre
Selenium, 86
Serum glutamate oxaloacetic transaminase (SGOT), 200
Serum glutamic pyruvate transaminase (SGPT), 200
SGOT, *see* Serum glutamate oxaloacetic transaminase
SGPT, *see* Serum glutamic pyruvate transaminase
Shooting season, 40
SHRS, *see* Spontaneously hypersensitive rats
Silicon, 83–84
Soaking, 133
Sodium, 82–83
Solar-drying, 123, 130, 133, 139, 148
Soluble dietary fibre (SDF), 98, 105
Spontaneously hypersensitive rats (SHRS), 67
Starch
 flour utilization, 180
 macro-nutrients, 73–75, 140–141
 nutrient content, processing, 146, 147
 shoot quality, 175
 tannins, 115
Steroid products, 96
Sulphur, 83
Sun-drying, 126–127
Superfoods, 204
Sympodial bamboo, 17, 18, 119

T

Tabasheer, 4–5, 32, 55, 84
Tabaxir, 4
Takenoko-no-tosani, 52
Tannins, 115, 135–136
Taxiphyllin, 108
TBARS, *see* Thiobarbituric Acid Reactive Substances
TBS, *see* Tender bamboo shoot
Tender bamboo shoot (TBS), 185
Thiobarbituric Acid Reactive Substances (TBARS), 62
Traditional methods
 drying, 125–126
 fermentation, 127–128
 fermented shoots, 128–130
 heat treatment, 124–125
 oven-drying, 127
 soaking, 123–124
 sun-drying, 126–127
Tray-drying/hot air-drying, 130–131
True/pseudo spikelets, 17

V

Vacuum packaging, 173
Vitamin C (ascorbic acid), 86–87
Vitamin E (tocopherols), 87

W

Wakthou, 7
Water phase extract of bamboo shavings (WEBS), 65

Water-soluble hemicelluloses, 104
WEBS, *see* Water phase extract of bamboo shavings

X

XOS, *see* Xylo-oligosaccharides
X-ray fluorescence spectrometry, 81, 82
Xylo-oligosaccharides (XOS), 180

Y

Yenpak, 7

Z

Zinc, 85
Zong-zi, 31

For Product Safety Concerns and Information please contact our EU representative GPSR@taylorandfrancis.com
Taylor & Francis Verlag GmbH, Kaufingerstraße 24, 80331 München, Germany

www.ingramcontent.com/pod-product-compliance
Ingram Content Group UK Ltd.
Pitfield, Milton Keynes, MK11 3LW, UK
UKHW022016180926
475701UK00005B/868
* 9 7 8 0 3 6 7 4 6 7 4 1 8 *